# LEUKEMIA AND LYMPHOMA

# LEUKEMIA AND LYMPHOMA

*Detection of Minimal Residual Disease*

*Edited by*

## THEODORE F. ZIPF, PhD, MD
*Houston, TX*
*and*

## DENNIS A. JOHNSTON, PhD
*Department of Biomathematics, MD Anderson Cancer Center*
*Houston, TX*

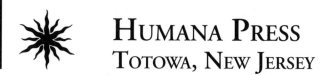

## HUMANA PRESS
### TOTOWA, NEW JERSEY

© 2003 Humana Press Inc.
999 Riverview Drive, Suite 208
Totowa, New Jersey 07512

For additional copies, pricing for bulk purchases, and/or information about other Humana titles, contact Humana at the above address or at any of the following numbers: Tel: 973-256-1699; Fax: 973-256-8341; E-mail: humana@humanapr.com or visit our website at http://www.humanapress.com

Due diligence has been taken by the publishers, editors, and authors of this book to assure the accuracy of the information published and to describe generally accepted practices. The contributors herein have carefully checked to ensure that the drug selections and dosages set forth in this text are accurate and in accord with the standards accepted at the time of publication. Notwithstanding, as new research, changes in government regulations, and knowledge from clinical experience relating to drug therapy and drug reactions constantly occurs, the reader is advised to check the product information provided by the manufacturer of each drug for any change in dosages or for additional warnings and contraindications. This is of utmost importance when the recommended drug herein is a new or infrequently used drug. It is the responsibility of the treating physician to determine dosages and treatment strategies for individual patients. Further it is the responsibility of the health care provider to ascertain the Food and Drug Administration status of each drug or device used in their clinical practice. The publisher, editors, and authors are not responsible for errors or omissions or for any consequences from the application of the information presented in this book and make no warranty, express or implied, with respect to the contents in this publication.

This publication is printed on acid-free paper. ⊚
ANSI Z39.48-1984 (American National Standards Institute)
Permanence of Paper for Printed Library Materials.
Cover design by Patricia F. Cleary.

**Photocopy Authorization Policy:**
Authorization to photocopy items for internal or personal use, or the internal or personal use of specific clients, is granted by Humana Press Inc., provided that the base fee of US $10.00 per copy, plus US $00.25 per page, is paid directly to the Copyright Clearance Center at 222 Rosewood Drive, Danvers, MA 01923. For those organizations that have been granted a photocopy license from the CCC, a separate system of payment has been arranged and is acceptable to Humana Press Inc. The fee code for users of the Transactional Reporting Service is: [0-89603-966-8/03 $10.00 + $00.25].

Printed in the United States of America.  10 9 8 7 6 5 4 3 2 1

Library of Congress Cataloging-in-Publication Data

Leukemia and lymphoma: detection of minimal residual disease / edited by Theodore F. Zipf and Dennis A. Johnston.
          p.;cm.
     Includes bibliographical references and index.
     ISBN 0-89603-966-8 (alk. paper)
     1. Leukemia–Molecular diagnosis. 2. Lymphomas–Molecular diagnosis. I. Zipf, Theodore F.
     II. Johnston, Dennis A.
     [DNLM: Neoplasm, Residual–diagnosis. 2. Leukemia. 3. Lymphoma. QZ 202 L652 2003]
     RC643.L3724 2003
     616.99'419075–dc21                                           2002024349

# PREFACE

*Leukemia and Lymphoma: Detection of Minimal Residual Disease* is being published at a time when the detection of microscopically unobservable disease in the leukemias and lymphomas is leaving its adolescent stage and entering the early stages of maturity. Detection of disease at levels almost four orders of magnitude below detection by light microscopy has now been accomplished and many of the methods have been shown to provide reproducible results. The groundwork has thus been laid for future construction of a methodology superior to the present methods of outcome prediction. Results of this nature will undoubtedly be necessary to justify the expense of future large-scale clinical trials using the various minimal residual disease (MRD) techniques that have been developed during the past decade. This places the burden of proof on those clinical investigators, statisticians, and basic scientists who are convinced that such measurements have an important role in producing future advances in treatment outcome.

As editors we have chosen contributors who have been successful in applying their chosen technique to the particular diseases that are their interests. We have especially tried to select those authors who were responsible for developments in the technique they used to make residual disease measurements. For this reason, we have encouraged them to give their insights into the methodology used in their research. As a result the reader will find several different descriptions of similar laboratory and analysis techniques, each of which we hope will prove helpful. We have taken advantage of the expertise of Professor Ludwig and Dr. Ratei to include a separate chapter on flow cytometry techniques. This addition should facilitate understanding the chapters on the use of flow cytometry to detect residual disease in the lymphoid and myeloid leukemias. In addition, one of us (DAJ) has written a rigorous mathematical description of an approach to the analysis of the predictive capabilities of an MRD detection system that accompanies a clinical trial. There is also a section of Editor's Notes at the end of this volume that contains comments on portions of each chapter. We hope that these comments will be found helpful to readers.

The chapter by Dr. Dario Campana describes the use of a patient-specific immunophenotype to identify residual leukemia in patients who are in remission. He carefully describes the different categories of leukemia-associated immunophenotypes and shows how they are used to follow patients in remission. His research has shown that he can detect one leukemia cell among ten thousand normal marrow cells.

Dr. Geoffrey Neale, a veteran contributor to the study of Childhood Acute Lymphocytic Leukemia using polymerase chain reaction (PCR)-based methods, describes the original methods for the detection of residual disease using PCR. He then progresses to a discussion of the various methods of quantitation of the level of disease. He completes his chapter with a description of real-time quantitative PCR (RQ-PCR). Throughout the chapter he gives the outcome of clinical studies of MRD in patients during remission.

Following Dr. Johnston's chapter on the analysis of MRD studies, we both have written a brief discussion on the evaluation of these techniques when used in clinical trials. In particular we address the question of assessing the predictive capability of a study that follows patients during and after therapy. We use simple arithmetic methods of performing these evaluations.

The predictive properties of semiquantitative PCR measurements of MRD prior to and after allogeneic stem cell transplantation of children with ALL are described by Moppet et al., who outline their experience with the technique in this setting. This chapter provides the reader with many possible routes for future MRD studies of allogeneic transplantation.

Drs. Foroni, Mortuza, and Hoffbrand give a detailed summary of the high sensitivity monitoring of adult patients with ALL. They review the approaches used to detect residual leukemia during remission. They define high and low risk groups according to the measured response to therapy and also contrast MRD in adult and childhood ALL.

Professor San Miguel and his colleagues present an extensive discussion of the immunophenotypes observed in patients with Acute Myeloid Leukemia (AML) and the frequent occurrence of asynchronous antigen expression in this disease. This chapter gives an excellent presentation of the methods of confirming the detection sensitivity of the flow cytometry–based assay. The results of clinical studies using this method to identify risk groups are presented.

The chapter presented by Drs. Marcucci and Caligiuri discusses the nonrandom chromosomal abnormalities in AML that lead to chimeric fusion genes thought to be leukemia-specific. Reverse transcription PCR (RT-PCR) is capable of detecting these transcripts with high sensitivity and thereby allows monitoring of the leukemia during remission. The authors review the results of clinical studies that detect these fusion transcripts and the use of their data in stratifying patients during remission according to the risk of relapse. They also discuss the importance of high sensitivity, as well as the associated hidden risks.

Dr. Lo Coco and Ms. Diverio discuss detection of MRD in Acute Promyelocytic Leukemia (APL), a subtype of AML that is associated with a specific chromosomal translocation, the t(15;17). The detection of the reverse transcription product of this fusion gene using RT-PCR has become an important aspect of both the diagnosis and monitoring during remission of this leukemia. The authors present a comprehensive review of the laboratory and clinical aspects of this endeavor.

The detection of MRD in Chronic Myelogenous Leukemia (CML) is described in the chapter of Drs. Cross and Hochhaus. Their discussion begins with the molecular genetics of the CML-associated t(9;22) chromosomal translocation and the BCR-ABL fusion gene. This is followed immediately by a section on the methods used to detect CML cells and leads to the application of RT-PCR to detect the BCR-ABL fusion transcript. The presentation of qualitative RT-PCR to detect the presence of the leukemia-associated transcript is closely followed by a thorough discussion of the methods for quantitation of the number of BCR-ABL transcripts. The chapter concludes with a critical discussion of the results of BCR-ABL detection in patients with CML. The problems associated with defining molecular relapse is presented in addition to a brief discussion about the presence of the BCR-ABL transcript in normal individuals.

Drs. Krackhardt and Gribben describe the detection of the t(14;8), t(11;14), t(8;14), t(2;5), t(11;18), and the antigen receptor gene rearrangements. They then present quantitation strategies based upon competitive PCR. They then apply the PCR technique to detection of these translocations in bone marrow and peripheral blood of patients with Non-Hodgkin's Lymphoma who have been treated with autologous bone marrow stem cell transplantation. The issue of whether or not "molecular complete remission" is the goal of therapy is presented in an unambiguous manner.

Tsimberidou et al. summarize the literature regarding the use of real-time and conventional PCR in patients with Non-Hodgkin's Lymphoma and t(14;18). They then describe real-time PCR, as they apply it in their laboratory, to specimens from patients with follicular lymphoma. They studied peripheral blood and bone marrow in these patients, as well as peripheral blood from normal donors. Their technique employs the simultaneous amplification of an internal beta actin sequence for quantitation and comparison.

Drs. Lee and Cabanillas describe the application of PCR to monitoring follicular lymphoma in patients with all stages of disease during remission. They use PCR results to define molecular nonresponders and develop a multivariate analysis of these patients. There was a high complete remission rate for patients who were molecular responders and a low rate for the non-responders. They extend this work to patients treated with bone marrow transplantation.

Throughout this book there are several issues that reappear frequently. They represent uncertainties about MRD that must be resolved before these assays achieve status as a reliable tool for clinical decision-making. Since these issues are essentially of equal importance, the following is not in any particular order of impact: (1) Some investigators have observed persistent low levels of detectable disease in patients who remain in clinical remission. This observation is closely coupled to the question of the optimal (most cost effective?) detection sensitivity. It also raises the question of interference by normal background. (2) The capability of detecting disease at submicroscopic levels has given rise to the real possibility of new definitions of the clinical terms remission and relapse.

These new definitions might allow improvements in treatment outcomes if they were properly established. For example, a reliable definition of molecular remission applied in cases where it was found persistently could lead to decreased treatment morbidity. There are two possible benefits of a reliable definition of molecular relapse. First, the signal for molecular relapse would, optimally, appear when the disease level is quite low and, at this level, the disease may be sensitive to many innovative therapeutic interventions. Second, prior to clinical relapse the patient is probably better able to tolerate intensive therapy than after clinical relapse. The actual implementation of these new criteria would provide an entrée to a completely new area of clinical investigation that could be very beneficial to patient care. (3) Many authors have noted that standardization is necessary. This standardization must include not only laboratory methods, but also the statistical methods used to analyze the data. This is an absolute requirement for the comparison of data from different institutions. (4) Finally, the emergence of the RQ-PCR technique as the method of choice is quite apparent in these chapters and in the recent literature. It seems probable that this development will facilitate the standardization of detection and quantitation techniques. We make these observations here so that the reader may keep them in mind as he/she reads the following chapters. If this book is to have any impact, it will hopefully inspire its readers to find solutions to the problems that now face the field.

The editors would like to thank the authors for the variety of their excellent chapters. More important, we would like to thank them and the many others working with MRD for the lively and impassioned discussions of MRD and their willingness to share their technical methods and ideas for the direction, use, and application of MRD. This has advanced the techniques and applications far beyond what we could have done working individually.

The editors would also like to thank Walter Pagel for his technical assistance and encouragement on this project, and Connie Siefert and Candy Schuenenman for their excellent editorial assistance. And last but most important, we would like to thank our wives, Maureen and Janice, for their support and patience throughout this project.

*Theodore F. Zipf, PhD, MD*
*Dennis A. Johnston, PhD*

# CONTENTS

# CONTRIBUTORS

AMOS BURKE, MD, Bristol Children's Hospital and Department of Pathology and Microbiology, Bristol, UK

FERNANDO CABANILLAS, MD, Department of Lymphoma and Myeloma, The University of Texas M. D. Anderson Cancer Center, Houston, TX

MICHAEL A. CALIGIURI, MD, Associate Director for Clinical Research, Comprehensive Cancer Center, and the Division of Hematology and Oncology, Department of Internal Medicine, The Ohio State University, Columbus, OH

DARIO CAMPANA, MD, PhD, Departments of Hematology/Oncology and Pathology, St. Jude Children's Hospital, Memphis, TN, and University of Tennessee College of Medicine, Memphis, TN

NICHOLAS C. P. CROSS, MA, PhD, Wessex Regional Genetics Laboratory, Salisbury District Hospital and Human Genetics Division, University of Southampton School of Medicine, UK

DANIELA DIVERIO, MSc, Department of Cellular Biotechnologies and Hematology, University La Sapienza, Rome, Italy

RICHARD J. FORD, MD, PhD, Department of Hematology, The University of Texas M. D. Anderson Cancer Center, Houston, TX

LETIZIA FORONI, MD, PhD, Haematology Department, Royal Free and University College School of Medicine, Royal Free Hospital NHS Hampstead Trust, London, UK

NICHOLAS J. GOULDEN, MD, PhD, Bristol Children's Hospital and Department of Pathology and Microbiology, Bristol, UK

JOHN G. GRIBBEN, MD, DSC, Department of Adult Oncology, Dana Farber Cancer Institute, and Department of Medicine, Brigham and Women's Hospital, Harvard Medical School, Boston, MA

ANDREAS HOCHHAUS, DM, FRCP, FRCPath, DSC III. Medizinische Klinik, Klinikum Mannheim der Universität Heidelberg, Mannheim, Germany

A. VICTOR HOFFBRAND, Haematology Department, Royal Free and University College School of Medicine, Royal Free Hospital NHS Hampstead Trust, London, UK

YUNFANG JIANG, MD, PhD, Department of Lymphoma and Myeloma, The University of Texas M. D. Anderson Cancer Center, Houston, TX

DENNIS A. JOHNSTON, PhD, Department of Biomathematics, University of Texas M. D. Anderson Cancer Center, Houston, TX

CHRISTOPHER KNECHTLI, MD, PhD, Bristol Children's Hospital and Department of Pathology and Microbiology, Bristol, UK

ANGELA M. KRACKHARDT, MD, III. Medizinische Klinik, Hämatologie, Onkologie und Transfusionmedizin, Universitätsklinikum Benjamin Franklin, Berlin, Germany

MING-SHENG LEE, MD, Molecular Diagnostics Laboratory in the Division of Pathology and Laboratory Medicine, The University of Texas M. D. Anderson Cancer Center, Houston, TX

FRANCESCO LO COCO, MD, Department of Cellular Biotechnologies and Hematology, Unversity La Sapienza, Rome, Italy

WOLF-DIETER LUDWIG, MD, PhD, Robert-Rössle Klinik, Department of Hematology, Oncology and Tumor Immunology, Charité Campus Berlin-Buch, Humboldt University, Berlin, Germany

GUIDO MARCUCCI, MD, Division of Hematology and Oncology, Department of Internal Medicine, and The Comprehensive Cancer Center, The Ohio State University, Columbus, OH

JOHN MOPPETT, MD Bristol Children's Hospital and Department of Pathology and Microbiology, Bristol, UK

FORIDA Y. MORTUZA, PhD, Haematology Department, Royal Free and University College School of Medicine, Royal Free Hospital NHS Hampstead Trust, London, UK

GEOFFREY NEALE, PhD, Departments of Hematology/Oncology and Pathology, St. Jude Children's Hospital, Memphis, TN, and University of Tennessee College of Medicine, Memphis, TN

ANTHONY OAKHILL, MD, Bristol Children's Hospital and Department of Pathology and Microbiology, Bristol, UK

ALBERTO ORFAO, MD, PhD, Centro de Investigación del Cancer, Salamanca, Spain, and Department of Cytometry, University of Salamanca, Spain

RICHARD RATEI, MD, Robert-Rössle Klinik, Department of Hematology, Oncology and Tumor Immunology, Charité Campus Berlin-Buch, Humboldt University, Berlin, Germany

JESÚS F. SAN MIGUEL, MD, PhD, Department of Hematology, University Hospital, Salamanca, Spain, and Centro de Investigación del Cancer, Salamanca, Spain

ANDREAS H. SARRIS, MD, PhD, Department of Lymphoma and Myeloma, The University of Texas M. D. Anderson Cancer Center, Houston, TX

COLIN STEWARD, MD, PhD, Bristol Children's Hospital and Department of Pathology and Microbiology, Bristol, UK

APOSTOLIA-MARIE TSIMBERIDOU, MD, PhD, Department of Leukemia, The University of Texas M. D. Anderson Cancer Center, Houston, TX

MARÍA B. VIDRIALES, MD, PhD, Department of Hematology, University Hospital, Salamanca, Spain

THEODORE F. ZIPF, PhD, MD, Houston, TX

# 1 Flow-Cytometry Methods for the Detection of Residual Leukemia

## Richard Ratei and Wolf-Dieter Ludwig

### INTRODUCTION

The diagnosis and classification as well as the evaluation of therapy response and the estimation of residual disease in acute leukemias depend on the detection and description of the leukemic cell clone. The phenotype can be assessed with morphology, cytochemistry, immunohistochemistry, fluorescence microscopy, and flow cytometry. The genotype is studied with cytogenetic and molecular techniques (e.g., banding techniques, polymerase chain reaction [PCR], or fluorescence *in situ* hybridization [FISH]) (Table 1).

Usually, these methods have to be applied exclusively and only a few studies have described methods that detect phenotypic and genotypic features simultaneously *(1–3)*. Each of these methods puts a spotlight on the disease according to its inherent ability to detect a certain feature of the leukemic clone. This is limited, of course, by the specificity and sensitivity of the method that is applied for the diagnosis or the detection of minimal residual disease. Each of these methods describes biological components of the disease that can be assembled by the clinician to compose a detailed picture for disease monitoring, thus forming the rational ground for the earlier and better distinction of patients with "poor risk" features, who require a more intensive therapy, from patients with "good risk" features, who probably do not need any additional treatment to reach a cure and remain in remission *(4–9)*.

Flow cytometry has been available for almost three decades and has evolved to a sophisticated and indispensable tool in various fields of biology and medicine, with a significant impact in hematology, especially for the diagnosis and classification of leukemias *(10–12)*. The intriguing possibility of detecting

From: *Leukemia and Lymphoma: Detection of Minimal Residual Disease*
Edited by: T. F. Zipf and D. A. Johnston © Humana Press Inc., Totowa, NJ

Table 1
Methods for Detecting Phenotypic and Genotypic Features of Leukemic Cells

| Phenotype | Genotype | Phenotype/Genotype |
|---|---|---|
| Morphology | Cytogenetics | "Fiction" |
| Immunohistochemistry | Banding techniques | |
| Fluorescence microscopy | Fluorescence in situ hybridization (FISH) | |
| Flow cytometry | Molecular biology | (FISH and immunophenotype) |

phenotypic features on a single-cell level in large cell populations forms the rational basis for flow cytometry to be used in the evaluation of minimal residual leukemia *(4,13,14)*. Recent developments in modern technologies, including fluidics, lasers, optics, analog and digital electronics, computers, software, fluorochromes, and antibodies have been utilized, so that flow cytometry has evolved from a one-color, three-parameter technique to a three-color, five-parameter method (multiparametric flow cytometry, MFC), and, more recently, to the so-called polychromatic flow cytometry (PFC) featuring 9 colors and 11 parameters *(15,16)*. In addition, it gives the clinician a fast, reliable, and sensitive method for disease monitoring at hand.

This chapter is intended as a technical overview on the flow-cytometric methodology that is used to diagnose minimal residual disease in acute leukemias. In the chapters by San Miguel et al. (Chapter 8) and Campana (Chapter 2), the focus is more on the clinical application and evaluation of minimal residual disease in acute myeloid lymphoblastic and acute leukemias, respectively.

## FUNDAMENTAL FLOW CYTOMETRY

In order to understand the technical problems and difficulties that inevitably come along with the new technological developments of multiparametric flow cytometry, a short summary of the characteristics of flow cytometers and fluorochromes is necessary *(17,18)*.

### *Optical System*

Almost all commercially available flow cytometers use essentially the same optical layout with an orthogonal configuration of the three main axes of the instrument. The sample flow, the laser beam, and the optical axis of scatter light and fluorescence detection are arranged at right angles to each other. The laser light has to be focused in the direction of the sample flow, which is usually achieved with one or two lenses. Thereby, the width of the focus is a compromise between the need for high sensitivity and for high resolution. High sensitivity requires a narrow focus to concentrate as much light as possible on the sample, and high resolution calls for a broader focus allowing a larger beam width.

In some instruments, two or three lasers are employed, with the laser beams closely adjacent but separately focused, so that particles or cells are excited sequentially with two or three different wavelengths. This arrangement makes it possible to detect multiple cellular components stained with dyes that are excited at different wavelengths, but it requires an exact time delay calibration to ensure that the emitted light signals are recognized as belonging to one and the same cell.

Emitted light is detected at right angles to the laser beam, either through standard microscope objectives or a specially designed lens. In analogy to the optics in microscopy, the amount of light or fluorescence collected depends on the numerical aperture of the lens and the medium from which the light source originates. With the light source in water, as is the case with most currently used flow cytometers, the collection efficiency is low; hence, only a small fraction of the fluorescence is actually detected.

In order to eliminate light from sources other than the cells that pass through the laser beam, it is necessary to position an opaque screen with a "pinhole" in the image plane of the detection optics. This aperture has an important function in reducing the signal-to-noise ratio. After the elimination or reduction of noise signals, the emitted light is still heterogeneous after passing the pinhole aperture, containing scattered light of the same wavelength as the laser light and emissions of the different fluorescences, which are always shifted toward higher wavelengths as the scatter light. The right-angle scatter light with the same wavelength as the laser light is a measure of the granularity of the cell passing through the laser beam. To separate scattered light from fluorescence, dichroic mirrors are situated at 45° angles to the light beam behind the pinhole aperture. They reflect the scatter light onto one detector, whereas the higher-wavelength fluorescence light is transmitted to other detectors. The separation of colors by dichroic mirrors does not always prevent the light emitted by fluorochrome from entering the detector for another fluorochrome. Therefore, additional bandpass filters are used in front of each detector. Because of spectral overlap, the spillover of fluorescences into different detectors cannot be eliminated completely and requires compensation between the different fluorochromes and detectors for the analysis of samples stained with multiple dyes. Such an arrangement of dichroic mirrors, specific bandpass filters, and detectors can be extended and stacked behind each other, so that usually two to four fluorescences excited by one or two laser beams are measured simultaneously.

## *Light Sources*

Basically, lasers and arc lamps are the possible light sources used in flow cytometers. The older gas ion lasers are now almost all completely replaced by the newer diode lasers that, in contemporary instruments, have at least 50 mW

Table 2
Commonly Used Laser Lines and Fluorochrome Combinations
for Multicolor Flow Cytometry

| Laser | Dye | Fluorochrome combination |
|-------|-----|--------------------------|
| 2 (488 nm + 647 nm) | 4 | FITC, PE, Cy5.5PE or Cy7PE, APC |
|  |  | FITC, PE, Cy5PE, Cy5.5APC or Cy7PE |
|  |  | FITC, PE, Cy5PE, APC |
|  |  | FITC, PE, TRPE, APC |
| 1 (488 nm) | 4 | FITC, PE, Cy5PE, Cy5.5PE or Cy7PE |
|  |  | FITC, PE, ECD, Cy5PE |

[a]See Editors' comments in the Appendix for further identification of fluorochromes and lasers and wavelengths.

of power. Usually, the lasers in commercially available flow cytometers used for the immunophenotyping of hematological neoplasias are air-cooled argon lasers with a power of 10–50 mW and an emission line that is tuned to 488 nm. Some flow cytometers are provided with a second laser, which may be another argon laser or a krypton laser. It is crucial to remember that the fluorescence signal increases with laser power, but that more than 50 mW of power does not necessarily produce more fluorescence signal. Indeed, most fluorochromes will saturate with higher power, actually reducing relative signal-to-background staining. Some of the commonly used lasers, dyes, and fluorochrome combinations for the detection of minimal residual disease (MRD) in acute leukemias are listed in Table 2.

## Detectors

Fluorescence and right-angle light scatter (RALS) are detected by photomultiplier tubes (PMTs). Photomultipliers are current amplifiers that transform pulses of light into equivalent electrical pulses. They contain a light-sensitive photocathode within a vacuum tube, which, when hit by a photon, releases an electron with a certain probability (quantum yield).

## Flow Chambers

Flow cells are the most critical component of a flow cytometer. They have to fulfill two tasks: maintenance of laminar flow and hydrodynamic focusing. In a flow cell, the dispersed sample is directed in a single file along a narrow path that intersects the laser beam such that single cells are passing the excitation beam sequentially. This narrow path is obtained by using two concentric laminar-flow columns. The outer column of diluent is referred to as the sheath column, where the flow usually travels faster than the inner flow core column containing the sample. The differential flow rates of the inner and outer columns control the diameter of the core path. Laminar smooth flow has to be maintained to confine the sample flow to the inner core.

The orifice of the flow chamber is usually of a larger diameter (70–100 μm) than the excitation beam (30–50 μm). In order to prevent cells from wandering in and out of the excitation beam, the sample flow has to be focused to ensure that each cell will travel at the same velocity and that each cell will get the same amount of exposure from the excitation beam. This process is referred to as "hydrodynamic focusing" and is achieved by injecting the sample flow into the middle of the sheath stream. Most of the flow cytometers currently in the clinic have a closed flow chamber of the "stream-in-cuvet" type, with the laser beam exciting the sample through the wall of the flow chamber, whereas most sorting flow cytometers use "stream-in-air" configurations, with the laser beam striking the sample streams in open air after they have left the flow cell. This usually results in a higher noise level than closed instruments, but provides the ability to form droplets that can be charged that allows sorting.

### *Fluorochromes*

For the right choice of a fluorochrome or a fluorochrome combination, several criteria have to be taken into consideration. First, the expected expression levels for the markers of interest should be known, thus ensuring that weakly expressed antigens can be stained with an antibody conjugated to one of the brightest fluorochromes like PE, Cy5PE or APC, and strongly expressed antigens with antibodies conjugated to less bright fluorochromes like fluorescein-isothiocyanate (FITC). Therefore, weak coexpression of myeloid markers like CD33 or CD13 on blast cells of acute lymphoblastic leukemias (ALL) can only be identified if bright fluorochromes are used for aberrant expressed markers in combination with less bright fluorochromes for the lineage-specific markers like CD3 for T-lineage ALL and CD19 or CD22 for B-lineage ALL.

Another crucial point is made by the spectral overlaps that exist between the various dyes used in staining. Although hardware or software compensation can eliminate some of the spectral spillovers, careful combination of fluorochromes must take into account that bright fluorochromes with a large spectral overlap used for the detection of strongly expressed antigens can blanket the dim fluorescence of weakly coexpressed markers despite an appropriate compensation procedure and filters.

Furthermore, fluorochromes have to fulfill several conditions. These include biological inertness, a prerequisite for a fluorochrome to be used for diagnostic purposes in flow cytometry because any interaction with cellular components hampers the specific detection of an antigen. Most currently available fluorochromes do not interact with cellular components, but exceptions have to be kept in mind, for example, the most common is the background binding of cyanine tandem dyes like Cy5PE on monocytes and B-cells. Another point that has to be kept in mind when using tandem conjugates, especially with Cy5PE , is that the chemical composition of these molecules differs between manufacturers and even between lots from the same manufacturer. Thus, a different ratio of donor and acceptor dye within a tandem conjugate can result in different spectral behavior, which influences instrument settings and compensation and may require several different compensation settings for a particular application.

## *Instrument Setup and Compensation*

The instrument setup and the calibration of the flow cytometer for multicolor immunophenotyping should satisfy three main objectives. First, optimal positioning of the window of analysis in the sample space must be achieved. The sample space is defined by the physical properties of the sample (e.g., the cell characterized by its diameter as measured by forward-angle light scatter [FALS], its granularity as measured by RALS, and its excitation and emission spectra as measured by the fluorescence detectors). Amplifier gain or PMT settings have to be adjusted in such a way that each parameter appears in the appropriate range of histogram channels for that parameter.

Second, it should be verified that the spectral overlap between the fluorochromes used is correct. Compensation is the process by which spectral overlaps between different fluorochromes are eliminated or, at least, minimized. This can be performed by hardware after the signal is detected but before its logarithmic conversion and/or digitization, or after data collection by using software algorithms. Especially for the monitoring of minimal residual disease (MRD), it is of utmost importance to know that a certain population cannot be clearly distinguished or even disappear from the "window of analysis" because of false compensation settings. Therefore, the compensation settings should be ascertained by using a sample that matches the "sample space" of the probe as closely as possible or even use part of the probe material for the compensation setup.

Third, standardized beads or lymphocytes from normal individuals are commonly used for setting up a multicolor compensation matrix. However, in the case of acute myeloid leukemias, these compensation settings often are not adequate because of the differences in the physical properties of the myeloid leukemia cells, not only in RALS and FALS but also in its differences because of background staining and autofluorescence compared to lymphocytes or beads. For a two-color analysis, the pairwise compensation between the two fluorochromes is sufficient and complete. However, with the introduction of more and more fluorochromes in a stain, the interactions and spectral overlaps become so complex and numerous that a fully corrected compensation cannot be achieved manually anymore. It is beyond the scope of this chapter to outline the different approaches and algorithms for achieving optimal compensation settings for two-, three-, or multicolor stainings. The reader is referred to excellent reviews by Stewart and Stewart *(19)* and Roederer et al. (http://www.drmr.com/compensation).

## QUALITY CONTROL

The performance of the instrument for fluorescence measurements must be controlled and documented. Each laboratory participating in MRD studies should have a quality control program that ascertains the reliability and reproducibility of the major instrument parameters over time. This is a prerequisite for the longitudinal analyses aimed at the monitoring of therapy response. Multiple samples from the same patient have to be analyzed over a period of time, which can be weeks, months, or years, and the measurements should be undertaken within established tolerance limits. Quality control measures should include the examination of the optical alignment, including the efficiency and performance of the laser tube, the optical filters, and the photomultiplier tubes. Several consensus recommendations on the immunophenotypic analysis of hematological neoplasias, including validation and control procedures, have been published in recent years *(20–24)*. These recommendations apply to the diagnosis of acute leukemias as well as to the detection of MRD and should form the basis for a valid assessment of minimal residual disease.

## SAMPLE CHOICE AND SAMPLE PREPARATION

Bone marrow or, in the case of a leukemia, peripheral blood is used for the initial diagnosis of the leukemia. With flow cytometry the leukemia-associated immunophenotype (LAIP) is characterized and the best combination of fluorochromes and antibodies is identified for follow-up investigations. In the initial samples, the leukemic cell count is usually high and makes up more than 80–90% of all nucleated cells in the sample, so that, normally, a homogeneous distribution of blast cells is present independent of the aspiration technique and the frequency of aspiration during one bone marrow puncture. Follow-up bone marrow samples might be heterogeneous with regard to the distribution of blast cells, especially if multiple aspirations during one bone marrow puncture are undertaken. If the last aspiration available is submitted to the flow-cytometric MRD laboratory, a nonrepresentative distribution of residual blast cells in bone marrow blood may occur.

In the case of peripheral blood samples, the constant vascular flow almost always ensures a homogeneous distribution of blood cells and blast cells independent of aspiration technique and multiple aspirations during one puncture, unless the blood is drawn inappropriately from an infusion line or directly behind it, thus diluting the sample. Therefore, peripheral blood samples are more consistent and homogeneous in their composition and less susceptible to disturbances of composition than bone marrow samples. In terms of sensitivity, there are studies using PCR suggesting that peripheral blood samples might have a sufficient sensitivity compared to bone marrow samples for the monitoring of MRD, but no studies have been undertaken comparing the sensitivity of MRD detection by flow cytometry in bone marrow and peripheral blood samples *(25,26)*.

## STAINING

For surface staining of *whole-blood* cell samples, we prefer the *stain/lyse/wash* procedure without fixation because this method achieves a better reduction of background staining than the *stain/lyse/no-wash* method. Monoclonal antibodies and whole blood are mixed in an appropriate ratio, usually $(0.5–1.0) \times 10^6$ cells per 10–15 µL of monoclonal antibody. After incubation of the sample–antibody mixture, the lysis reagent is added and the sample is vortexed and incubated. Afterward, the sample is centrifuged, the supernatant discarded, and the cell pellet washed in buffer and, finally, resuspended in buffer again to be measured immediately.

The simultaneous staining of membrane and intracellular antigens requires a slightly more elaborate procedure because cells have to be fixed after the membrane staining. The addition of the lysis reagent can be omitted from the procedure because the permeabilization reagent added together with the antibody for the intracellular antigen sufficiently lyses red blood cells. The additional washing procedure can lead to a little more loss of cells; thus, it is advisable to use a higher cell input, especially if a large amount of cells are to be acquired and analyzed. The staining and fixation procedures alter the light-scatter properties and even shift fluorochrome intensities, so that different instrument settings might be necessary for samples with intracellular staining. Many protocols and reagents for intracellular staining are commercially available. A careful and meticulous evaluation of reagents and procedures has been presented recently *(27,28)*.

In the whole-blood staining procedure, elimination of interfering red blood cells is achieved with a lysing reagent usually containing ammonium chloride, but debris usually remains in the sample. Another possibility for clearing the sample of red blood cells and debris is given by density gradient centrifugation. After isolation of the mononuclear cells from the gradient, subsequent staining procedures do not differ from the above-described method, except for the omission of the lysis reagent. With regard to antigen expression as measured by the percentage of positive cells or fluorescence intensity, measured as mean expression, we have seen no significant differences for both methods, as illustrated in Fig. 1. Of course, certain cell populations can be lost during gradient centrifugation, so that the flow-cytometric data should be compared and controlled by morphological examination of bone marrow or peripheral blood smears. In this way, incorrect interpretations because of sample preparation can be avoided in most cases.

For any staining procedure, the optimal concentration of each antibody has to be titrated carefully before the set up of a definite antibody panel and for every

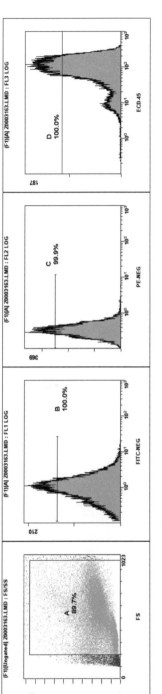

## Density Gradient Centrifugation

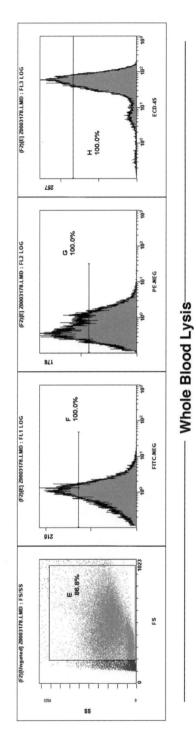

## Whole Blood Lysis

**Fig. 1.** Analysis of a peripheral blood sample of a patient with acute myeloid leukemia after density gradient centrifugation or whole blood lysis stained with a three-color panel did not show any great differences, either in the light-scatter properties or in the fluorescence characteristics.

combination of antibodies in each tube. Staining properties can be influenced by a variety of factors, including temperature, pH, ratio of cells and antibodies, and the fluorochrome combination mixed in a stain. Despite the optimal modulation of all of these factors and the consistent performance, the upgrading of a two-color stain to a three- or four-color stain can lead to slightly different staining properties (*see* Figs. 2 and 3), so that it is mandatory to apply the same antibodies under the same conditions on initial diagnosis and during follow-up investigations.

## RATIONALE FOR THE CHOICE OF ANTIBODIES AND COMPILATION OF AN ANTIBODY PANEL

As described in depth in the chapters by Campana and San Miguel, the precise identification of the leukemic cell depends on the clear distinction of the leukemic and normal immunophenotype *(31–33)*. This presupposes an exact knowledge of the immunophenotypic pattern displayed with a certain antibody panel not only in normal hematopoiesis but also in conditions of a reconstituting hematopoiesis, e.g., after chemotherapy or under the influence of growth factors (e.g., granulocyte colony-stimulating factor [G-CSF]) *(23,24,34)*.

A universal common denominator in the pathogenesis of acute leukemias is that the immunophenotype of the leukemic clone resembles that of their normal counterparts. However, many immunophenotypic studies with an increasingly sophisticated approach have shown that this does not always hold true *(11,35–46)*. Instead, with the use of multiparametric flow cytometry, numerous studies have shown that it is possible to define certain criteria that can be applied to characterize a leukemia-associated immunophenotype (LAIP) (*see* Table 3) *(4,33,38,47–50)*. Examples of aberrant antigen expressions for acute myeloid and acute lymphoblastic leukemias are given in the chapters by Campana and San Miguel et al.

These criteria for the detection of the LAIP are directed by the characteristics of antigen expression (weak or strong) and fluorochrome properties (e.g., brightness, spectral overlap) that have to be carefully evaluated to compose the best possible combination of fluorochromes and markers for a reproducible and valid assay.

---

**Fig. 2.** *(opposite page)* Differences of fluorescences for CD34-FITC, CD2-PE, CD33-PE/CD33-Cy5PE, and CD45PE/CD45-ECD according to three different staining procedures. All samples were stained after cells were isolated with Ficoll gradient centrifugation. Two-color stainings were performed with FITC and PE, three-color stainings with FITC, PE, and PC5, the four-color stain with FITC, PE, ECD and PC5. CD45 staining was not included in the three-color analysis.

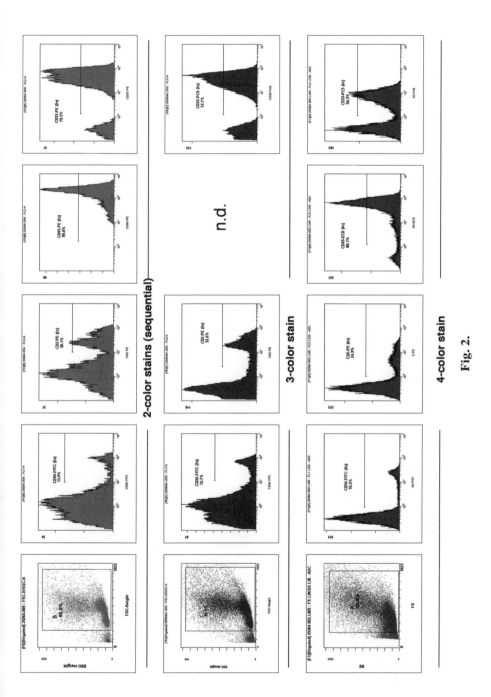

Fig. 2.

11

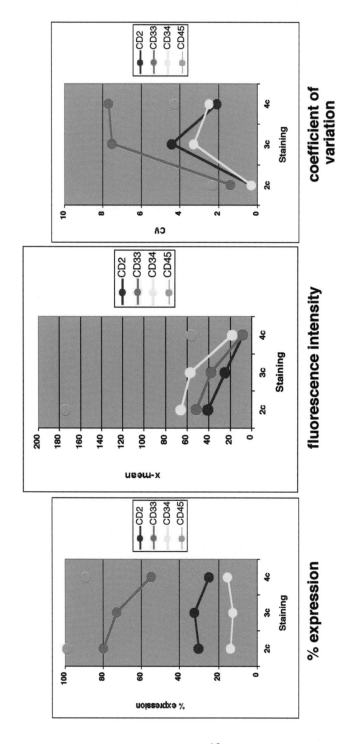

**Fig. 3.** Changes of fluorescence features measured as percentage of expression in all analyzed cells (% expression), fluorescence intensity (x-mean), and fluorescence distribution (coefficient of variation [cv]). The decrease of % expression of CD33 can be attributed either to fluorochrome switch (PE to Cy5PE) or to fluorochrome interferences in the four-color stain. Fluorescence intensity (x-mean) decreases for all fluorochrome–antibody combinations in the three- and four-color stain.

Table 3
Characterization of Leukemia-Associated Immunophenotypes

| Criteria | Example |
|---|---|
| Cross-lineage antigen expression | Expression of lymphoid antigens on myeloid blast or vice versa |
| Asynchronous antigen expression | Coexpression of antigens that correspond to different maturational stages |
| Antigen overexpression | Abnormally high expression of a certain antigens |
| Abnormal light scatter | High FSC and high SSC of lymphoid cells |
| Differentially expressed antigens | Expression of molecules associated with chromosomal abnormalities, e.g., NG2 molecule (moAb 7.1) in leukemic cells with 11q23 rearrangements (35) |

In Figs. 2 and 3, an example of an acute myeloid leukemia is given to illustrate the changes in expression (%), fluorescence intensity ($x$-mean), and coefficient of variation (CV) according to different staining procedures (two-color, three-color, and four-color staining). Despite the use of identical antibody clones in the different stainings, optimal instrument setup and compensation, variations in the percentage of expression are seen. Especially, for CD33, which is conjugated to PE in the two-color stain and conjugated to Cy5PE in the three- and four-color stains, a decrease is noted. The $x$-mean as a measure for fluorescence intensity decreases in the multicolor stains despite constant or even higher PMT settings in the three- and four-color assays.

Thus, the qualities of a multiparameter flow-cytometric analysis have to accept the disadvantages concerning percentage expression, fluorescence intensity, and coefficient of variation restricted by the best available antibody and fluorochrome combination and the best possible instrument setup and compensation.

## HOW MANY COLORS, HOW MANY PARAMETERS?

In the beginning of monoclonal antibody and flow-cytometric technology, the detection of immunophenotypic features was confined to the use of unconjugated primary antibodies directed against a specific antigen and a second-layer antibody directed against the Fc part of the specific antibody conjugated to a certain fluorochrome. This procedure did not allow multiple stainings on one cell, thus the two light-scatter parameters could only be analyzed in combination with one fluorescence. With this approach, the exact definition of subpopulations expressing a distinct phenotype is not possible, although weakly expressed antigens can be detected more precisely than with direct conjugated antibodies.

Table 4
Number of Population Discernible by Multicolor Systems

| | No. of fluorochromes | | |
| --- | --- | --- | --- |
| No. of conditions | Two-color | Three-color | Four-color |
| 2 | 4 | 8 | 16 |
| 3 | 9 | 27 | 108 |
| 4 | 16 | 64 | 256 |

With the availability of direct fluorochrome-conjugated monoclonal antibodies, double, triple, and multiple stainings have become increasingly possible. Thus, with an increasing number of separable fluorochromes applied to a stain, the number of populations that can be detected increases geometrically according to the formula

$$p = n_1 x\, n_2\, x\, ...xn_k$$

$$p = n^k$$

where p is the number of possible populations defined, $k$ is the number of fluorochromes used in a stain, and $n$ $(n_1..., n_k)$ is defined by the number of presumed conditions separable by each fluorochrome. With the most commonly used and commercially available flow cytometers, three- or four-color stains are routinely applied. Expression of a certain antigen is normally assessed on the basis of a single cutoff level, usually negative if expression is below 20% and positive if expression is measured above 20%, e.g., the number of presumed conditions is two, leading to either eight (three-color analysis) or 16 (four-color analysis) discernible populations (see Table 4).

The simultaneous use of multiple colors tremendously enhances the amount of information that can be obtained from one stain. Only this multicolor approach can clearly reveal abnormalities in antigen expression on subpopulations that could not have been detected from any panel of sequential one- or two-color analysis (see Figs. 4 and 5). Especially in the diagnosis of MRD, the conclusions drawn from a series of one- or two-color stains by comparing the percentages of expression in a bulk population are not sufficient to define a certain LAIP that can be used to monitor the disease.

---

Fig. 4. *(opposite page)* The two-color four-parameter analysis allows for the distinction of four populations. There are two CD34+ populations, one with coexpression of CD56 (red, population C) and one without the coexpression of CD56 (blue, population D). The bulk of the remaining blast cells in this acute myeloid leukemia are CD56+ without coexpression of CD34 (yellow, population B).

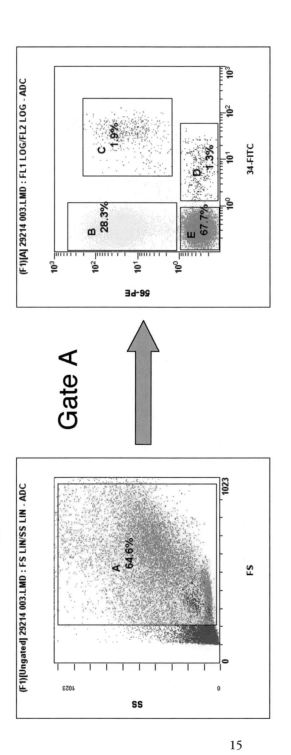

Fig. 4.

15

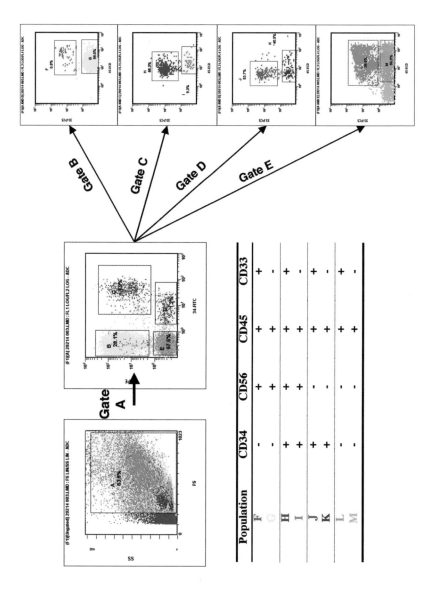

**Fig. 5.** With a four-color six-parameter analysis eight populations are discernible. Although small, they characterize the heterogeneity of the leukemic and normal populations. There are four subpopulations of CD34+ cells from which population H and I certainly constitute the leukemic clone and population J and K probably belong to residual normal precursors.

16

# OUTLOOK

Multiparametric flow cytometry has evolved to a powerful and indispensable tool for the detection of MRD in acute leukemias. The application requires a certain knowledge of the characteristics of the individual fluorochromes, fluorochrome–antibody combinations, and marker expressions in different disease entities and in normal conditions to choose appropriate reagents, reagent combinations, and fluorochrome–antibody pairings. New developments in software and amplifier technology will improve and simplify the instrument setup as well as compensation algorithms for multiparameter flow cytometry, so that a multitude of reproducible and valid assays can be investigated to provide the clinician with the most important information for disease monitoring and MRD.

# REFERENCES

1. Weber Matthiesen K, Deerberg J, Poetsch M, Grote W, and Schlegelberger B. Clarification of dubious karyotypes in Hodgkin's disease by simultaneous fluorescence immunophenotyping and interphase cytogenetics (FICTION), *Cytogenet. Cell Genet.*, **70** (1995) 243–245.
2. Weber Matthiesen K, Deerberg J, Wittram J, Rosenwald A, Poetsch M, Grote W, et al. Translocation t(2;5) is not a primary event in Hodgkin's disease. Simultaneous immunophenotyping and interphase cytogenetics, *Am. J. Pathol.*, **149** (1996) 463–468.
3. Zhang Y, Poetsch M, Weber Matthiesen K, et al. Secondary acute leukaemias with 11q23 rearrangement: clinical, cytogenetic, FISH and FICTION studies, *Br. J. Haematol.*, **92** (1996) 673–680.
4. Campana D and Coustan-Smith E. Detection of minimal residual disease in acute leukemia by flow cytometry, *Cytometry* **38** (1999) 139–152.
5. Campana D and Coustan-Smith E. The use of flow cytometry to detect minimal residual disease in acute leukemia, *Eur. J. Histochem.*, **40(Suppl. 1)** (1996) 39–42.
6. Yin JA and Tobal K. Detection of minimal residual disease in acute myeloid leukaemia: methodologies, clinical and biological significance, *Br. J. Haematol.*, **106** (1999) 578–590.
7. Coustan-Smith E, Sancho J, Hancock ML, et al. Clinical importance of minimal residual disease in childhood acute lymphoblastic leukemia, *Blood*, **96** (2000) 2691–2696.
8. Campana D, Neale GAM, Coustan-Smith E, and Pui CH. Detection of minimal residual disease in acute lymphoblastic leukemia: the St. Jude experience, *Leukemia*, **15** (2001) 278–279.
9. Pui CH. Recent advances in the biology and treatment of childhood acute lymphoblastic leukemia, *Curr. Opin. Hematol.*, **5** (1998) 292–301.
10. Bene MC, Castoldi G, Knapp W, et al. Proposals for the immunological classification of acute leukemias. European Group for the Immunological Characterization of Leukemias (EGIL), *Leukemia*, **9** (1995) 1783–1786.
11. Bene MC, Bernier M, Castoldi G, et al. Impact of immunophenotyping on management of acute leukemias, *Haematologica*, **84** (1999) 1024–1034.
12. Jennings CD and Foon KA. Recent advances in flow cytometry: application to the diagnosis of hematologic malignancy, *Blood*, **90** (1997) 2863–2892.
13. Ludwig WD, van Dongen JJ, Thiel E, Teichmann JV, Hofmann J, and Riehm H. Possibilities and limitations of immunological marker analyses for the detection of minimal residual disease in childhood acute lymphoblastic leukemia, *Onkologie*, **13** (1990) 166–174.
14. Macedo A, Orfao A, Gonzalez M, et al. Immunological detection of blast cell subpopulations in acute myeloblastic leukemia at diagnosis: implications for minimal residual disease studies, *Leukemia*, **9** (1995) 993–998.

15. Herzenberg LA and De Rosa SC. Monoclonal antibodies and the FACS: complementary tools for immunobiology and medicine, *Immunol. Today*, **21** (2000) 383–390.
16. Roederer M, De Rosa S, Gerstein R, et al. 8-color, 10-parameter flow cytometry to elucidate complex leukocyte heterogeneity, *Cytometry*, **29** (1997) 328–339.
17. Melamed MR, Lindmo T, and Mendelsohn ML. *Flow Cytometry and Sorting*. New York: Wiley–Liss.
18. Shapiro HM. *Practical Flow Cytometry*. New York: Wiley–Liss.
19. Stewart CC and Stewart SJ. Four color compensation. *Cytometry*, **38** (1999) 161–175.
20. Borowitz MJ, Bray R, Gascoyne R, et al. U.S.–Canadian Consensus recommendations on the immunophenotypic analysis of hematologic neoplasia by flow cytometry: medical indications, *Cytometry*, **30** (1997) 249–263.
21. Braylan RC, Atwater SK, Diamond L, et al. U.S.–Canadian Consensus recommendations on the immunophenotypic analysis of hematologic neoplasia by flow cytometry: data reporting, *Cytometry*, **30** (1997) 245–248.
22. Davis BH, Foucar K, Szczarkowski W, et al. U.S.–Canadian Consensus recommendations on the immunophenotypic analysis of hematologic neoplasia by flow cytometry: medical indications, *Cytometry*, **30** (1997) 249–263.
23. Rothe G and Schmitz G. Consensus protocol for the flow cytometric immunophenotyping of hematopoietic malignancies. Working Group on Flow Cytometry and Image Analysis, *Leukemia*, **10** (1996) 877–895.
24. Stewart CC, Behm FG, Carey JL, et al. U.S.–Canadian Consensus recommendations on the immunophenotypic analysis of hematologic neoplasia by flow cytometry: selection of antibody combinations, *Cytometry*, **30** (1997) 231–235.
25. Pallisgaard N, Clausen N, Schroder H, and Hokland P. Rapid and sensitive minimal residual disease detection in acute leukemia by quantitative real-time RT-PCR exemplified by t(12;21) TEL-AML1 fusion transcript, *Genes Chromosomes Cancer*, **26** (1999) 355–365.
26. Pongers Willemse MJ, Seriu T, Stolz F, et al. Primers and protocols for standardized detection of minimal residual disease in acute lymphoblastic leukemia using immunoglobulin and T cell receptor gene rearrangements and TAL1 deletions as PCR targets: report of the BIOMED-1 CONCERTED ACTION: investigation of minimal residual disease in acute leukemia, *Leukemia*, **13** (1999) 110–118.
27. Groeneveld K, te Marvelde JG, van den Beemd MW, Hooijkaas H, and van Dongen JJ. Flow cytometric detection of intracellular antigens for immunophenotyping of normal and malignant leukocytes, *Leukemia*, **10** (1996) 1383–1389.
28. Van Lochem EG, Groeneveld K, Te Marvelde JG, Van den Beemd MW, Hooijkaas H, and Van Dongen JJ. Flow cytometric detection of intracellular antigens for immunophenotyping of normal and malignant leukocytes: testing of a new fixation-permeabilization solution [letter], *Leukemia*, **11** (1997) 2208–2210.
29. Koester SK and Bolton WE. Intracellular markers, *J. Immunol. Methods*, **243** (2000) 99–106.
30. Koester SK and Bolton WE. Strategies for cell permeabilization and fixation in detecting surface and intracellular antigens, *Methods Cell Biol.*, **63** (2001) 253–268.
31. Babustkova O, Glasova M, Konikova E, and Kusenda J. Leukemia-associated phenotypes: their characteristics and incidence in acute leukemia, *Neoplasma*, **443** (1996) 67–72.
32. Baer MR. Assessment of minimal residual disease in patients with acute leukemia, *Curr. Opin. Oncol.*, **10** (1998) 17–22.
33. San Miguel JF, Martinez A, Macedo A, et al. Immunophenotyping investigation of minimal residual disease is a useful approach for predicting relapse in acute myeloid leukemia patients, *Blood*, **90** (1997) 2465–2470.
34. Reading CL, Estey EH, Huh YO, et al. Expression of unusual immunophenotype combinations in acute myelogenous leukemia, *Blood*, **81** (1993) 3083–3090.

35. Wuchter C, Harbott J, Schoch C, et al. Detection of acute leukemia cells with mixed lineage leukemia (MLL) gene rearrangements by flow cytometry using monoclonal antibody 7.1, *Leukemia*, **14** (2000) 1232–1238.
36. van Dongen JJ, Breit TM, Adriaansen HJ, Beishuizen A, and Hooijkaas H. Immunophenotypic and immunogenotypic detection of minimal residual disease in acute lymphoblastic leukemia, *Recent Results Cancer Res.*, **131** (1993) 157–184.
37. van Dongen JJ, Breit TM, Adriaansen HJ, Beishuizen A, and Hooijkaas H. Detection of minimal residual disease in acute leukemia by immunological marker analysis and polymerase chain reaction, *Leukemia*, **6(Suppl. 1)** (1992) 47–59.
38. Terstappen LW and Loken MR. Myeloid cell differentiation in normal bone marrow and acute myeloid leukemia assessed by multi-dimensional flow cytometry, *Anal. Cell Pathol.*, **2** (1990) 229–240.
39. Terstappen LW, Konemann S, Safford M, et al. Flow cytometric characterization of acute myeloid leukemia. Part 1. Significance of light scattering properties, *Leukemia*, **5** (1991) 315–321.
40. Terstappen LW, Safford M, Konemann S, et al. Flow cytometric characterization of acute myeloid leukemia. Part II. Phenotypic heterogeneity at diagnosis [corrected and republished article originally printed in Leukemia 1991 Sep;5(9):757–767], *Leukemia*, **6** (1992) 70–80.
41. Schwartz S, Heinecke A, Zimmermann M, et al. Expression of the C-kit receptor (CD117) is a feature of almost all subtypes of de novo acute myeloblastic leukemia (AML), including cytogenetically good-risk AML, and lacks prognostic significance, *Leuk. Lymphoma*, **34** (1992) 85–94.
42. Weinkauff R, Estey EH, Starostik P, et al. Use of peripheral blood blasts vs bone marrow blasts for diagnosis of acute leukemia, *Am. J. Clin. Pathol.*, **111** (1999) 733–740.
43. Langerak AW, Wolvers Tettero IL, van den Beemd MW, et al. Immunophenotypic and immunogenotypic characteristics of TCRgammadelta+ T cell acute lymphoblastic leukemia, *Leukemia*, **13** (1999) 206–214.
44. Bene MC, Bernier M, Casasnovas RO, et al. The reliability and specificity of c-kit for the diagnosis of acute myeloid leukemias and undifferentiated leukemias. The European Group for the Immunological Classification of Leukemias (EGIL), *Blood*, **92** (1998) 596–599.
45. Ludwig WD, Rieder H, Bartram CR, et al. Immunophenotypic and genotypic features, clinical characteristics, and treatment outcome of adult pro-B acute lymphoblastic leukemia: results of the German multicenter trials GMALL 03/87 and 04/89, *Blood*, **92** (1998) 1898–1909.
46. Schott G, Sperling C, Schrappe M, et al. Immunophenotypic and clinical features of T-cell receptor gammadelta+ T-lineage acute lymphoblastic leukaemia, *Br. J. Haematol.*, **101** (1998) 753–755.
47. Venditti A, Buccisano F, Del Poeta G, et al. Level of minimal residual disease after consolidation therapy predicts outcome in acute myeloid leukemia, *Blood*, **96** (2000) 3948–3952.
48. Wormann B, Safford M, Konemann S, Buchner T, Hiddemann W, and Terstappen LW. Detection of aberrant antigen expression in acute myeloid leukemia by multiparameter flow cytometry, *Recent Results Cancer Res.*, **131** (1993) 185–196.
49. Pui CH, Behm FG, and Crist WM. Clinical and biologic relevance of immunologic marker studies in childhood acute lymphoblastic leukemia, *Blood*, **82** (1993) 343–362.
50. Sperling C, Schwartz S, Buchner T, Thiel E, and Ludwig WD. Expression of the stem cell factor receptor C-KIT (CD117) in acute leukemias, *Haematologica*, **82** (1997) 617–621.

# 2

# Flow-Cytometry–Based Studies of Minimal Residual Disease in Children with Acute Lymphoblastic Leukemia

## Dario Campana

## INTRODUCTION

A central problem in childhood acute lymphoblastic leukemia (ALL) is the identification of patients who require more aggressive therapy to avert relapse. Although clinical (e.g., white blood cell count, age) and biologic (e.g., immunophenotype, ploidy, structural chromosomal abnormalities, and gene rearrangements) parameters can be used for treatment stratification, none of these prognostic factors is ideal. A proportion of patients with "good risk" features relapse, whereas others may receive more intensive treatment than is necessary. Studies of minimal residual disease (MRD) aim at improving estimates of the total burden of leukemic cells during clinical remission. This information provides an indicator of the aggressiveness and drug sensitivity of the disease and helps in the selection of appropriate therapeutic strategies.

Reliable MRD assays would allow not only the early identification of patients at a higher risk of relapse and detection of impending clinical relapse, but would also provide a powerful tool for assessing bone marrow or peripheral blood that has been harvested for autologous hematopoietic stem cell transplantation and for determining the efficacy of "purging" procedures (1). In addition, MRD measurements could be used as end points to rapidly compare the effectiveness of different chemotherapeutic regimens.

The main purpose of MRD assays is to be clinically useful. Therefore, methods must be robust, reliable, rapid, and suitable for a clinical laboratory. Numerous methods of monitoring MRD in acute leukemia have been developed and are

From: *Leukemia and Lymphoma: Detection of Minimal Residual Disease*
Edited by: T. F. Zipf and D. A. Johnston © Humana Press Inc., Totowa, NJ

discussed extensively in this book. The following sections review the methodologic and clinical advances in the detection and measurement of MRD in childhood ALL based on immunophenotype.

## IMMUNOPHENOTYPIC IDENTIFICATION OF LEUKEMIA CELLS

### *Rationale*

In general, the immunophenotype of leukemic cells reflect that of their normal counterparts. The normal equivalents of T-lineage ALL cells are immature T-cells, which expand in the thymus and are confined to this organ *(2)*. Therefore, in patients with this subtype of leukemia, detection of MRD in the bone marrow or in the peripheral blood is relatively straightforward: It consists in the identification of immunophenotypically immature T-cells *(3)*. For example, the combination CD3/TdT is expressed by most T-lineage ALL cells and by developing T-cells in the thymus, but it is never observed among normal peripheral blood or bone marrow cells *(4)*. Other similar thymus-restricted immunophenotypic combinations can also be used *(5)*. In the case of B-lineage ALL cells, the normal equivalent cells are the B-cell progenitors, which normally reside in the bone marrow *(6)*. These cells are particularly abundant in samples from young children or in bone marrow regenerating after chemotherapy and bone marrow transplantation *(7)* and can also be found, albeit in low proportions, in the peripheral blood *(8)*. Therefore, in patients with this subtype of leukemia, detection of MRD by immunophenotypic criteria depends on the identification of molecules differentially expressed in normal and leukemic cells.

Differentially expressed molecules that constitute leukemia-associated immunophenotypes in B-lineage ALL can be classified in three broad categories. The first category includes the product of gene fusions that accompany chromosomal translocations such as *BCR-ABL*, *E2A-PBX1*, *MLL-AF4*, and *TEL-AML1*. The encoded chimeric proteins are genuine tumor-associated markers, and antibodies specific for these tumor markers should be useful for studies of MRD. Unfortunately, it has been difficult to produce monoclonal antibodies that would allow reliable detection of these proteins by immunofluorescence, although one such reagent, which reacts with the *E2A-PBX1* chimeric protein, has been described *(9)*.

A second category is represented by molecules whose expression becomes dysregulated by the leukemic process. For example, the human homolog of the rat chondroitin sulfate proteoglycan (NG2), recognized by the antibody 7.1, is expressed by leukemic lymphoblasts (generally those with 11q23 abnormalities) but not by normal hematopoietic cells *(10,11)*. Another molecule, CD66c, is expressed in approximately one-third of B-lineage ALL cases, but it is not expressed in normal B-cell progenitors *(12–15)*. Because this antibody also reacts with myeloid cells, it must be used in combination with reagents that identify lymphoid progenitors.

A third category of immunophenotypic features that can be used to distinguish B-lineage ALL cells from normal B-cell progenitors is represented by molecules that are expressed during normal B-cell development but are relatively underexpressed or overexpressed in leukemic cells *(16–18)*. For example, normal CD19$^+$CD34$^+$ B-cell progenitors lack CD21, a marker expressed later during differentiation, but cells in a proportion of B-lineage ALL cases are CD19$^+$ CD34$^+$CD21$^+$. In addition, a number of quantitative differences in antigen expression can be used to distinguish leukemic blast cells from subsets of normal cells with similar phenotypes. Thus, the expression of CD19, CD10, and CD34 in some cases of B-lineage ALL can be more than 10-fold greater than that of normal B-cell progenitors *(16–19)*. Underexpression of CD45 and CD38 is also an abnormal feature in some B-lineage ALL cases *(16–20)*. Other markers, such as CD45RA, CD11a, and CD44 may also be overexpressed or underexpressed *(21)*. Overexpression of WT1 in ALL *(22,23)* could also, in principle, be exploited for MRD studies.

## Flow Cytometry

In theory, the availability of antibodies to true tumor antigens (e.g., proteins product of gene fusions) would allow identification of residual leukemic cells. Even in this case, however, it seems likely that focusing the analysis on selected cell subsets identified by other markers would increase the reliability and sensitivity of the assay. Current immunologic strategies for detecting residual disease rely on combinations of multiple markers; hence, they cannot be performed by immunohistochemistry. They require immunofluorescence techniques that allow the simultaneous application of antibodies conjugated to different fluorochromes. Early MRD studies were performed by fluorescence microscopy *(3–24)*. However, microscopic screening of a large number of cells is tedious and time-consuming. The automation of this process by computerized image analysis is desirable, but we have not yet encountered a sufficiently sensitive and accurate instrument that we could recommend for reliable MRD detection. Virtually all laboratories currently prefer flow cytometry, which allows multiparameter analysis, antigen quantitation, and rapid screening of large numbers of cells. Additional capabilities of flow cytometry, such as cell sorting followed by fluorescence *in situ* hybridization (FISH) *(25)* or simultaneous analysis of phenotype and DNA content *(26)*, may also aid MRD studies, but have not been used extensively for this purpose.

Currently, most laboratories use three-color analysis for MRD studies, including antibodies conjugated to FITC, PE, and PerCP. Dual-laser flow cytometers that allow the detection of other fluorochromes such as antigen-presenting cells (APC) and permit four-color analysis appear to be ideally suited for these studies.

In addition, this approach potentially allows a reduction in the number of individual test tubes per sample, thus employing reagents and cells more efficiently.

## Sensitivity and Precision

The sensitivity of detecting rare cells by flow cytometry is determined by the degree of difference in the features of the target population as compared to the remaining cells and by the number of cells that can be counted. As discussed in this chapter, ALL cells do express markers in combinations that are not found in normal hematopoietic cells. Thus, the main limitation in sensitivity for all MRD detection methods is the number of cells that can be analyzed. A marrow sample taken from a child with acute leukemia in clinical remission typically yields $5 \times 10^7$ or fewer mononuclear cells, and technical constraints may limit the number of cells available for study to less than $1 \times 10^6$. Flow cytometry allows the detection of 1 target cell in $10^8$ or more cells, providing that a large number of cells is studied (e.g., $10^8$ or more) and the fluidics system is exhaustively cleansed *(27–30)*. Because such large samples are rarely available during routine MRD studies in patients with leukemia, a more reasonable sensitivity for practical applications is approximately 1 target cell in $10^4$–$10^5$ cells.

To determine the precision of flow-cytometric detection of rare cells, we prepared mixtures of leukemic and normal cells and compared the results of multiple measurements of residual leukemia in identical cell preparations. The results demonstrated that this assay is highly precise: in 23 tests of mixtures containing 1 leukemic cell in $10^4$ normal cells, results were remarkably similar (coefficient of variation = 15%); in 22 tests of mixtures containing 1 leukemic cell in $10^3$ cells, the coefficient of variation was 10% *(31)*.

## Methodological Approach

The methodological approach that we use in our laboratory has previously been described in detail *(16)*. Briefly, we first perform a detailed analysis of the immunophenotype of the leukemic blasts at diagnosis or at relapse. The results from the patients' cells are then compared to previously obtained results of an identical immunophenotypic analysis of normal bone marrow and peripheral blood samples. The most distinctive marker combinations in each case are thus selected. If the immunophenotype of the leukemic cells were not known, one would have to apply the full range of potentially useful markers for MRD studies in remission samples. This not only would be expensive and time-consuming, but it may still fail to identify residual disease.

At the time of MRD analysis, cells are labeled with the selected antibody combinations, and the light-scattering and immunophenotypic features of 10,000 cells are recorded *(16)*. We then selectively store and examine the information for cells that fulfill the predetermined morphologic and immunophenotypic criteria, from a total of over $2 \times 10^5$ bone marrow mononuclear cells.

At least 10–20 dots expressing the leukemia-associated features must be captured to interpret a cluster of abnormal flow cytometric events.

## Selection of Markers

To date, leukemia-specific phenotypes have been searched by systematically comparing the immunophenotypes of leukemic cells with those of normal bone marrow cells *(16)*. This approach has identified phenotypic features that are uniquely associated with leukemic cells and are never expressed during normal hematopoietic cell development, even during chemotherapy or after bone marrow transplantation. Unfortunately, this process is slow and largely based on trial and error.

We have recently used cDNA arrays to identify immunophenotypic differences between ALL cells and normal lymphoid progenitors *(32)*. By cDNA array analysis, 334 of 4132 genes studied were expressed 1.5-fold to 5.8-fold higher in leukemic cells relative to both normal samples; 238 of these genes were also overexpressed in the leukemic cell line RS4;11. We selected 9 genes among the 274 overexpressed in at least two leukemic samples and measured expression of the encoded proteins by flow cytometry. Seven proteins (CD58, creatine kinase B, ninjurin1, Ref1, calpastatin, HDJ-2, and annexin VI) were expressed in B-lineage ALL cells at higher levels than in normal $CD19^+CD10^+$ B-cell progenitors ($p < 0.05$ in all comparisons). Because of its abundant and prevalent overexpression, CD58 was chosen for further analysis. An anti-CD58 antibody identified residual leukemic cells (0.01–1.13%, median 0.03%) in 9 of 104 bone marrow samples from children with ALL in clinical remission. MRD estimates by CD58 staining correlated well with those of polymerase chain reaction (PCR) amplification of immunoglobulin genes.

The identification of immunophenotypic differences between normal bone marrow cells and leukemic cells in diagnostic samples is just a starting point. It is then important to test the expression of the selected markers on normal bone marrow cells under different conditions. In particular, it is crucial to establish whether levels of expression remain consistent in leukemic cells of patients undergoing chemotherapy and in normal cells actively proliferating after chemotherapy or bone marrow transplantation. Investigators planning to test samples after several hours from collection (e.g., those shipped from other centers) should ensure that the leukemia-associated immunophenotypes are stable. In addition, experiments with mixtures of leukemic and normal cells are required to test the sensitivity afforded by the new immunophenotypic combination.

## ANTIBODY PANELS

Table 1 summarizes the phenotypic combinations currently used in our laboratory. We use only immunophenotypes that allow us to detect 1 leukemic cell

Table 1
Immunophenotypic Markers Currently Used to Study MRD in Children with ALL

| ALL lineage | Type of phenotypic abnormality | Markers | Frequency (%)[a] |
|---|---|---|---|
| B | Overexpression | CD19/CD34/CD10/TdT | 30–50 |
|   | or under expression | CD19/CD34/CD10/CD22 | 20–30 |
|   | of markers also expressed | CD19/CD34/CD10/CD38 | 30–50 |
|   | in normal B-cell progenitors | CD19/CD34/CD10/CD45 | 30–50 |
|   |   | CD19/CD34/CD10/CD58 | 40–60 |
|   | Expression of markers | CD19/CD34/CD10/**CD13** | 10–20 |
|   | not expressed | CD19/CD34/CD10/**CD15** | 5–10 |
|   | in normal B-cell progenitors | CD19/CD34/CD10/**CD33** | 5–10 |
|   | (**aberrant marker**) | CD19/CD34/CD10/**CD65** | 5–10 |
|   |   | CD19/CD34/CD10/**CD56** | 5–10 |
|   |   | CD19/CD34/CD10/**CD66c** | 10–20 |
|   |   | CD19/CD34/CD10/**7.1** | 3–5 |
|   | Expression of markers expressed | CD19/CD34/CD10/CD21 | 5–10 |
|   | at different stages | CD19/CD34/TdT/cytopl.μ | 10–20 |
|   | of normal B-cell maturation |   |   |
| T | Phenotypes normally confined | TdT/CD3 | 90–95 |
|   | to the thymus | CD34/CD3 | 30–50 |

[a]Proportion of childhood ALL cases in which 1 leukemic cell in $10^4$ normal bone marrow cells can be detected with the listed immunophenotypic combination. Most cases express more than one combination useful for MRD studies (16).

in $10^4$ or more normal cells. We use the combination of nuclear TdT with T-cell markers, such as cytoplasmic or surface CD3 or CD5, in virtually all cases of T-ALL. In cases with weak or negative TdT expression, we used CD34 instead, if this marker is found to be expressed at diagnosis. CD19 and HLA-Dr, which are not usually expressed on T-ALL blasts but are strongly positive on most normal bone marrow TdT$^+$ cells, can be used to further distinguish normal from leukemic cells. By this approach, MRD can be studied in virtually all cases of T-ALL.

Detection of MRD in B-lineage ALL requires a larger panel of antibodies. We usually identify immature B-cells by the simultaneous expression of CD19, CD10, and CD34 or TdT. Quantitative differences in antigenic expression between leukemic and normal cells in the expression of these markers can be used in approx 30–50% of cases. Other useful markers whose expression may differ quantitatively in leukemic and normal immature B-cells are CD38, CD45, CD22, and the recently identified CD58. Qualitative differences between normal and leukemic cells can be detected by using antibodies to myeloid- and NK-associated molecules or to molecules expressed by mature normal B-cells.

CD66c and anti-NG2 (7.1), as mentioned above, are two additional informative markers. With all of these marker combinations, approx 90% of B-lineage ALL cases can be studied at the 1 in $10^4$ level of sensitivity.

## Flow Cytometry Compared to PCR

Each method of MRD detection has specific advantages and potential pitfalls *(33)*. For example, immunologic techniques yield a more accurate quantitation of MRD and can discriminate viable from dying cells, whereas PCR may have superior sensitivity. In any case, neither immunologic nor molecular techniques can, at present, be applied to all patients, which is a prerequisite for the introduction of MRD monitoring in clinical protocols. To determine how well measurements obtained by flow cytometry and PCR amplification of IgH genes were correlated, we tested serial dilutions of normal and leukemic cells by both methods *(34)*. We found the two methods to be highly sensitive ($10^{-4}$ or greater sensitivity), accurate ($r^2$ was 0.999 for flow cytometry and 0.960 for PCR by regression analysis), and concordant ($r^2 = 0.962$). We then used both methods to examine 62 bone marrow samples collected from children with ALL in clinical remission *(34)*. In 12 samples, both techniques detected MRD levels $>10^{-4}$. The percentages of leukemic cells measured by the two methods were highly correlated ($r^2 = 0.978$). Of the remaining 50 samples, 48 had MRD levels $<10^{-4}$. Results were discordant in only two of these samples: PCR detected 2 in $10^4$ and 5 in $10^4$ leukemic cells, whereas the results of the flow-cytometric assays were negative; both patients remain in remission by clinical, flow-cytometric, and molecular criteria, 22 and 32 mo after remission.

We also compared the results of flow cytometry to those of reverse transcription (RT)-PCR amplification of fusion transcripts (*BCR-ABL* and *MLL-AF4*; Coustan-Smith et al., unpublished results). In 25 of 27 bone marrow samples collected during remission, the methods gave concordant results (10 were MRD$^+$ and 15 were MRD$^-$). Of the two remaining samples, one was negative by flow cytometry but positive ($10^{-5}$) by PCR; the other was positive by flow cytometry but negative by PCR (MRD was detectable by both methods in prior and subsequent samples from this patient). These results indicate that measurements of MRD by our flow-cytometric method and by PCR assay are comparable and that levels of MRD associated with a higher risk of relapse (i.e., $>10^{-4}$) can be detected by either technique.

## Potential Sources of Error

Detection of rare events by flow cytometry requires meticulously clean and precise procedures *(16)*. False-positive results can be caused by sample contamination, dirty reagents, and imperfect cleansing of the fluidics system. False-positive results can be caused by using antibodies that react nonspecifically. We strongly recommend the use of isotype-matched nonreactive antibodies as controls and careful titration of all antibodies. The sequence in which antibodies are added to cells and the times of incubation must be rigorously standardized, because variations in these procedures can alter the intensity of cell labeling. Variations resulting from changes between different batches of antibodies must be monitored by frequent staining of normal samples. It goes without saying that the instrument should be maintained in excellent condition, with frequent calibration and periodic servicing.

A small fraction of patients has a recurrence of acute leukemia whose cellular features are unlike those determined at diagnosis. In the majority of cases, these leukemias are unrelated to the original leukemic clone and represent secondary malignancies, which are often caused by the mutagenic effects of leukemia treatment (35,36). Clearly, secondary leukemias cannot be anticipated by currently available methods for monitoring MRD. In a proportion of cases, recurrent leukemia has genetic features that confirm its relationship to the original leukemic clone, but has the phenotype of a different lineage (lineage switch). There have been reports of leukemias morphologically and immunophenotypically characterized as ALL that relapse as AML, while retaining the karyotypic and molecular features of the original clone (37–39). Such "lineage switch" relapses may be detected early by molecular methods such as including PCR amplification of chromosomal breakpoints or antigen-receptor gene rearrangements, but not by flow cytometry.

Another cause of false-negative results during monitoring for residual leukemia is clonal evolution during and after treatment, which may cause the disappearance of one or more of the markers detected at diagnosis—a phenomenon already noted in early studies (40–46). The impact of immunophenotypic changes on MRD monitoring with multiple markers is related to the number of marker combinations that can be applied to each patient.

## CLINICAL STUDIES OF MRD IN ALL BY FLOW CYTOMETRY

### *Correlation Between MRD and Treatment Outcome*

Immunophenotyping was the first method to be productively used to study MRD (3). Several earlier studies demonstrated the potential usefulness of this approach (24,47,48). Despite promising initial results, interest in this approach was somewhat diverted by the advent of PCR in the late 1980s. Many investigators, startled by the novelty and elegance of PCR, began regarding almost any other existing laboratory technique as a relic of another era. However, when we directly compared the two methods over a decade ago (49), we emerged with the impression that flow cytometry would remain a valid, informative, and clinically applicable approach to study MRD. This impression was corroborated by the consistent improvement in antibody and fluorochrome quality and variety and by the relentless refinement of flow cytometers and analytical hardware and software.

Our findings on monitoring residual disease in children with ALL have been summarized in a recent publication *(50)*. We prospectively studied MRD in 195 children with newly diagnosed ALL in clinical remission. Bone marrow aspirates ($n = 629$) were collected at the end of remission induction therapy and at three intervals thereafter. Detectable MRD (i.e., ≥0.01% leukemic mono-nuclear cells) at each time-point was associated with a higher relapse rate ($p < 0.001$); patients with high levels of MRD at the end of the induction phase (≥1%) or at wk 14 of continuation therapy (≥0.1%) had a particularly poor outcome. The incidence of relapse among patients with MRD at the end of the induction phase was 68±16% (SE) if they remained MRD$^+$ (18 patients) through wk 14 of continuation therapy, compared with 7±7% if MRD became undetectable (14 patients) ($p = 0.035$). The persistence of MRD until wk 32 was highly predictive of relapse (all four MRD$^+$ patients relapsed versus two of the eight who converted to undetectable MRD status; $p = 0.021$).

Residual disease was significantly more frequent in infants and patients ≥10 yr of age than in children of intermediate ages ($p = 0.007$). Notably, four of six infants had ≥0.01% leukemic cells at the end of remission induction. Among cellular features, rates of detection did not differ significantly in comparisons based on cell lineage, but there was a strong association between MRD detection and the Philadelphia chromosome: All eight cases with this abnormality had positive findings ($p < 0.001$). This contrasts with MRD positivity in 2 of 15 cases with a *TEL* gene rearrangement and 8 of 42 cases with hyperdiploid (>50 chromosomes) B-lineage ALL, both considered favorable prognostic signs *(51–55)*.

The predictive strength of MRD remained significant even after adjusting for adverse presenting features. It also remained significant in analyses that excluded patients at very high or very low risk of relapse by St. Jude criteria *(56)* or that focused on patients with high risk of relapse by NCI criteria *(57)*. Because persistence of circulating lymphoblasts after the first week of treatment identifies children with ALL at a higher risk of relapse *(58–62)*, we also determined whether MRD studies at the end of remission induction would add to the prognostic information provided by the earlier morphologic assessment of circulating lymphoblasts. MRD findings at the end of the induction phase correlated well with treatment outcome in patients with or without circulating blasts.

Additional findings demonstrating the value of immunologic MRD monitoring in patients with ALL were reported by Farahat et al. *(63)*, who used antibodies to TdT, CD10, and CD19 to detect MRD in six of nine patients 5–15 wk before relapse. By contrast, 43 patients who remained in continuous complete remission, with a median follow-up of 23 mo, were consistently free of MRD by flow cytometry. In a study of 53 ALL patients (37 B-lineage and 16 T-lineage ALL), Ciudad et al. *(64)* used three-color flow cytometry to study MRD. Patients who had a gradual increase in MRD levels showed a higher relapse rate (90% vs 22%) and shorter median relapse-free survival than those with stable or decreasing

MRD levels. The adverse predictive value of MRD was also observed when children and adults were analyzed separately.

## Bone Marrow Versus Peripheral Blood for MRD Studies

Practical and ethical considerations limit the acquisition of sequential bone marrow samples from children. The use of peripheral blood rather than bone marrow may provide additional opportunities for MRD studies, but little is known about the clinical significance of studying MRD in peripheral blood. The existing studies on the subject have used PCR and produced discordant results. Brisco et al. used quantified MRD in 35 paired blood and bone marrow samples from 15 children with B-lineage ALL receiving induction therapy and found that the level of MRD in peripheral blood was approx 10-fold lower than in marrow (65). Van Rhee et al., in a study of Ph+ ALL, had similar findings in 3 of 18 patients, while in the remainder, there was no significant difference in MRD detected in blood and marrow (66). Martin et al. also found that MRD levels in marrow exceeded those in blood by a factor of 10 or more in six patients (67). However, more recently, Donovan et al. used PCR amplification of antigen-receptor genes to compare MRD in 801 paired blood and bone marrow samples obtained from 165 patients; findings in 82% of the pairs were concordant (68).

We studied 90 pairs of bone marrow and peripheral blood samples. Of these, 69 were negative in both marrow and blood and 10 were positive in both. In the remaining 11 samples, leukemic cells were detected in the bone marrow but not in peripheral blood. Interestingly, all five patients with T-lineage ALL who had detectable MRD in the bone marrow had an approximately equal proportion of leukemic cells in the peripheral blood. By contrast, only 5 of the 16 patients with B-lineage ALL who had detectable MRD in the bone marrow also had detectable circulating blast cells (Coustan-Smith et al., unpublished results). Taken together, the available evidence suggests that the correlation between levels of MRD in the peripheral blood and bone marrow may vary with the time of measurement, the subtype of ALL, and, possibly, the type of treatment.

## FUTURE PERSPECTIVES

The studies of MRD in childhood ALL reported to date collectively indicate that measurements of MRD provide a powerful and independent prognostic indicator of treatment outcome in children with ALL and are likely to have a consequential impact on the clinical management of these patients. The results of MRD studies during the early phases of therapy in this disease are consistent with, and add to, the predictive value of other measurements of early response to therapy, such as the presence of circulating blast cells at d 7 of therapy (59), the degree of response to prednisone (61), and the morphologic detection of blast cells in the bone marrow on d 15 and 21 (69).

It remains to be decided how MRD assays should be used to guide treatment. Based on the existing evidence, it seems reasonable to intensify therapy for those patients who have a slow early response to treatment and have detectable MRD during clinical remission. Conversely, the excellent clinical outcome of MRD-negative cases raises the possibility of using MRD assays to identify candidates for experimenting reductions in treatment intensity. However, it may be argued that studies of MRD are unlikely to substantially improve clinical strategies in a disease such as childhood ALL, in which approximately three-fourths of patients can be cured and for which several risk factors strongly predictive of outcome are already guiding therapy (70). However, known prognostic factors are not 100% predictive, and MRD studies might well complement and enhance their informative value. Moreover, oncologists may be reluctant to abandon clinical and biologic parameters, such as age, leukocyte counts, and genetic features, whose relation with treatment response has been repeatedly confirmed, even within different treatment protocols, and there are only a few informative (but not nearly as extensive) clinical studies of MRD. Therefore, at present, it seems prudent to combine MRD with clinical and biologic parameters for a comprehensive risk assignment in children with ALL.

We still do not know whether early detection of relapse and subsequent changes in therapeutic strategies will improve cure rates, but there is reason to believe that this might be the case. First, it is well established that the tumor burden and the curability of cancer are related. In ALL, for example, a large tumor mass at diagnosis as demonstrated by high leukocyte counts and high serum lactate dehydrogenase activity is an indicator of poor prognosis (56). Second, the likelihood of the emergence of drug-resistant malignant cells by mutation increases as the number of cell divisions increases and, hence, relates to the total tumor burden (71).

The use of MRD studies may benefit treatment of childhood ALL beyond risk assignment. For example, the utility of autologous transplantation could conceivably be improved by the development of effective techniques for purging the graft of leukemic cells, coupled with sensitive methods for detection of MRD. In addition, testing of new treatment approaches, such as tyrosine kinase inhibitors, cytokines, immunotoxins, adoptive T-cells, compounds interfering with oncogenic molecular aberrations, and inhibitors of angiogenic growth factors, may necessitate modifying the way in which anticancer treatments have traditionally been tested. MRD measurements may serve as surrogate end points in the clinical testing of these novel therapeutic approaches.

One has to recognize that none of the methods developed to date to study MRD is perfect and that existing techniques have advantages and disadvantages. Therefore, our approach is to combine two methods in efforts to study all patients. By using flow cytometry and PCR amplification of antigen-receptor genes simultaneously, we have been able to study 96 consecutive cases. This approach should also prevent false-negative results because of changes in immuno-phenotype or predominant antigen-receptor gene clone during the course of the disease.

## ACKNOWLEDGMENTS

This work was supported by grants CA60419, CA52259, CA21765, and CA20180 from the National Cancer Institute, by the Rizzo Memorial Grant from the Leukemia Research Foundation, and by the American Lebanese Syrian Associated Charities (ALSAC).

## REFERENCES

1. Rambaldi A, Borleri G, Dotti G, Bellavita P, Amaru R, Biondi A, et al. Innovative two-step negative selection of granulocyte colony-stimulating factor-mobilized circulating progenitor cells: adequacy for autologous and allogeneic transplantation, *Blood*, **91** (1998) 2189–2196.
2. Bradstock KF, Janossy G, Pizzolo G, Hoffbrand AV, McMichael A, Pilch JR, et al. Subpopulations of normal and leukemic human thymocytes: an analysis with the use of monoclonal antibodies, *J. Natl. Cancer Inst.*, **65** (1980) 33–42.
3. Bradstock KF, Janossy G, Tidman N, Papageorgiou ES, Prentice HG, Willoughby M, et al. Immunological monitoring of residual disease in treated thymic acute lymphoblastic leukaemia, *Leuk. Res.*, **5** (1981) 301–309.
4. Campana D, Thompson JS, Amlot P, Brown S, and Janossy G. The cytoplasmic expression of CD3 antigens in normal and malignant cells of the T lymphoid lineage, *J. Immunol.*, **138** (1987) 648–655.
5. Porwit-MacDonald A, Bjorklund E, Lucio P, van Lochem EG, Mazur J, Parreira A, et al. BIOMED-1 concerted action report: flow cytometric characterization of CD7+ cell subsets in normal bone marrow as a basis for the diagnosis and follow-up of T cell acute lymphoblastic leukemia (T-ALL), *Leukemia*, **14** (2000) 816–825.
6. Janossy G, Bollum FJ, Bradstock KF, and Ashley J. Cellular phenotypes of normal and leukemic hemopoietic cells determined by analysis with selected antibody combinations, *Blood*, **56** (1980) 430–441.
7. Asma GE, van den Bergh RL, and Vossen JM. Regeneration of TdT+, pre-B, and B cells in bone marrow after allogeneic bone marrow transplantation, *Transplantation*, **43** (1987) 865–870.
8. Froehlich TW, Buchanan GR, Cornet JA, Sartain PA, and Smith RG. Terminal deoxynucleotidyl transferase-containing cells in peripheral blood: implications for the surveillance of patients with lymphoblastic leukemia or lymphoma in remission, *Blood*, **58** (1981) 214–220.
9. Sang BC, Shi L, Dias P, Liu L, Wei J, Wang ZX, et al. Monoclonal antibodies specific to the acute lymphoblastic leukemia t(1;19)-associated E2A/pbx1 chimeric protein: characterization and diagnostic utility, *Blood*, **89** (1997) 2909–2914.
10. Smith FO, Rauch C, Williams DE, March CJ, Arthur D, Hilden J, et al. The human homologue of rat NG2, a chondroitin sulfate proteoglycan, is not expressed on the cell surface of normal hematopoietic cells but is expressed by acute myeloid leukemia blasts from poor-prognosis patients with abnormalities of chromosome band 11q23, *Blood*, **87** (1996) 1123–1133.
11. Behm FG, Smith FO, Raimondi SC, Pui CH, and Bernstein ID. Human homologue of the rat chondroitin sulfate proteoglycan, NG2, detected by monoclonal antibody 7.1, identifies childhood acute lymphoblastic leukemias with t(4;11)(q21;q23) or t(11;19)(q23;p13) and MLL gene rearrangements, *Blood*, **87** (1996) 1134–1139.

12. Hanenberg H, Baumann M, Quentin I, Nagel G, Grosse-Wilde H, von Kleist S, et al. Expression of the CEA gene family members NCA-50/90 and NCA-160 (CD66) in childhood acute lymphoblastic leukemias (ALLs) and in cell lines of B-cell origin, *Leukemia*, **8** (1994) 2127–2133.

13. Mori T, Sugita K, Suzuki T, Okazaki T, Manabe A, Hosoya R, et al. A novel monoclonal antibody, KOR-SA3544 which reacts to Philadelphia chromosome-positive acute lymphoblastic leukemia cells with high sensitivity, *Leukemia*, **9** (1995) 1233–1239.

14. Sugita K, Mori T, Yokota S, Kuroki M, Koyama TO, Inukai T, et al. The KOR-SA3544 antigen predominantly expressed on the surface of Philadelphia chromosome-positive acute lymphoblastic leukemia cells is nonspecific cross-reacting antigen-50/90 (CD66c) and invariably expressed in cytoplasm of human leukemia cells, *Leukemia*, **13** (1999) 779–785.

15. Carrasco M, Munoz L, Bellido M, Bernat S, Rubiol E, Ubeda J, et al. CD66 expression in acute leukaemia, *Ann. Hematol.*, **79** (2000) 299–303.

16. Campana D and Coustan-Smith E. Detection of minimal residual disease in acute leukemia by flow cytometry, *Cytometry*, **38** (1999) 139–152.

17. Lucio P, Parreira A, van den Beemd MW, van Lochem EG, Van Wering ER, Baars E, et al. Flow cytometric analysis of normal B cell differentiation: a frame of reference for the detection of minimal residual disease in precursor-B-ALL, *Leukemia*, **13** (1999) 419–427.

18. Ciudad J, San Miguel JF, Lopez-Berges MC, Garcia MM, Gonzalez M, et al. Detection of abnormalities in B-cell differentiation pattern is a useful tool to predict relapse in precursor-B-ALL, *Br. J. Haematol.*, **104** (1999) 695–705.

19. Lavabre-Bertrand T, Janossy G, Ivory K, Peters R, Secker-Walker L, and Porwit-MacDonald A. Leukemia-associated changes identified by quantitative flow cytometry: I. CD10 expression, *Cytometry*, **18** (1999) 209–217.

20. Behm FG, Raimondi SC, Schell MJ, Look AT, Rivera GK, and Pui CH. Lack of CD45 antigen on blast cells in childhood acute lymphoblastic leukemia is associated with chromosomal hyperdiploidy and other favorable prognostic features, *Blood*, **79** (1992) 1011–1016.

21. Dworzak MN, Fritsch G, Fleischer C, Printz D, Froschl G, Buchinger P, et al. Comparative phenotype mapping of normal vs. malignant pediatric B-lymphopoiesis unveils leukemia-associated aberrations, *Exp. Hematol.*, **26** (1998) 305–313.

22. Inoue K, Ogawa H, Sonoda Y, Kimura T, Sakabe H, Oka Y, et al. Aberrant overexpression of the Wilms tumor gene (WT1) in human leukemia, *Blood*, **89** (1997) 1405–1412.

23. Menssen HD, Renkl HJ, Rodeck U, Kari C, Schwartz S, and Thiel E. Detection by monoclonal antibodies of the Wilms' tumor (WT1) nuclear protein in patients with acute leukemia, *Int. J. Cancer*, **70** (1997) 518–523.

24. van Dongen JJ, Breit TM, Adriaansen HJ, Beishuizen A, and Hooijkaas H. Detection of minimal residual disease in acute leukemia by immunological marker analysis and polymerase chain reaction, *Leukemia*, **6** (1992) 47–59.

25. Engel H, Goodacre A, Keyhani A, Jiang S, Van NT, Kimmel M, et al. Minimal residual disease in acute myelogenous leukaemia and myelodysplastic syndromes: a follow-up of patients in clinical remission, *Br. J. Haematol.*, **99** (1997) 64–75.

26. Nowak R, Oelschlaegel U, Schuler U, Zengler H, Hofmann R, Ehninger G, et al. Sensitivity of combined DNA/immunophenotype flow cytometry for the detection of low levels of aneuploid lymphoblastic leukemia cells in bone marrow, *Cytometry*, **30** (1997) 47–53.

27. Gross HJ, Verwer B, Houck D, and Recktenwald D. Detection of rare cells at a frequency of one per million by flow cytometry, *Cytometry*, **14** (1993) 519–526.

28. Gross HJ, Verwer B, Houck D, Hoffman RA, and Recktenwald D. Model study detecting breast cancer cells in peripheral blood mononuclear cells at frequencies as low as $10(-7)$, *Proc. Natl. Acad. Sci. USA*, **92** (1995) 537–541.

29. Rosenblatt JI, Hokanson JA, McLaughlin SR, and Leary JF. Theoretical basis for sampling statistics useful for detecting and isolating rare cells using flow cytometry and cell sorting, *Cytometry*, **27** (1997) 233–238.

30. Rehsem MA, Corpuzm S, Heimfeldm S, Minie M, and Yachimiak D. Use of fluorescence threshold triggering and high-speed flow cytometry for rare event detection, *Cytometry*, **22** (1995) 317–322.
31. Coustan-Smith E, Behm FG, Sanchez J, Boyett JM, Hancock ML, Raimondi SC, et al. Immuno-logical detection of minimal residual disease in children with acute lymphoblastic leukaemia, *Lancet*, **351** (1998) 550–554.
32. Chen J-S, Coustan-Smith E, Suzuki T, Neale GA, Mihara K, Pui C-H, et al. Identification of novel markers for monitoring minimal residual disease in acute lymphoblastic leukemia, *Blood*, **97** (2001) 2115–2120.
33. Campana D and Pui CH. Detection of minimal residual disease in acute leukemia: methodologic advances and clinical significance, *Blood*, **85** (1995) 1416–1434.
34. Neale GA, Coustan-Smith E, Pan Q, Chen X, Gruhn B, Stow P, et al. Tandem application of flow cytometry and polymerase chain reaction for comprehensive detection of minimal residual disease in childhood acute lymphoblastic leukemia, *Leukemia*, **13** (1999) 1221–1226.
35. Neglia JP, Meadows AT, Robison LL, Kim TH, Newton WA, Ruymann FB, et al. Second neo-plasms after acute lymphoblastic leukemia in childhood, *N. Engl. J. Med.*, **325** (1991) 1330–1336.
36. Pui CH, Ribeiro RC, Hancock ML, Rivera GK, Evans WE, Raimondi SC, et al. Acute myeloid leukemia in children treated with epipodophyllotoxins for acute lymphoblastic leukemia, *N. Engl. J. Med.*, **325** (1991) 1682–1687.
37. Stass S, Mirro J, Melvin S, Pui CH, Murphy SB, and Williams D. Lineage switch in acute leukemia, *Blood*, **64** (1984) 701–706.
38. Gagnon GA, Childs CC, LeMaistre A, Keating M, Cork A, Trujillo JM, et al. Molecular heterogeneity in acute leukemia lineage switch, *Blood*, **74** (1989) 2088–2095.
39. Beishuizen A, Verhoeven MA, Van Wering ER, Hahlen K, Hooijkaas H, and van Dongen JJ. Analysis of Ig and T-cell receptor genes in 40 childhood acute lymphoblastic leukemias at diagnosis and subsequent relapse: implications for the detection of minimal residual disease by polymerase chain reaction analysis, *Blood*, **83** (1994) 2238–2247.
40. Borella L, Casper JT, and Lauer SJ. Shifts in expression of cell membrane phenotypes in childhood lymphoid malignancies at relapse, *Blood*, **54** (1979) 64–71.
41. Greaves M, Paxton A, Janossy G, Pain C, Johnson S, and Lister TA. Acute lymphoblastic leukaemia associated antigen. III Alterations in expression during treatment and in relapse, *Leuk. Res.*, **4** (1980) 1–14.
42. Lauer S, Piaskowski V, Camitta B, and Casper J. Bone marrow and extramedullary variations of cell membrane antigen expression in childhood lymphoid neoplasias at relapse, *Leuk. Res.*, **6** (1982) 769–774.
43. Pui CH, Raimondi SC, Head DR, Schell MJ, Rivera GK, et al. Characterization of childhood acute leukemia with multiple myeloid and lymphoid markers at diagnosis and at relapse, *Blood*, **78** (1991) 1327–1337.
44. Raghavachar A, Thiel E, and Bartram CR. Analyses of phenotype and genotype in acute lymphoblastic leukemias at first presentation and in relapse, *Blood*, **70** (1987) 1079–1083.
45. Abshire TC, Buchanan GR, Jackson JF, Shuster JJ, Brock B, Head D, et al. Morphologic, immunologic and cytogenetic studies in children with acute lymphoblastic leukemia at diag-nosis and relapse: a Pediatric Oncology Group study, *Leukemia*, **6** (1992) 357–362.
46. Van Wering ER, Beishuizen A, Roeffen ET, van der Linden-Schrever BE, Verhoeven MA, Hahlen K, et al. Immunophenotypic changes between diagnosis and relapse in childhood acute lymphoblastic leukemia, *Leukemia*, **9** (1995) 1523–1533.
47. Campana D, Coustan-Smith E, and Janossy G. The immunologic detection of minimal residual disease in acute leukemia, *Blood*, **76** (1990) 163–171.
48. Drach J, Drach D, Glassl H, Gattringer C, and Huber H. Flow cytometric determination of atypical antigen expression in acute leukemia for the study of minimal residual disease, *Cytometry*, **13** (1992) 893–901.

49. Campana D, Yokota S, Coustan-Smith E, Hansen-Hagge TE, Janossy G, and Bartram CR. The detection of residual acute lymphoblastic leukemia cells with immunologic methods and polymerase chain reaction: a comparative study, *Leukemia*, **4** (1990) 609–614.

50. Coustan-Smith E, Sancho J, Hancock ML, Boyett JM, Behm FG, Raimondi SC, et al. Clinical importance of minimal residual disease in childhood acute lymphoblastic leukemia, *Blood*, **96** (2000) 2691–2696.

51. Rubnitz JE, Downing JR, Pui CH, Shurtleff SA, Raimondi SC, Evans WE, et al. TEL gene rearrangement in acute lymphoblastic leukemia: a new genetic marker with prognostic significance, *J. Clin. Oncol.*, **15** (1997) 1150–1157.

52. Rubnitz JE, Behm FG, Wichlan D, Ryan C, Sandlund JT, Ribeiro RC, et al. Low frequency of TEL-AML1 in relapsed acute lymphoblastic leukemia supports a favorable prognosis for this genetic subgroup, *Leukemia*, **13** (1999) 19–21.

53. Secker-Walker LM, Swansbury GJ, Hardisty RM, Sallan SE, Garson OM, Sakurai M, et al. Cytogenetics of acute lymphoblastic leukaemia in children as a factor in the prediction of long-term survival, *Br. J. Haematol.*, **52** (1982) 389–399.

54. Williams DL, Tsiatis A, Brodeur GM, Look AT, Melvin SL, Bowman WP, et al. Prognostic importance of chromosome number in 136 untreated children with acute lymphoblastic leukemia, *Blood*, **60** (1982) 864–871.

55. Trueworthy R, Shuster J, Look T, Crist W, Borowitz M, Carroll A, et al. Ploidy of lymphoblasts is the strongest predictor of treatment outcome in B-progenitor cell acute lymphoblastic leukemia of childhood: a Pediatric Oncology Group study, *J. Clin. Oncol.*, **10** (1992) 606–613.

56. Pui CH and Evans WE. Drug therapy: acute lymphoblastic leukemia, *N. Engl. J. Med.*, **339** (1998) 605–615.

57. Smith M, Arthur D, Camitta B, Carroll AJ, Crist W, Gaynon P, et al. Uniform approach to risk classification and treatment assignment for children with acute lymphoblastic leukemia, *J. Clin. Oncol.*, **14** (1996) 18–24.

58. Riehm H, Reiter A, Schrappe M, Berthold F, Dopfer R, Gerein V, et al. Corticosteroid-dependent reduction of leukocyte count in blood as a prognostic factor in acute lymphoblastic leukemia in childhood (therapy study ALL-BFM 83), *Klin. Padiatr.*, **199** (1987) 151–160.

59. Gajjar A, Ribeiro R, Hancock ML, Rivera GK, Mahmoud H, Sandlund JT, et al. Persistence of circulating blasts after 1 week of multiagent chemotherapy confers a poor prognosis in childhood acute lymphoblastic leukemia, *Blood*, **86** (1995) 1292–1295.

60. Lilleyman JS, Gibson BE, Stevens RF, Will AM, Hann IM, Richards SM, et al. Clearance of marrow infiltration after 1 week of therapy for childhood lymphoblastic leukaemia: clinical importance and the effect of daunorubicin. The Medical Research Council's Working Party on Childhood Leukaemia, *Br. J. Haematol.*, **97** (1997) 603–606.

61. Schrappe M, Arico M, Harbott J, Biondi A, Zimmermann M, Conter V, et al. Philadelphia chromosome-positive (Ph+) childhood acute lymphoblastic leukemia: good initial steroid response allows early prediction of a favorable treatment outcome, *Blood*, **92** (1998) 2730–2741.

62. Dordelmann M, Reiter A, Borkhardt A, Ludwig WD, Gotz N, Viehmann S, et al. Prednisone response is the strongest predictor of treatment outcome in infant acute lymphoblastic leukemia, *Blood*, **94** (1999) 1209–1217.

63. Farahat N, Morilla A, Owusu-Ankomah K, Morilla R, Pinkerton CR, Treleaven JG, et al. Detection of minimal residual disease in B-lineage acute lymphoblastic leukaemia by quantitative flow cytometry, *Br. J. Haematol.*, **101** (1998) 158–164.

64. Ciudad J, San Miguel JF, Lopez-Berges MC, Vidriales B, Valverde B, Ocqueteau M, et al. Prognostic value of immunophenotypic detection of minimal residual disease in acute lymphoblastic leukemia, *J. Clin. Oncol.*, **16** (1998) 3774–3781.

65. Brisco MJ, Sykes PJ, Hughes E, Dolman G, Neoh SH, Peng LM, et al. Monitoring minimal residual disease in peripheral blood in B-lineage acute lymphoblastic leukaemia, *Br. J. Haematol.*, **99** (1997) 314–319.

66. van Rhee F, Marks DI, Lin F, Szydlo RM, Hochhaus A, Treleaven J, et al. Quantification of residual disease in Philadelphia-positive acute lymphoblastic leukemia: comparison of blood and bone marrow, *Leukemia*, **9** (1995) 329–335.
67. Martin H, Atta J, Bruecher J, Elsner S, Schardt C, Stadler M, et al. In patients with BCR-ABL-positive ALL in CR peripheral blood contains less residual disease than bone marrow: implications for autologous BMT, *Ann. Hematol.*, **68** (1994) 85–87.
68. Donovan JW, Poor C, Bowers D, Waters S, Zou G, Neuberg D, et al. Concordance of MRD results in matched bone marrow and peripheral blood samples indicate the peripheral blood could be a sole sample source for MRD detection in pediatric acute lymphoblastic leukemia, *Blood*, **94(Suppl. 1)** (1999) 626a.
69. Sandlund JT, Harrison P, Rivera GK, Behm FG, Head D, Boyett JM, et al. Persistence of lymphoblasts in bone marrow on day 15 and day 22–25 of remission induction predicted a poorer treatment outcome in children with acute lymphoblastic leukemia, *Blood*, **90(Suppl. 1)** (1997) 560a–560a.
70. Pui CH, Ribeiro RC, Campana D, Raimondi SC, Hancock ML, Behm FG, et al. Prognostic factors in the acute lymphoid and myeloid leukemias of infants, *Leukemia*, **10** (1996) 952–956.
71. Goldie JH and Coldman AJ. Application of theoretical models to chemotherapy protocol design, *Cancer Treat. Rep.*, **70** (1986) 127–131.

# 3 PCR Methods for the Detection of Minimal Residual Disease in Childhood Acute Lymphoblastic Leukemia

*Geoffrey Neale*

## PROGNOSTIC VALUE OF MRD IN ALL

Acute lymphoblastic leukemia (ALL) is the most common form of cancer in children. The main cause of treatment failure, which occurs in approx 20% of patients, is relapse arising from outgrowth of residual leukemic cells that are refractory to therapy. ALL is a heterogeneous disease, characterized by stage of differentiation and by a spectrum of recurrent chromosomal abnormalities *(1–5)*. Thus, ALL is not a single entity, and uniform therapy is not ideal. Children at high risk require intensive treatment, whereas others have an excellent prognosis with less toxic therapies. The question remains: How best to identify the patients with ALL who are at high risk of relapse?

As the cure rate of ALL now approaches 80%, many clinical and biologic features once considered important in risk assignment have lost their predictive value. Clinical features that predict relapse are patient age and leukocyte count. Patients with the t(9;22) translocation or rearrangement of the MLL locus at chr11q23 have an overall unfavorable outcome. Some genetic abnormalities, however, are associated with good prognosis. These include hyperdiploidy (51–65 chromosomes per cell) and the t(12;21) translocation. None of these features, however, is 100% predictive *(1,2)*.

To find better predictors of patient outcome, investigators have examined the in vivo response of leukemic cells during therapy by using sensitive assays to investigate subclinical levels of leukemic cells (minimal residual disease [MRD]) in patient samples during clinical remission *(6–20)*. There are four major conclusions from MRD studies *(21)*. First, quantitative assessment of

From: *Leukemia and Lymphoma: Detection of Minimal Residual Disease*
Edited by: T. F. Zipf and D. A. Johnston © Humana Press Inc., Totowa, NJ

MRD, as opposed to qualitative assessment, is necessary. Second, high levels of MRD after induction therapy are associated with poor prognosis, whereas low (<0.01%) or undetectable levels are associated with excellent outcome. Third, persistence of MRD at two or more time-points during therapy is associated with a particularly poor prognosis. Fourth, MRD is an independent predictor of patient outcome.

## CLONAL MARKERS FOR MRD ASSESSMENT IN ALL

### *Fusion Genes*

There are two types of clone-specific markers that can be used for MRD assessment in ALL. These are the breakpoint fusion regions of chromosomal abnormalities found in ALL and the junction regions of antigen-receptor gene rearrangements that arise during normal lymphoid development. A large number of recurrent chromosomal abnormalities have been characterized in ALL *(1,4,5)*. One example is the *SIL-TAL1* fusion gene *(TAL-1* deletion) that is found in leukemic cells, but not in normal cells. This genetic lesion is generated by site-specific recombination on chromosome 1p32, and the genomic sequence of this gene fusion can be used as a leukemia-specific target in approx 25% of T-lineage ALL cases *(22–24)*. Other leukemia-specific lesions, such as the *TEL-AML1*, *BCR-ABL*, *E2A-PBX1*, and *MLL-AF4* fusion genes, arise from chromosomal translocations. However, in contrast to the *SIL-TAL1* fusion, the genomic breakpoints of these fusion genes are spread over large distances within each gene locus. This makes it difficult to precisely identify the genomic regions fused together. Consequently, genomic sequences from these chromosomal translocations are not amenable for routine MRD assessment. This shortcoming, however, can be overcome by the observation that although the genomic breakpoints differ from case to case, the fusion transcripts arising from a particular chromosomal translocation are virtually identical. Therefore, these fusion transcripts may be used as leukemia-specific targets for MRD assessment in ALL *(25–28)*.

There are drawbacks, however, in using fusion transcripts for assessment of MRD. A prerequisite for clinical monitoring is that every patient should be evaluated for residual leukemic cells. Because well-defined chromosomal translocations are found in only 35–40% of ALL cases *(1,4,5)*, fusion transcripts can be used to monitor MRD only in the minority of cases. Potential problems also arise when using RNA as a molecular target. RNA is more susceptible to degradation than DNA, and the possibility exists that the number of mRNA transcripts per cell might fluctuate during therapy.

### *Antigen-Receptor Gene Rearrangements*

Because of the limited applicability of fusion transcripts, the most common method for investigating MRD in ALL is polymerase chain reaction (PCR)

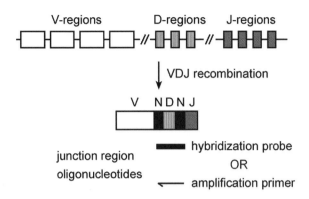

**Fig. 1.** Generation of clone-specific markers of lymphoid cells by antigen-receptor gene rearrangement. During the process of VDJ recombination, V (variable), D (diversity), and J (joining) regions, normally interspersed along the chromosome, are randomly joined. This joining is imprecise, and random nucleotides (N nucleotides) are incorporated among the V, D, and J segments. The diversity of the VDJ junction permits synthesis of a complementary oligonucleotide that is specific for each lymphoid cell. This oligonucleotide is used as a hybridization probe or an amplification primer for clone-specific detection.

amplification of clone-specific immunoglobulin (Ig) and T-cell receptor (TCR) gene rearrangements *(29)*. As part of normal development, lymphoid cells rearrange their antigen-receptor gene segments (V, D, and J regions) to create an amazingly diverse repertoire of receptors for antigen recognition *(30–32)*. This process provides a unique genetic "fingerprint" for each lymphoid cell, and this fingerprint can be used as a monoclonal marker for MRD detection.

Because each lymphoid cell has its own unique fingerprint, the sequence of the Ig/TCR gene rearrangement present in the leukemic clone must be identified for each patient. To facilitate this identification, DNA from the diagnostic sample is amplified using sets of consensus primers to the V-, D-, and J-region gene segments *(33,34)*. After amplification, the clonal PCR products are sequenced directly to precisely identify the VDJ-junction region nucleotides. From this sequence, an oligonucleotide complementary to the unique junction region sequence is synthesized. This clone-specific oligonucleotide is then used to detect leukemic cells among normal hematopoietic and lymphoid cells, either as a hybridization probe or as a primer to specifically amplify the rearrangement of the leukemic clone *(see* Fig. 1).

Antigen-receptor gene rearrangements are readily identified in ALL *(see* Table 1). Rearrangements of the IgH, Igκ, TCR-δ, and TCR-γ loci are common and at least one is found in virtually all cases. Notably, cross-lineage rearrangements, such as TCR-δ and TCR-γ rearrangements in B-precursor ALL, are frequently found in ALL *(35,36)*. These rearrangements, not detected in mature lymphoid cells,

Table 1
Incidence of Ig and TCR Gene Rearrangements in Childhood ALL

|                 | IgH | Igκ | TCR-δ | TCR-γ | TCR-β |
|-----------------|-----|-----|-------|-------|-------|
| B-Precursor ALL | 95% | 30% | 55%   | 60%   | 30%   |
| T-Lineage ALL   | 20% | 0%  | 70%   | 95%   | 90%   |
| Total ALL       | 85% | 25% | 60%   | 65%   | 45%   |

*Source*: Data from ref. *35*.

increase the probability of finding an Ig/TCR clonal marker. In B-precursor ALL, the IgH, Igκ, TCR-δ, and TCR-γ are rearranged in 95%, 30%, 55%, and 60% of cases, respectively. In T-lineage ALL, the TCR-δ and TCR-γ loci are rearranged in 70% and 95% of cases, respectively. Although the TCR-β locus is frequently rearranged in T-lineage ALL, this locus is rarely used for MRD assessment because of the high frequency of TCR-γ and TCR-δ rearrangements and the difficulty in identifying TCR-β rearrangements from genomic DNA. Overall, the high incidence of Ig/TCR gene rearrangements permits the design of assays for their detection in approx 90% of ALL cases.

Choosing an Ig/TCR clonal marker is balanced between two issues: the sensitivity of residual disease detection and the likely stability of the gene rearrangement. In general, the junction sequences of the Igκ and TCR-γ gene rearrangements are less diverse than those of the IgH and TCR-δ loci. This is because Igκ and TCR-γ rearrangements lack D-region segments and because the VJ junctions usually contain only a small number of random nucleotides (*N* nucleotides). This restricted diversity can prevent the design of assays that distinguish the rearrangement found in the leukemic clone from those found in polyclonal cells.

However, rearrangements of the Igκ and TCR-γ loci are favored by some investigators (*17,18*) for clinical studies because they are the most stable. Rearrangement of the Igκ or TCR-γ loci represent "end points" of VDJ recombination, and these loci rarely undergo secondary rearrangement during disease progression (*37*). In contrast, rearrangements of the IgH and TCR-δ loci frequently undergo continuing gene rearrangement (*38–41*). In the IgH locus, VH replacement, as well as VH to DJ joining, can occur (*42,43*). In the TCR-δ locus, incomplete rearrangements (V–D, D–D, and D–J) are frequently found in ALL (*35*). These partial rearrangements can undergo secondary rearrangement or they can be deleted (*40,44*). This process of continuing rearrangement, referred to as "clonal evolution," poses problems for MRD assessment because loss of the clonal marker identified at diagnosis can lead to false-negative results.

Although clonal evolution occurs in approx 30% of ALL (*38–41*), studies have shown that at least one of the Ig/TCR gene rearrangements present at diagnosis is retained in 90–95% of cases at relapse (*42,44*). Because of this finding, investigators have used a strategy of monitoring MRD by using two independent gene rearrangements *(17,18)*. This should limit the possibility of false negatives arising from clonal evolution. Those investigators found that the data from independent clonal markers were concordant *(17,18)*. However, this strategy was applicable to only 28% of cases *(17)* and 60% of cases *(18)*, respectively. An alternative strategy to reduce false negatives has been suggested. The most common mechanisms of clonal evolution occurs via VH replacement (V to VDJ joining) or VH addition to existing DJ rearrangements *(38,41)*. The molecular mechanisms of VH replacement and VH addition do not usually alter the nucleotides between the D and J regions *(42,44,45)*. Therefore, the design of junction region oligonucleotides complementary to the stable DJ sequences should further reduce the chance of false negative results because of clonal evolution.

## QUANTIFICATION OF CLONAL MARKERS BY PCR

Once a clonal Ig/TCR target has been identified, a PCR assay is developed for quantifying leukemic cells harboring that gene rearrangement. This is not a simple task because of the exponential amplification of targets that occurs during the PCR. Although it is relatively easy to quantify the amount of product after amplification, it is far more difficult to calculate the number of targets that gave rise to that product. This is especially problematic when the starting number is very low or very high. Under these conditions, PCR quantification can result in large errors resulting from inefficient amplification of the target sequence. Thus, over the past decade, investigators have used various approaches to quantify MRD by PCR. Of these methods, three have been used the most and they are summarized below. As indicated, each of these methods has inherent advantages and drawbacks. The disadvantages associated with the "classical" methods might soon be overcome by recent improvements in MRD assessment using real-time quantitative PCR. An outline of this method and its application to assessment of MRD in childhood ALL is also described.

### *Classical Methods of MRD Detection by PCR*

#### COMPARATIVE HYBRIDIZATION

This semiquantitative method has been used in the majority of MRD studies *(8,9,11,13,15,18,46–51)*. In this method, the oligonucleotide complementary to the junction region is used as a radiolabeled hybridization probe to detect the clone-specific gene rearrangement. For quantification of MRD, DNA from an unknown sample is amplified using the set of consensus primers that identified the gene rearrangement at diagnosis. Polyclonal DNA (negative controls) and a set of standards, made by serial dilution of the diagnostic DNA, are amplified using the same primers in separate reaction tubes. After amplification, aliquots from each reaction are blotted and hybridized to the clone-specific junction region probe. The level of MRD is estimated by comparing the hybridization signal of the unknown sample to those of the standards. Thus, the standards serve two purposes. They establish the sensitivity of detection for each assay and they provide reference values for quantifying the number of leukemic cells in the unknown sample.

Although this method is relatively simple to perform in most research laboratories, it is also the most time-consuming, taking 2–3 d to complete. Data from this method are semiquantitative because it is difficult, if not impossible, to establish PCR conditions where targets over a 5-log range are amplified equally and where PCR products do not reach a plateau. The sensitivity of this method is quite variable, ranging from $10^{-6}$ to $10^{-3}$, although the majority of assays *(18)* have a sensitivity of detection at least $10^{-4}$. This variability can be attributed to several factors. One factor is the efficiency of hybridization of the junction region probe. This will vary from patient to patient because no two junction probes are the same. Another factor is the composition of the junction region probe. Probes containing mostly germ-line sequences can not provide sensitive discrimination of the leukemic gene rearrangement from those found in nonleukemic polyclonal cells. Yet another factor is the design of the PCR amplification. By using consensus primers that amplify both the leukemic and nonleukemic gene rearrangements, the efficiency of leukemic target amplification can vary considerably at low target doses.

## COMPETITIVE PCR

Competitive PCR has also been used extensively in MRD studies of childhood ALL *(7,17,52–54)*. In this method, an unknown sample is amplified in a PCR reaction containing an internal standard of known amount. The internal standard has identical V- and J-region sequences to those of the leukemic gene rearrangement *(7)*. Thus, in the PCR, the internal standard is a competitor and it is amplified at the same time as the leukemic target. In order to be used as an internal standard, the competitor must be distinguishable from the leukemic gene rearrangement either by size or by hybridization with a junction region probe. Following amplification, the initial copy number of the leukemic target is calculated by comparing the signal of the unknown sample with the signal of the internal competitor. Similar to comparative hybridization, the sensitivity of MRD detection using competitive PCR varies among patients. In one report *(7)*, the sensitivity ranged between $1 \times 10^{-5}$ and $2.5 \times 10^{-4}$, whereas another study by the same researchers *(17)* had a median sensitivity of $5 \times 10^{-5}$.

Because the ratio of competitor to leukemic target can vary dramatically in an unknown sample, a calibration curve is required to correlate the signal of the unknown with that of the competitor. In this method *(7)*, standards containing different amounts of the diagnostic leukemia DNA and a fixed amount of competitor are prepared. After amplification, the ratio of the leukemic signal to the competitor signal is plotted against the number of leukemic targets. This calibration curve is then used to calculate the number of leukemic cells in the unknown sample.

Several conditions must be met for competitive PCR to provide accurate results. First, the efficiency of amplification must be the same for the leukemic target and the competitor target. This efficiency must be constant over a wide range of starting concentrations. Second, the number of PCR cycles must be calibrated carefully to ensure that the signal of each product in the reaction does not reach a plateau during amplification. Third, detection of the competitor signal must have the same efficiency as the detection of the leukemic target. This problem is readily avoided when using ethidium bromide staining or fluorescence detection. However, when using junction region probes to visualize reaction products, the use of standards is recommended to overcome different hybridization efficiencies arising from oligonucleotide probes of different lengths and/or composition.

## LIMITING DILUTION

This technique has been used in many MRD studies *(6,12,14,55–57)*. In this method, the junction region oligonucleotide is used as an amplification primer, and amplification is optimized using two rounds of PCR to provide an "all-or-none" readout. Amplification conditions are established so that as little as a single copy of the leukemic gene rearrangement will generate a PCR product that can be visualized on a gel stained with ethidium bromide. In the first round, samples are amplified by using two consensus primers (e.g., V- and J-region primers) or by using one consensus primer and one patient-specific primer. Following this preamplification, the first reaction is diluted and then reamplified using one consensus primer in combination with a nested patient-specific primer. The net result of this process is that a reaction containing one or more leukemic genomes will be positive, whereas a reaction that contains polyclonal or nonleukemic DNA will be negative when analyzed on an agarose or acrylamide gel. Accurate quantification is achieved by performing multiple replicates of serial dilutions of the unknown sample. At the limiting dilution, where replicate assays are either positive or negative, the MRD level is calculated from the fraction of negative assays by using Poisson statistics *(58)*.

There are several advantages to using limiting dilution for MRD assessment. These include (1) an end point that does not require quantitation or radioactivity, (2) a uniform sensitivity of detection (approx $10^{-6}$) that is unsurpassed by other techniques *(59)*, and (3) MRD levels quantified in the absence of standards and with statistical confidence. However, there is a major drawback to this method. It is very laborious because of the preparation of sample dilutions and the analysis of multiple replicates by using two rounds of PCR. This is mitigated somewhat in that this process need only be performed once at the original development of the patient's PCR test.

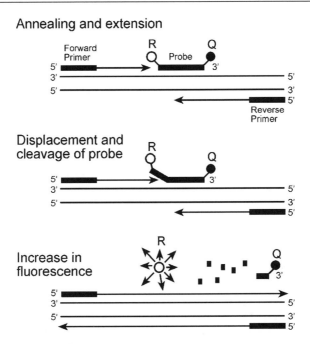

**Fig. 2.** Schematic depiction of RQ-PCR using TaqMan probes. The TaqMan probe hybridizes to sequences between the two amplification primers (top panel). During synthesis of the new DNA strand, the TaqMan probe is displaced (middle panel) and cleaved (bottom panel). Cleavage of the probe separates the reporter dye (R) from the quencher (Q), resulting in increased fluorescence in the reaction (bottom panel).

## *Real-Time Quantitative PCR*

As described above, the "classical" PCR methods are too time-consuming or laborious for routine quantification of MRD. Recent advances in quantitative PCR technology, however, promise to eliminate those problems. Of the available automated methods, real-time quantitative PCR (RQ-PCR) using TaqMan probes *(60)* appears to have the greatest potential (*see* Fig. 2). TaqMan technology requires a reporter probe, containing a fluorescent dye and a quencher, to hybridize between two amplification primers. This probe is cleaved during the amplification only when the primers direct amplification to the target sequence. When the TaqMan probe is hydrolyzed, the fluorescent dye is separated from the quencher and an increase in fluorescence is detected in the reaction. The increase in fluorescence is proportional to the amount of product synthesized in the PCR. Thus, the TaqMan probe provides both the sensitivity and the specificity required for MRD assessment. A set of standards, made from serial dilutions of diagnostic DNA, is used for quantification purposes. By monitoring the accumulation of fluorescence in "real time," data from the standards and the unknown sample are

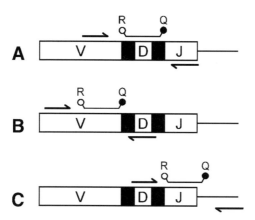

**Fig. 3.** Three possible locations of TaqMan probes for detection of Ig/TCR gene rearrangements. TaqMan probes may be complementary to the VDJ junction (**A**), the V region (**B**), or the J region (**C**). Amplification primers in each scenario are indicated by half arrows.

obtained from the exponential phase of the reaction, and the initial target amount is extrapolated from the standard curve.

TaqMan probes can be designed to detect Ig/TCR gene rearrangements at three possible locations (*see* Fig. 3). First, the probe can be synthesized complementary to the unique junction region (*see* Fig. 3A). This approach has been used with some success *(61)*. However, as in comparative hybridization methods, the sensitivity of junction region TaqMan probes can vary *(61)*. A further complication is that unique junction region probes would be required for every patient. This would add considerable time and expense to the routine monitoring of MRD. The second potential location of the TaqMan probe is within the V region (*see* Fig. 3B). In this case, the specificity of leukemic cell detection comes from using the junction region oligonucleotide as an amplification primer. Initial studies have reported considerable success using this strategy *(62–64)*. However, there are potential pitfalls in using TaqMan probes directed to the V region and the junction region. As described earlier, clonal evolution of the Ig/TCR gene rearrangement can cause the loss of V-region and VD sequences. Therefore, TaqMan probes to these regions could generate false negative results.

The third location for TaqMan probes is the J region (*see* Fig. 3C). This approach is particularly advantageous for quantification of IgH rearrangements *(65,66)*. There are only 6 JH regions as compared to approx 50 VH regions and, therefore, only a limited number of TaqMan probes need be synthesized. The sequence homology between the JH regions permits a further reduction in the number of TaqMan probes needed for quantification of IgH gene rearrangements. Another advantage of JH-region probes is that clonal evolution is less

## TaqMan vs Limiting dilution

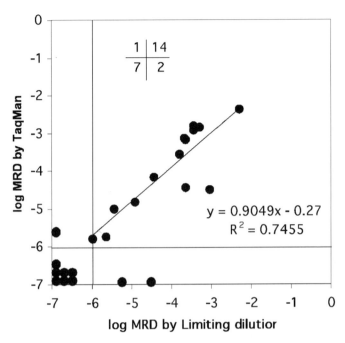

**Fig. 4.** Concordance between RQ-PCR data and limiting dilution data in B-precursor ALL. Twenty-four samples from 14 patients were analyzed by RQ-PCR and by limiting dilution. Seven samples had undetectable leukemic cells by both methods.

likely to result in false-negative results. When VH replacement or VH to DJ joining occurs, the DJ portion of the rearrangement usually remains intact. Therefore, leukemia-specific primers designed in the DJ portion of the rearrangement will still detect the original leukemic clone. A further benefit is that J-region probes permit design of assays for detection of partial IgH gene rearrangements.

Several studies have reported successful use of TaqMan technology for quantification of leukemic cells in ALL *(61–67)*. Few studies, however, have investigated the sensitivity of RQ-PCR assays relative to other methods *(61,67)*. Our experience *(67)* using RQ-PCR to detect the *TAL-1* deletion in T-lineage ALL shows that extremely sensitive detection of leukemic cells ($10^{-5}$ or better) is possible using TaqMan probes. In addition, we found that limiting dilution data and RQ-PCR data were highly concordant *(67)*.

We are currently evaluating a small number of JH-region probes for RQ-PCR detection of MRD in B-precursor ALL. In our hands, these probes routinely detect a single copy of the leukemic genome among $10^5$ normal genomes. Thus, by using multiple replicates, the sensitivity of RQ-PCR detection can be equivalent to that of limiting dilution—the most sensitive MRD technique (*see* Fig. 4; Neale et al., unpublished data). Overall, these findings strongly indicate that RQ-PCR will soon replace previous time-consuming or laborious MRD assays.

## SUMMARY

The prognostic value of MRD assessment during therapy has recently been established in several large prospective studies. These studies have shown the value of quantitative, as opposed to qualitative, evaluation of MRD levels. However, a major obstacle to the routine MRD assessment in clinical studies has been the lack of rapid and accurate methods for detection of residual leukemic cells. Now, new RQ-PCR technology promises to improve MRD detection and to accelerate the availability of routine MRD evaluation in clinical studies. Rapid and accurate monitoring of MRD will permit the opportunity for timely therapeutic intervention in those patients who have persistent leukemia.

## ACKNOWLEDGMENTS

This work was supported in part by the following grants: NIH CA52259, NIH CA21765, by a Center of Excellence grant from the State of Tennessee, and by the American Lebanese Syrian Associated Charities (ALSAC).

## REFERENCES

1. Pui CH and Evans WE. Acute lymphoblastic leukemia, *N. Engl. J. Med.*, **339** (1998) 605–615.
2. Pui CH. Acute lymphoblastic leukemia in children, *Curr Opin. Oncol.*, **12** (2000) 3–12.
3. Rubnitz JE and Look AT. Molecular genetics of childhood leukemias, *J. Pediatr. Hematol. Oncol.*, **20** (1998) 1–11.
4. Rabbitts TH. Chromosomal translocations in human cancer, *Nature*, **372** (1994) 143–149.
5. Look AT. Oncogenic transcription factors in the human acute leukemias, *Science*, **278** (1997) 1059–1064.
6. Brisco MJ, Condon J, Hughes E, Neoh SH, Sykes PJ, Seshadri R, et al. Outcome prediction in childhood acute lymphoblastic leukaemia by molecular quantification of residual disease at the end of induction, *Lancet*, **343** (1994) 196–200.
7. Cave H, Guidal C, Rohrlich P, Delfau MH, Broyart A, Lescoeur B, et al. Prospective monitoring and quantitation of residual blasts in childhood acute lymphoblastic leukemia by polymerase chain reaction study of delta and gamma T-cell receptor genes, *Blood*, **83** (1994) 1892–1902.
8. Seriu T, Yokota S, Nakao M, Misawa S, Takaue Y, Koizumi S, et al. Prospective monitoring of minimal residual disease during the course of chemotherapy in patients with acute lymphoblastic leukemia, and detection of contaminating tumor cells in peripheral blood stem cells for autotransplantation, *Leukemia*, **9** (1995) 615–623.
9. Steenbergen EJ, Verhagen OJ, van Leeuwen EF, van den Berg H, Behrendt H, Slater RM, et al. Prolonged persistence of PCR-detectable minimal residual disease after diagnosis or first relapse predicts poor outcome in childhood B-precursor acute lymphoblastic leukemia, *Leukemia*, **9** (1995) 1726–1734.

10. Brisco J, Hughes E, Neoh SH, Sykes PJ, Bradstock K, Enno A, et al. Relationship between minimal residual disease and outcome in adult acute lymphoblastic leukemia, *Blood*, **87** (1996) 5251–5256.
11. Foroni L, Coyle LA, Papaioannou M, Yaxley JC, Sinclair MF, Chim JS, et al. Molecular detection of minimal residual disease in adult and childhood acute lymphoblastic leukaemia reveals differences in treatment response, *Leukemia*, **11** (1997) 1732–1741.
12. Roberts WM, Estrov Z, Ouspenskaia MV, Johnston DA, McClain KL, and Zipf TF. Measurement of residual leukemia during remission in childhood acute lymphoblastic leukemia, *N. Engl. J. Med.*, **336** (1997) 317–323.
13. Jacquy C, Delepaut B, Van Daele S, Vaerman JL, Zenebergh A, Brichard B, et al. A prospective study of minimal residual disease in childhood B-lineage acute lymphoblastic leukaemia: MRD level at the end of induction is a strong predictive factor of relapse, *Br. J. Haematol.*, **98** (1997) 140–146.
14. Gruhn B, Hongeng S, Yi H, Hancock ML, Rubnitz JE, Neale GA, et al. Minimal residual disease after intensive induction therapy in childhood acute lymphoblastic leukemia predicts outcome, *Leukemia*, **12** (1998) 675–681.
15. Goulden NJ, Knechtli CJ, Garland RJ, Langlands K, Hancock JP, Potter MN, et al. Minimal residual disease analysis for the prediction of relapse in children with standard-risk acute lymphoblastic leukaemia, *Br. J. Haematol.*, **100** (1998) 235–244.
16. Evans PA, Short MA, Owen RG, Jack AS, Forsyth PD, Shiach CR, et al. Residual disease detection using fluorescent polymerase chain reaction at 20 weeks of therapy predicts clinical outcome in childhood acute lymphoblastic leukemia, *J. Clin. Oncol.*, **16** (1998) 3616–3627.
17. Cave H, van dèr Werff ten Bosch J, Suciu S, Guidal C, Waterkeyn C, Otten J, et al. Clinical significance of minimal residual disease in childhood acute lymphoblastic leukemia. European Organization for Research and Treatment of Cancer—Childhood Leukemia Cooperative Group, *N. Engl. J. Med.*, **339** (1998) 591–598.
18. van Dongen JJ, Seriu T, Panzer-Grumayer ER, Biondi A, Pongers-Willemse MJ, Corral L, et al. Prognostic value of minimal residual disease in acute lymphoblastic leukaemia in childhood, *Lancet*, **352** (1998) 1731–1738.
19. Coustan-Smith E, Behm FG, Sanchez J, Boyett JM, Hancock ML, Raimondi SC, et al. Immunological detection of minimal residual disease in children with acute lymphoblastic leukaemia, *Lancet*, **351** (1998) 550–554.
20. Coustan-Smith E, Sancho J, Hancock ML, Boyett JM, Behm FG, Raimondi SC, et al. Clinical importance of minimal residual disease in childhood acute lymphoblastic leukemia, *Blood*, **96** (2000) 2691–2696.
21. Pui CH and Campana D. New definition of remission in childhood acute lymphoblastic leukemia, *Leukemia*, **14** (2000) 783–785.
22. Brown L, Cheng JT, Chen Q, Siciliano MJ, Crist W, Buchanan G, et al. Site-specific recombination of the tal-1 gene is a common occurrence in human T cell leukemia, *EMBO. J.*, **9** (1990) 3343–3351.
23. Bash RO, Crist WM, Shuster JJ, Link MP, Amylon M, Pullen J, et al. Clinical features and outcome of T-cell acute lymphoblastic leukemia in childhood with respect to alterations at the TAL1 locus: a Pediatric Oncology Group study, *Blood*, **81** (1993) 2110–2117.
24. Breit TM, Beishuizen A, Ludwig WD, Mol EJ, Adriaansen HJ, van Wering ER, et al. tal-1 deletions in T-cell acute lymphoblastic leukemia as PCR target for detection of minimal residual disease, *Leukemia*, **7** (1993) 2004–2011.
25. Gehly GB, Bryant EM, Lee AM, Kidd PG, and Thomas ED. Chimeric BCR-abl messenger RNA as a marker for minimal residual disease in patients transplanted for Philadelphia chromosome-positive acute lymphoblastic leukemia, *Blood*, **78** (1991) 458–465.
26. Miyamura K, Tanimoto M, Morishima Y, Horibe K, Yamamoto K, Akatsuka M, et al. Detection of Philadelphia chromosome-positive acute lymphoblastic leukemia by polymerase chain

reaction: possible eradication of minimal residual disease by marrow transplantation, *Blood*, **79** (1992) 1366–1370.

27. Radich J, Gehly G, Lee A, Avery R, Bryant E, Edmands S, et al. Detection of bcr-abl transcripts in Philadelphia chromosome-positive acute lymphoblastic leukemia after marrow transplantation, *Blood*, **89** (1997) 2602–2609.

28. Hunger SP, Fall MZ, Camitta BM, Carroll AJ, Link MP, Lauer SJ, et al. E2A-PBX1 chimeric transcript status at end of consolidation is not predictive of treatment outcome in childhood acute lymphoblastic leukemias with a t(1;19)(q23;p13): a Pediatric Oncology Group study, *Blood*, **91** (1998) 1021–1028.

29. Campana D and Pui CH. Detection of minimal residual disease in acute leukemia: methodologic advances and clinical significance, *Blood*, **85** (1995) 1416–1434.

30. Tonegawa S. Somatic generation of antibody diversity, *Nature*, **302** (1983) 575–581.

31. Davis MM and Bjorkman PJ. T-Cell antigen receptor genes and T-cell recognition, *Nature*, **334** (1988) 395–402.

32. Chen J and Alt FW. Gene rearrangement and B-cell development, *Curr. Opin. Immunol.*, **5** (1993) 194–200.

33. Deane M and Norton JD. Immunoglobulin gene "fingerprinting": an approach to analysis of B lymphoid clonality in lymphoproliferative disorders, *Br. J. Haematol.*, **77** (1991) 274–281.

34. Pongers-Willemse MJ, Seriu T, Stolz F, d'Aniello E, Gameiro P, Pisa P, et al. Primers and protocols for standardized detection of minimal residual disease in acute lymphoblastic leukemia using immunoglobulin and T cell receptor gene rearrangements and TAL1 deletions as PCR targets: report of the BIOMED-1 CONCERTED ACTION: investigation of minimal residual disease in acute leukemia, *Leukemia*, **13** (1999) 110–118.

35. Szczepanski T, Pongers-Willemse MJ, Langerak AW, and van Dongen JJ. Unusual immunoglobulin and T-cell receptor gene rearrangement patterns in acute lymphoblastic leukemias, *Curr. Topies Microbiol. Immunol.*, **246** (1999) 205–213.

36. Szczepanski T, Beishuizen A, Pongers-Willemse MJ, Hahlen K, Van Wering ER, Wijkhuijs AJ, et al. Cross-lineage T cell receptor gene rearrangements occur in more than ninety percent of childhood precursor-B acute lymphoblastic leukemias: alternative PCR targets for detection of minimal residual disease, *Leukemia*, **13** (1999) 196–205.

37. Taylor JJ, Rowe D, Kylefjord H, Chessells J, Katz F, Proctor SJ, et al. Characterisation of non-concordance in the T-cell receptor gamma chain genes at presentation and clinical relapse in acute lymphoblastic leukemia, *Leukemia*, **8** (1994) 60–66.

38. Steenbergen EJ, Verhagen OJ, van Leeuwen EF, von dem Borne AE, and van der Schoot CE. Distinct ongoing Ig heavy chain rearrangement processes in childhood B-precursor acute lymphoblastic leukemia, *Blood*, **82** (1993) 581–589.

39. Baruchel A, Cayuela JM, MacIntyre E, Berger R, and Sigaux F. Assessment of clonal evolution at Ig/TCR loci in acute lymphoblastic leukaemia by single-strand conformation polymorphism studies and highly resolutive PCR derived methods: implication for a general strategy of minimal residual disease detection, *Br. J. Haematol.*, **90** (1995) 85–93,

40. Steenbergen EJ, Verhagen OJ, van Leeuwen EF, van den Berg H, von dem Borne AE, and van der Schoot CE. Frequent ongoing T-cell receptor rearrangements in childhood B-precursor acute lymphoblastic leukemia: implications for monitoring minimal residual disease, *Blood*, **86** (1995) 692–702.

41. Davi F, Gocke C, Smith S, and Sklar J. Lymphocytic progenitor cell origin and clonal evolution of human B-lineage acute lymphoblastic leukemia, *Blood*, **88** (1996) 609–621.

42. Beishuizen A, Verhoeven MA, van Wering ER, Hahlen K, Hooijkaas H, and van Dongen JJ. Analysis of Ig and T-cell receptor genes in 40 childhood acute lymphoblastic leukemias at diagnosis and subsequent relapse: implications for the detection of minimal residual disease by polymerase chain reaction analysis, *Blood*, **83** (1994) 2238–2247.

43. Choi Y, Greenberg SJ, Du TL, Ward PM, Overturf PM, Brecher ML, et al. Clonal evolution in B-lineage acute lymphoblastic leukemia by contemporaneous VH-VH gene replacements and VH-DJH gene rearrangements, *Blood*, **87** (1996) 2506–2512.

44. Steward CG, Goulden NJ, Katz F, Baines D, Martin PG, Langlands K, et al. A polymerase chain reaction study of the stability of Ig heavy-chain and T-cell receptor delta gene rearrangements between presentation and relapse of childhood B-lineage acute lymphoblastic leukemia, *Blood*, **83** (1994) 1355–1362.

45. Rosenquist R, Thunberg U, Li AH, Forestier E, Lonnerholm G, Lindh J, et al. Clonal evolution as judged by immunoglobulin heavy chain gene rearrangements in relapsing precursor-B acute lymphoblastic leukemia, *Eur. J. Haematol.*, **63** (1999) 171–179.

46. d'Auriol L, Macintyre E, Galibert F, and Sigaux F. In vitro amplification of T cell gamma gene rearrangements: a new tool for the assessment of minimal residual disease in acute lymphoblastic leukemias, *Leukemia*, **3** (1989) 155–158.

47. Hansen-Hagge TE, Yokota S, and Bartram CR. Detection of minimal residual disease in acute lymphoblastic leukemia by in vitro amplification of rearranged T-cell receptor delta chain sequences, *Blood*, **74** (1989) 1762–1767.

48. Yamada M, Hudson S, Tournay O, Bittenbender S, Shane SS, Lange B, et al. Detection of minimal disease in hematopoietic malignancies of the B-cell lineage by using third-complementarity-determining region (CDR-III)-specific probes, *Proc. Natl. Acad. Sci. USA*, **86** (1989) 5123–5127.

49. Neale GA, Menarguez J, Kitchingman GR, Fitzgerald TJ, Koehler M, Mirro J Jr, et al. Detection of minimal residual disease in T-cell acute lymphoblastic leukemia using polymerase chain reaction predicts impending relapse, *Blood*, **78** (1991) 739–747.

50. Nizet Y, Van Daele S, Lewalle P, Vaerman JL, Philippe M, Vermylen C, et al. Long-term follow-up of residual disease in acute lymphoblastic leukemia patients in complete remission using clonogeneic IgH probes and the polymerase chain reaction, *Blood*, **82** (1993) 1618–1625.

51. van Dongen JJ, Breit TM, Adriaansen HJ, Beishuizen A, and Hooijkaas H. Immunophenotypic and immunogenotypic detection of minimal residual disease in acute lymphoblastic leukemia, *Recent Results Cancer Res.*, **131** (1993) 157–184.

52. Hosler GA, Bash RO, Bai X, Jain V, and Scheuermann RH. Development and validation of a quantitative polymerase chain reaction assay to evaluate minimal residual disease for T-cell acute lymphoblastic leukemia and follicular lymphoma, *Am. J. Pathol.*, **154** (1999) 1023–1035.

53. Potter MN, Cross NC, van Dongen JJ, Saglio G, Oakhill A, Bartram CR, et al. Molecular evidence of minimal residual disease after treatment for leukaemia and lymphoma: an updated meeting report and review, *Leukemia*, **7** (1993) 1302–1314.

54. van Rhee F, Marks DI, Lin F, Szydlo RM, Hochhaus A, Treleaven J, et al. Quantification of residual disease in Philadelphia-positive acute lymphoblastic leukemia: comparison of blood and bone marrow, *Leukemia*, **9** (1995) 329–335.

55. Brisco MJ, Condon J, Sykes PJ, Neoh SH, and Morley AA. Detection and quantitation of neoplastic cells in acute lymphoblastic leukaemia, by use of the polymerase chain reaction, *Br. J. Haematol.*, **79** (1991) 211–217.

56. Brisco MJ, Sykes PJ, Hughes E, Dolman G, Neoh SH, Peng LM, et al. Monitoring minimal residual disease in peripheral blood in B-lineage acute lymphoblastic leukaemia, *Br. J. Haematol.*, **99** (1997) 314–319.

57. Ouspenskaia MV, Johnston DA, Roberts WM, Estrov Z, and Zipf TF. Accurate quantitation of residual B-precursor acute lymphoblastic leukemia by limiting dilution and a PCR-based detection system: a description of the method and the principles involved, *Leukemia*, **9** (1995) 321–328.

58. Taswell C. Limiting dilution assays for the determination of immunocompetent cell frequencies. I. Data analysis, *J. Immunol.*, **126** (1981) 1614–1619.

59. Neale GA, Coustan-Smith E, Pan Q, Chen X, Gruhn B, Stow P, et al. Tandem application of flow cytometry and polymerase chain reaction for comprehensive detection of minimal residual disease in childhood acute lymphoblastic leukemia, *Leukemia*, **13** (1999) 1221–1226.
60. Heid CA, Stevens J, Livak KJ, and Williams PM. Real time quantitative PCR, *Genome Res.*, **6** (1996) 986–994.
61. Pongers-Willemse MJ, Verhagen OJ, Tibbe GJ, Wijkhuijs AJ, de Haas V, Roovers E, et al. Real-time quantitative PCR for the detection of minimal residual disease in acute lymphoblastic leukemia using junctional region specific TaqMan probes, *Leukemia*, **12** (1998) 2006–2014.
62. Donovan JW, Ladetto M, Zou G, Neuberg D, Poor C, Bowers D, et al. Immunoglobulin heavy-chain consensus probes for real-time PCR quantification of residual disease in acute lymphoblastic leukemia, *Blood*, **95** (2000) 2651–2658.
63. Kwan E, Norris MD, Zhu L, Ferrara D, Marshall GM, and Haber M. Simultaneous detection and quantification of minimal residual disease in childhood acute lymphoblastic leukaemia using real-time polymerase chain reaction, *Br. J. Haematol.*, **109** (2000) 430–434.
64. Eckert C, Landt O, Taube T, Seeger K, Beyermann B, Proba J, et al. Potential of LightCycler technology for quantification of minimal residual disease in childhood acute lymphoblastic leukemia, *Leukemia*, **14** (2000) 316–323.
65. Bruggemann M, Droese J, Bolz I, Luth P, Pott C, von Neuhoff N, et al. Improved assessment of minimal residual disease in B cell malignancies using fluorogenic consensus probes for real-time quantitative PCR, *Leukemia*, **14** (2000) 1419–1425.
66. Verhagen OJ, Willemse MJ, Breunis WB, Wijkhuijs AJ, Jacobs DC, Joosten SA, et al. Application of germline IGH probes in real-time quantitative PCR for the detection of minimal residual disease in acute lymphoblastic leukemia, *Leukemia*, **14** (2000) 1426–1435.
67. Chen X, Pan Q, Stow P, Behm FG, Goorha R, Pui CH, et al. Quantification of minimal residual disease in T-lineage acute lymphoblastic leukemia with the TAL-1 deletion using a standardized real-time PCR assay, *Leukemia*, **15** (2001) 166–170.

# 4

# Statistical Considerations in the Analysis of Minimal Residual Disease

*Dennis A. Johnston and Theodore F. Zipf*

## INTRODUCTION

This chapter presents statistical considerations used by many researchers and clinicians in the determination of minimal residual disease (MRD) in patients. Our developments were applied to polymerase chain reaction (PCR)-based measurement of MRD in patients with childhood acute lymphoblastic leukemia (ALL), but the methods and considerations are applicable to the other methods of determining MRD and to other disease diagnoses.

The methods discussed here are not new and have been borrowed from other fields, from vitamin research *(1,2)* to economics *(3)*. They are presented here in hopes of providing a framework for analysis and discussion of where the methods development can and needs to go from here.

There are at least three considerations that must be made when developing a new technique, such as MRD: (1) sensitivity, variability, and calibration of the technique; (2) verification that the technique can dependably distinguish the "target" groups; and (3) ability of the technique to predict the group into which an individual will eventually fall.

### Sensitivity, Variability, and Calibration

The first step in defining a new technique as it was in the development of MRD techniques, is to determine the sensitivity to change in the disease, including the minimal distinguishable level of the technique. Also, the variability on repeat samples as well as the variability from patient to patient needs to be determined. In the case of MRD, the method estimates the number of residual tumor cells in the bone marrow (BM) or peripheral blood (PB) without necessarily trying to

From: *Leukemia and Lymphoma: Detection of Minimal Residual Disease*
Edited by: T. F. Zipf and D. A. Johnston © Humana Press Inc., Totowa, NJ

count all of the tumor cells in the sample but rather based on counting the number of positive cells marked by a particular technique. The technique intends, either upon amplification or marking, to produce a "signal" that represents the current status of the patient. The variability from sample to sample even while just counting is a major concern. If the signal represents the number of cells by using the intensity of an actual signal, the correspondence between the magnitude of the signal and the number of cells must be determined, as well as the variability from sample to sample. This is known as calibration. The residual error from the calibration is a measure of the variability pooled from all sources. This is discussed in the next section.

The second step is to use the technique to measure residual disease in patients. The purpose here is to test and see if there are differences in the patient groups associated with the process of interest. With MRD, the interest is to see if there are differences between early-relapsing patients and those that remain in remission, either after therapy as the patient goes into remission or after bone marrow transplantation (BMT) to measure the reduction and possible return of the cancer clone as measured by MRD. The test can be merely a comparison of levels of residual disease compared between the groups of relapsing patients and those in long-term remission. Usually, either a continuous analysis of variance is performed or a threshold is defined and a chi-square or logistic regression analysis (e.g., positive MRD versus negative MRD at the number of cells tested and the sensitivity of the MRD technique) performed. Alternatively, survival analysis or Cox model proportion hazard analysis may be employed to test the length of remission versus level of MRD. These tests determine whether the population of early-relapse patients has a different level of MRD from those in long-term remission. If there is a separation of the patients groups, then MRD may be considered to be useful in distinguishing them. These statistical tests are discussed in the third section of this chapter.

The third step is to use the MRD to predict those patients who will relapse early. Often the results of the second step are considered as having a possible predictive value. If the threshold divides the patients into the desired groups (e.g., relapsing patients above the threshold and remission patients below the threshold), it can be used to predict the patient outcome. However, the tests are often statistically "significant" when there is still a substantial overlap in the two populations. If there is an overlap, two types of classification error occur. If the patients are to be further treated based on their classification as predicted to relapse (treated with a different therapeutic regimen or BMT) or predicted to continue in remission (no change in treatment), then these become two types of treatment errors. The first is that a patient predicted to relapse actually would not relapse and is, thus, exposed to the additional therapy needlessly. The other is that a patient classified as a long-term remission is destined to relapse and miss possibly live-saving therapy. The degree of overlap in the test is measured by calculating the sensitivity and specificity of the prediction. This sensitivity is a measure of the classification error and is not the same as the sensitivity of the MRD measurement. If the sensitivity or specificity of the test are low, the error in treatment is high. In the fourth section of this chapter, we present some alternative methods of predicting patient outcome when the threshold method has an unacceptably low sensitivity or specificity.

## DISEASE RESPONSE CURVE BY LIMITED DILUTION

In this section, we show our method of calibration of PCR-based markers. Although much of the method is specific to PCR, the limited dilution assay method *(4)* to obtain the response of the MRD technique and associate it to the proportion of positive cells based on samples of known numbers of cells (as measured in amount of DNA) is applicable to other techniques. Here, we present a generalized version of the limited dilution assay *(5,22)*. For other techniques, the exact form of the calibration curve may differ as a function of both the sensitivity of the technique and the response—in particular, in the upper (shoulder) and lower (heel) portions of the dose-response curve generated by the calibration.

### *Development of Known Dilutions*

Bone marrow samples from newly diagnosed leukemia patients who have the appropriate disease-associated genetic markers are used for the calibration. Each patient specimen used for calibration has >95% blasts and can be diluted in a 10-fold manner. The DNA is extracted from the mononuclear cells in the specimen and the number of cells is based on the total amount of DNA determined by spectrophotometry. Aliquots representing dilutions from 10 µg to 10 pg are prepared and these then divided into 10 aliquots per dilution. Nonleukemia cell DNA is added to each aliquot to bring the amount of DNA in each reaction to a total of 1 µg. The fraction of positive aliquots is the response, $y_i$, to the number of cells, $x_i$, in the $i$th calibration sample. In our hands, the relationship between the response and the number of cells was a typical sigmoid curve, as shown in Fig. 1. The expected log-linear relationship as it approaches saturation (shoulder of the curve) or the minimum detectable level (heel of the curve) is lost and, therefore, the rate of change in the observed signal with the change in number of cells flattens out. The lower end (heel) of the sigmoidal shape of the curve is a result of the fact that the number of potential positive cells is at least $10^7$ cells and the minimum detectable level of the PCR techniques is about 25 cells in $10^6$ cells ($2.5 \times 10^{-6}$ or about 15 pg DNA). As the fraction of actually positive cells nears this lower limit, the change in detection signal also decreases. A similar effect occurs on the upper end of the curve (shoulder) as the number of positive cells approaches 100% of the cells and saturates the signal. In many analyses, the heel

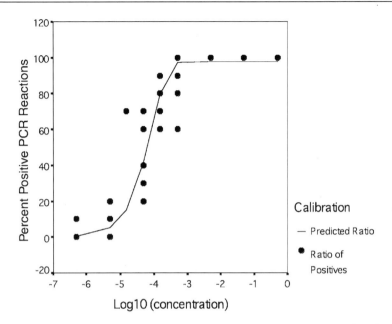

**Fig. 1.** The calibration of the PCR response curve using a second-order rational polynomial (Michaelis–Menton) function.

and shoulder regions are ignored and the body of the curve is used in the analysis as an approximate straight line producing a linear calibration curve. In the case of MRD, the heel and shoulder regions comprise too great a portion of the curve to ignore. By including the heel of the curve, we can add one to two orders of magnitude to the range of the test.

### Development of a Nonlinear Calibration Method

Because the curve of MRD PCR response versus actual numbers of leukemic cells is not linear, the inverse prediction method of linear limiting dilution assay proposed by Taswell (4) cannot be used directly. If the analysis was limited to the log-linear range, the standard method of Taswell could be used (22). We generalized the method of Taswell (5) that was based on the inverse prediction method of Fieller (1,2,6–8). The relationship of PCR response was fit to the number of cells using a nonlinear model. We tried several models, including the exponential model

$$f(x; A, a, b) = A(1 - e^{-ax}) + b$$

and the second-order rational function (second-order Michaelis–Menton) model

$$f(x; a_0, a_1, a_2, b_1, b_2) = \frac{a_0 + a_1 x + a_2 x^2}{1 + b_1 x + b_2 x^2}$$

using the NLR procedure in SPSS (SPSS, Inc, Chicago, IL). Both models include a minimal detectable level ($b$ or $a_0$, respectively) and a saturation level ($A + b$ or $a_2/b_2$, respectively). Both fit well and provided both estimates of the model parameters $\hat{\theta} = (A, a, b)$ or $\hat{\theta} = (a_0, a_1, a_2, b_1, b_2)$ and their respective asymptotic variance–covariance matrix $\hat{\Sigma}$.

To use the estimated model, for any value of PCR response, $y_0$, of an unknown sample, either estimated equation can be solved explicitly for the estimated number of cells, $x_0$, in the sample. More generally, either can be solved approximately to any degree of required accuracy by using a simple bisection technique (9, pp. 98, 261–262) only having the function and the estimated parameters. The method works for monotonic functions such as the ones used here for MRD and requires that the solution, $x_0$, be bracketed by estimated values, say, $x_1$ and $x_2$, and the corresponding functional values $f(x_1)$ and $f(x_2)$ calculated. The interval is bisected by calculating the midpoint and $x_m = (x_1 + x_2)/2$ and $f(x_m)$. The value of $y_0$ falls in the first half of the interval ($f(x_1), f(x_m)$) or the second half of the interval ($f(x_m), f(x_2)$) or exactly at $x_m$. If at $x_m$, the process stops. Otherwise, the upper or lower value of the outside interval is replaced with $x_m$, and the bisection proceeds until the difference between the lower and upper values of the interval is below a threshold. At that point, $x_0$ is assigned the midpoint of the final interval.

As fixed numbers of cells are possible for each sample using the 10-fold dilution method, a chart of response versus estimated number of positive cells can be provided for the assay. To determine the variability and the 95% confidence interval (called a fiducial interval by Fieller because the number of positive cells in the calibration assay is a fixed, not random, number), a generalization of Fieller's theorem to nonlinear models was developed. With either model, the estimated parameters of the model, designated as the vector $\hat{\theta}$, are approximately and asymptotically normally distributed with true mean $\theta$ and variance–covariance matrix $\Sigma$ (10). $\Sigma$ is estimated by the nonlinear regression (e.g., NLR in SPSS) by the unbiased estimator matrix in the output, designated as $\hat{\Sigma}$. A Monte Carlo simulation is performed that calculates estimators $\hat{\theta}_j$ from a multivariate normal distribution with mean $\theta$ and variance–covariance matrix $\hat{\Sigma}$ [$\hat{\theta}_j \sim MVN (\hat{\theta}, \hat{\Sigma})$] for $j = 1, \ldots, n$ using an eigenvector transformation $\hat{\Sigma}$ to transform to a diagonal matrix and then simulate independent normally distributed random variables, correlating them to match $\hat{\Sigma}$, producing the set of simulated solutions ($\hat{\theta}_j, j = 1, \ldots, n$). For each simulated $\hat{\theta}_j$, the inverse $x_{0,j}$ at $y_0$ is calculated by bisection. The $n$ must be sufficiently large that the order statistics needed to estimate the fiducial limits are defined. For example, $n$ must be at least 200 to estimate two-sided 95% fiducial limits [at percentiles 2.5% ($x_{0,(5)}$) and 97.5% ($x_{0,(195)}$), where the parentheses denotes the order statistics of the set of simulated solutions {$x_{0,j}$, $j = 1, \ldots, n$}]. This was accomplished using a custom program written in FORTRAN for the nonlinear regression estimates calculated by SPSS (access www.odin.mdacc.tmc.edu for a copy of the program).

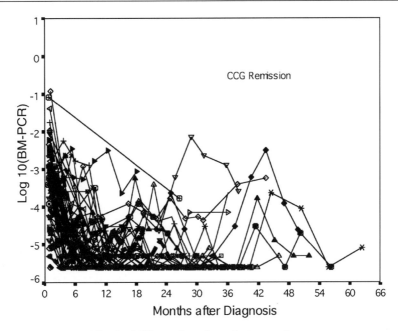

**Fig. 2.** CCG continued-remission patients.

## DATA ANALYSIS CONSIDERATIONS OF MRD DATA

In this section, we will illustrate the characteristics of MRD data obtained by the above methods. The data presented are from a study described in Roberts *(11)*. This study followed a subset of several Children's Cancer Group (CCG) protocols. Although other studies have more patients *(12–14)*, in this study the individual patient has a substantial number of follow-up bone marrows so that we can describe a range of outcomes and still see individual responses. We will describe the results of 69 patients who had serial follow-up. All patients achieved remission as defined by an end-induction bone marrow specimen with <5% blasts. Sixty-two patients remained in remission. Figure 2 is a scattergram of the CCG patients in continued remission with the serial determinations connected. The abscissa units are months after diagnosis, with a logarithm transformed bone marrow PCR [$\log_{10}(BM - PCR)$] for the ordinate. Observe that within a few months of diagnosis, $\log_{10}(BM - PCR)$ decreased. In some cases, the values initially decrease, then increase and decrease again. In others, the values decrease, remain low, then increase followed by a decline. The case represented with solid-angled triangles never decreases below $10^{-4}$. Figure 3 is a scattergram of patients who relapsed. These data include the data point prior to the diagnosis of relapse. Several of the patients show a decrease initially followed by a rapid rise, but others show a decrease in $\log_{10}(BM - PCR)$, followed by an increase to relapse

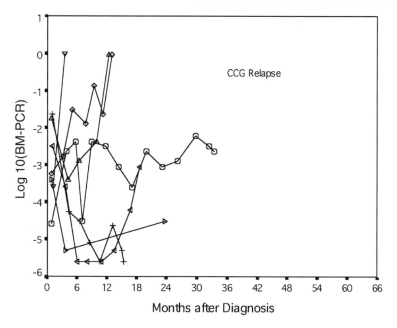

**Fig. 3.** CCG relapse patients.

(e.g., reverse open triangles) or a constant level of $\log_{10}(BM - PCR)$ (e.g., open circles).

## Population Analysis

Standard methods of analysis would suggest that the population of patients in continued remission be compared with the population of patients that relapse, comparing $\log_{10}(BM - PCR)$ levels. This is accomplished typically by a comparison of means either at each time of interest or looking at an interval of interest. Table 1 gives the means and standard deviations of the two groups at several times during the first year. After the $\log_{10}(BM - PCR)$ readings at 1 mo, the relapse patients have higher levels than the continued-remission patients through 1 yr. Beyond 1 yr, the trend continues but with a reduced number of patients in both groups. Two results bear further comment. The standard deviations of the relapse patients increase over time and are higher than the continued-remission patients from 6 mo on. The standard deviations of the continued-remission patients decrease over time. Both of these conditions are expected. The other result is that the means of the relapse patients decrease to mo 6 and then increase while the continued-remission patients decrease. This too is expected. Using both time interval and remission status in a two-factor analysis of variance analyzing $\log_{10}(BM - PCR)$, both remission status ($p < 0.001$) and time interval ($p < 0.001$) were highly significant, with a significant interaction

Table 1
Descriptive Statistics for the CCG Patient Example

| | $log_{10}(BM - PCR)$ | | | | |
| | Relapse | | Continued remission | | t-Test |
| Interval | Mean ± SD | N | Mean ± SD | N | p-Value |
|----------|-----------|---|-----------|---|---------|
| 1 mo | −2.96 ± 1.05 | 7 | −3.45 ± 1.09 | 58 | 0.265 |
| 3 mo | −2.95 ± 1.72 | 6 | −4.24 ± 0.92 | 55 | 0.005 |
| 6 mo | −3.67 ± 1.44 | 7 | −4.67 ± 0.89 | 45 | 0.014[a] |
| 9 mo | −3.04 ± 1.88 | 6 | −4.89 ± 0.83 | 50 | <0.001[a] |
| 12 mo | −2.57 ± 2.53 | 6 | −5.17 ± 0.59 | 44 | <0.001[a] |

[a]A t-test is a two-tailed pooled t-test with significant $F$-ratio of variances indicating that the standard deviation of the relapse patients is greater than that of the remission patients. The separate variance estimate t-test is not significant, partially as a result of an imbalance of sample size in the two groups.

($p = 0.013$) showing that the rates of change over time for continued-remission patients is different from that for relapse patients.

## *Prediction of Patient Relapse*

The ultimate intent and purpose of the PCR technique must be to predict early failure and eventual relapse of the patient, where relapse of the patient is defined clinically as a bone marrow with greater than 5% blast cells. Because the PCR technique estimates the proportion of cells from the leukemic clone, this estimate in some form or another should be predictive of eventual failure. Figure 4 shows the typical plot of mean ± standard error (SE) at 1, 3, 6, 9, and 12 mo following therapy. For the patients who relapsed, the penultimate bone marrow is the last marrow plotted. The conclusions of the previous section can be confirmed visually: The BM − PCR for continued remission patients continues to decrease with time, whereas the patients that will eventually relapse remain at an average of about $10^{-3}$, although the SE grows with time (fewer data points at each time). The plot would, however, suggest that a threshold level of $10^{-4}$ or $10^{-3}$ at 3 mo after the start of treatment would separate the patients who will relapse from those that will continue in remission. This suggestion of the separation of relapse and continued remission is overemphasized by the fact that there are fewer patients in the relapse group and many more in the remission group. A more correct plot to visually see if there is patient overlap would be either a mean ± standard deviation plot (*see* Fig. 5) or a box-plot (*see* Fig. 6), where the median is represented by the heavy bar in the middle of the box, the extent of the box includes the middle 50% of the patients in the group, and the whiskers above and below the box indicate the range. If there are data beyond 1.5 times the inter-quartile

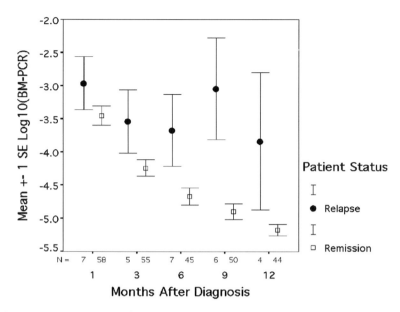

**Fig. 4.** Means ± standard error of CCG patients by interval after diagnosis and relapse status.

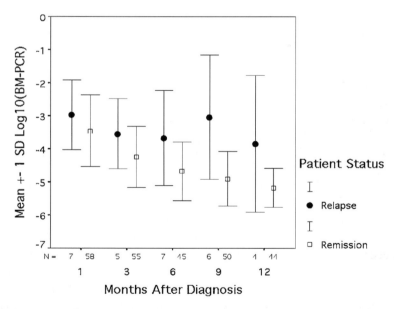

**Fig. 5.** Means ± standard deviation of CCG patients by interval after diagnosis and relapse status.

61

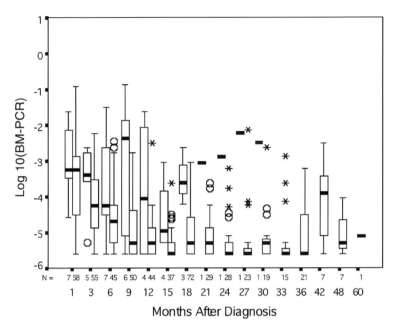

**Fig. 6.** Box-plot of CCG patients by interval after diagnosis and relapse status.

Table 2
$\log_{10}$(BM – PCR) with a Threshold of –3 at 3 mo Compared to Actual Patient Status

|  | Patient outcome | | |
|---|---|---|---|
|  | Relapse | Continued remission | Total |
| $\log_{10}$(BM – PCR) | | | |
| > –3 | 2 | 5 | 7 |
| ≤ –3 | 3 | 50 | 53 |
| Total | 5 | 55 | 60 |

*Note*: Fisher's exact test of association: $p = 0.099$.

range, then the whiskers indicate 1.5 times the interquartile range, with circles and asterisks indicating data beyond 1.5 times and 3 times the interquartile range, respectively. Relapse threshold levels at $10^{-4}$ and $10^{-3}$ have been proposed by several authors at various times after induction therapy (7, 14, and 28 d after completion of initial therapy being the most proposed) *(10,12,14)*. Tables 2 and 3 present the results of these threshold levels on the CCG data presented here. Because of the small number of patients, the Fisher's exact test of association is used instead of the customary chi-square approximate test. Neither Tables 2 nor 3 shows a significant association ($p = 0.099$ and $p = 0.091$, respectively), but

Table 3

$\log_{10}$(BM – PCR) with a Threshold of –4 at 3 mo Compared to Actual Patient Status

| | Patient outcome | | |
| --- | --- | --- | --- |
| | Relapse | Continued remission | Total |
| $\log_{10}$(BM – PCR) | | | |
| > –4 | 4 | 21 | 25 |
| ≤ –4 | 1 | 34 | 35 |
| Total | 5 | 55 | 60 |

*Note*: Fisher's exact test of association: $p = 0.091$.

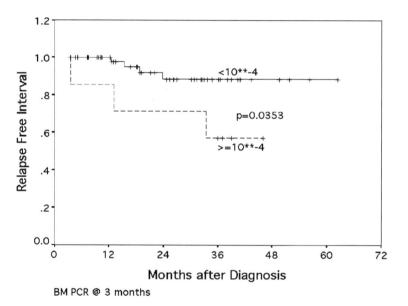

BM PCR @ 3 months

**Fig. 7.** Kaplan–Meier plot of relapse-free interval using the $10^{-4}$ threshold.

would if the number of patients were doubled with the same proportions ($p = 0.017$ and $p = 0.0128$, respectively). Note that if the $10^{-4}$ threshold is used to predict relapse, then 21 patients out of 55 that have remained in remission (38.2%) would have been classified as relapse patients that did not relapse and 1 patient out of 5 (20%) that actually relapsed would have been missed by the criterion. More will be said about this in the next section.

Another method that is often used is to calculate the time to relapse in the form of survival curves comparing the groups above and below the threshold. Although the patient size in this study is small for this method, the resultant Kaplan–Meier curves are shown in Fig. 7 using BM – PCR > $10^{-4}$ at approx 3 mo as the predictor

Table 4
General 2 × 2 Decision Table with Parameters at Two Levels

|  | True diagnosis | | |
|  | Relapse | Remission | Total |
|---|---|---|---|
| Decision |  |  |  |
| Relapse | A | B | A + B |
| Remission | C | D | C + D |
| Total | A + C | B + D | n |

of relapse. The patient count is slightly different in this analysis because several patients without 3 mo BM – PCR, but with bracketing values both below $10^{-4}$, were included as continued remission patients and one patient who relapsed at 90 d was included as a relapse that was not included in the previous analysis. The relapse-free interval of the BM – PCR > $10^{-4}$ group is significantly less ($p$ = 0.0353) than the BM – PCR ≤ $10^{-4}$ group. As in the table method above, we would have classified 4 patients who had continuous remission as going to relapse out of 57 total patients (7.0%), whereas 3 out of the 7 relapsing patients (42.9%) would have been missed.

## PREDICTIONS OF INDIVIDUAL PATIENT RELAPSE
### Sensitivity, Specificity, and the Decision Table

The decision table technique is used on everything from medical decision making to stock market and business predictions. Tables 3 and 4 are examples of contingency or decision tables. The analysis of these tables is used to determine the ability of a particular test to predict outcome. In our case, we want to use MRD to predict the occurrence of relapse in patients with acute leukemia. The structure of the problem is simple: There is an outcome (e.g., clinical relapse by a certain time after treatment and/or the determination that the patient is "disease free" or in remission) that is known on a set of patients. Parameters (e.g., MRD) have been taken that are thought to be predictive in some form for relapse or continued remission of the patients. A decision table is constructed, similar to Tables 2 and 3 using the prediction. If we restrict the parameters to two levels, the table looks like Table 4. The ability to predict relapse is termed the sensitivity and the ability of the parameter to predict continued remission is termed the specificity (15). Clearly, these definitions can be reversed, although sensitivity is usually reserved for the "positive condition," which, in this case, would be relapse. Sensitivity and specificity are defined in terms of Table 1 as

$$\text{Sensitivity} = s = \frac{A}{A + C}$$

$$\text{Specificity} = f = \frac{D}{B + D}$$

Sensitivity is then the estimated probability of deciding relapse when the patient truly relapsed. Specificity is then the estimated probability of deciding continued remission when the patient truly continues in remission. Accuracy of the prediction is given as

$$\text{Positive accuracy} = v = \frac{A}{A + B}$$

$$\text{Negative accuracy} = g = \frac{D}{C + D}$$

These are often called the positive predictive value (PPV) and the negative predictive value (NPV), respectively. For an ideal classification, $s = f = 1$ and there are no patients who are misclassified. However, as in Table 2, $s = 0.4$ and $f = 0.909$, or as in Table 3, $s = 0.80$ and $f = 0.618$. Whenever classification criteria are based on a continuous measure, as they are in the case of MRD, if the threshold point is changed, the sensitivity and specificity will change with one increasing and the other decreasing, depending on the direction of the change. In this case, moving the threshold from $10^{-3}$ to $10^{-4}$ increases the number of correctly classified as relapsing (1/5 to 4/5) but decreases the number correctly classified as remaining in remission (50/55 to 34/55); this is because the two populations, relapse and remission, are overlapping in MRD. This overlap is a feature of a classification based on a single threshold at a single time. The so-called optimum threshold can be calculated by minimizing a "cost or risk" function. If the patients classified as relapse were to be treated with additional therapy and those classified as remission were to be followed without additional treatment, we may wish to choose how the consequences of this decision are to be controlled. If we wish to minimize the number that would be treated unnecessarily, of the two thresholds we would choose $10^{-3}$. If we wanted to minimize the number of relapse patients to be missed for additional treatment, of the two thresholds we would choose $10^{-4}$. One purpose of this study would then be to establish a rule for future patients in the same diagnostic/treatment circumstance. Other thresholds can be established based on more complicated error criteria such as minimizing the dollar cost of therapy while treating the most patients who would relapse or minimizing the hazard of adverse outcome if the follow-on therapy had an increased risk of mortality or other adverse outcome.

We can set two thresholds, say above $10^{-3}$, $10^{-3}$–$10^{-4}$, and below $10^{-4}$. For our example, this yields Table 5. Here we can classify above $10^{-3}$ as relapse with sensitivity of 0.40 and below $10^{-4}$ as remission with specificity 0.618, but have the 18 patients between $10^{-4}$ and $10^{-3}$ as unclassified. We have several options

### Table 5
### Two Thresholds in MRD

|  | True diagnosis | | |
|---|---|---|---|
|  | Relapse | Remission | Total |
| $\log_{10}(BM - PCR)$ | | | |
| $> -3$ | 2 | 5 | 7 |
| $-3$ to $-4$ | 2 | 16 | 18 |
| $< -4$ | 1 | 34 | 35 |
| Total | 5 | 55 | 60 |

### Table 6
### Two Time-Point Measurements of MRD

| Degree of MRD at time 2 | Degree of MRD at time 1 | | | | |
|---|---|---|---|---|---|
|  | $\geq 10^{-2}$ | $10^{-3}$ | $\leq 10^{-4}$ | Negative | Total |
| $\geq 10^{-2}$ | 8/8 | 1/1 | C — | — | 9/9 |
| $10^{-3}$ | 3/5 | 3/5 | 0/2 | — E | 6/12 |
| $\leq 10^{-4}$ | 1/3 | 2/11 D | 2/6 | 0/1 | 5/21 |
| Negative | 1/2 | 1/13 | 5/17 B | 1/55 A | 8/87 |
| Total | 13/18 | 7/30 | 7/25 | 1/56 | 28/129 |

*Source*: Adapted from ref. *20*.

at this point: We could definitely decide that those above $10^{-3}$ will relapse, those below $10^{-4}$ will stay in remission while no decision is made on those between $10^{-4}$ and $10^{-3}$. This is the realm of so-called "fuzzy decision theory" *(16)*.

Another alternative is to add an additional evaluation point to the analysis. Several studies have reported using more than a single evaluation time, obtaining bone marrow aspirates at several distinct times *(12–14)*. Consider Table 5 from ref. *14* as an example of the situation adapted for our purposes as Table 6. At each time-point, the entries are divided into four groups according to MRD: (1) $\geq 10^{-2}$, (2) $10^{-3}$, (3) $\leq 10^{-4}$ but measurable, and (4) negative. This yields a $4 \times 4$ table with 3 empty cells and 5 cells with fewer than 5 patients, even though there are 129 patients total. This is typical of such a table where the times are not well separated and the patients are consistent over the time interval. The entries in Table 6 are the number of relapses divided by the number of cases in the cell of the table. Van Dongen collapses the table into five regions as designated in Table 6 with boxes and a letter to the right of the table. Table 7 gives a summary of the regions. There are three regions (B, D, E) that have approx 22% relapses

Table 7
Regional Analysis of Table 6

| Group | Total sample | Relative % relapses in group | Percent of total relapses |
|-------|-------------|------------------------------|---------------------------|
| A | 1/55 | 2.818% | 1/28 = 3.57% |
| B | 7/32 | 21.9% | 25% |
| C | 15/19 | 78.9% | 53.5% |
| D | 3/14 | 21.4% | 10.7% |
| E | 2/9 | 22.2% | 7.1% |
| Total | 28/129 | 21.7% | |

Table 8
Regional Analysis Combining Regions B, D, and E

| | True diagnosis of relapse | | |
|--------|---------|-----------|-------|
| Groups | Relapse | Remission | Total |
| C | 15 | 4 | 19 |
| B, D, E | 12 | 43 | 55 |
| A | 1 | 54 | 55 |
| Total | 28 | 101 | 129 |

within the region whereas group A (negative, negative) has the lowest percent relapses (1.18%) while Group C ($\geq 10^{-2}$, $\geq 10^{-2}$) has the highest percent. Groups such as A and C are expected. The middle group is intermediate, very much like the $10^{-4}$ to $10^{-3}$ group in the above CCG study. We can then calculate Table 8, summarizing these results. If groups B–E are combined and the sensitivity and specificity are calculated, $s = 0.964$ and $f = 0.535$. If A, B, D, and E are combined, $s = 0.536$ and $f = 0.96$.

With van Dongen's analysis, there were 2 times with 4 levels at each time, yielding 16 cells with 2 numbers in each cell (number relapses, number remissions) for a total of 32 numbers. In general, if there are $t$ times and $l$ levels at each time, there will be $2 \times l^t$ numbers, which means that most of the cells will be empty or a very large number of patients will have to be in the study. If more than two times are desired, the clinician/researcher must limit the number of levels to two or three. For $t = 2$, 2 levels implies 8 numbers and 3 levels implies 18 numbers. For $t = 3$, two levels implies 16 numbers and 3 levels implies 54 numbers.

## Practical Alternatives

There appears to be too much overlap of remission and relapse in the distributions of MRD using just one time-point because at least one of the sensitivities

and specificies are close to 50%. Although we would not like to establish what
an acceptable sensitivity/specificity combination should be for MRD, in general,
or even pediatric leukemia, in particular, we do believe that the level achieved
by our efforts and those around the world are not good enough to yield acceptable
levels. Just observing Figs. 2 and 3 shows visual heterogeneity in the response
of MRD in individual patients. This may be the result of either the heterogeneity
of the patients or the lack of leukemic clone specificity of the particular MRD
marker employed, or both.

Because the threshold or level method becomes impractical for more than two
times with more than two levels, other methods must be proposed to predict
patient relapse. We will illustrate our efforts to find an acceptable alternative in
the next few subsections.

### Autoregressive Methods

We first presented the autoregressive method approach in the article by Roberts *(11)*. The basic principle in these methods is to let the previous patient data
predict the future value of the MRD and then compare the actual value to
the prediction. If the observation was significantly higher than the prediction, the
patient showed an increase in MRD levels and, potentially, this is a precursor to
relapse. We will illustrate the prediction method first and then suggest scenarios
for prediction and possible early intervention.

Let the ordered set $\{t_j; j = 1, \ldots, i\}$ denote the times of measurement of a
particular patient up to the current time $i$ and $\{y_j; j = 1, \ldots, i\}$ denote the corresponding $\log_{10}(\text{BM} - \text{PCR})$ values. We use $\log_{10}(\text{BM} - \text{PCR})$ instead of BM –
PCR to stabilize the variance, as the calibration data have an exponential com-
ponent involved. The approach is to use the first $i$ $\log_{10}(\text{BM} - \text{PCR})$ values to
predict the $(i + 1)$ st $\log_{10}(\text{BM} - \text{PCR})$ value and then compare to the actual
observed value at $t_{i+1}$.

The simplest method of prediction is that of the weighted moving average.
Much as it is calculated for stocks, use

$$y_{mv,i+1} = \sum_{j=1}^{i} w_j y_j$$

where the weights $\{w_j\}$ sum to 1. Also, the sum is usually truncated at a reduced
number of terms, say $\tau$. The sample variance of $y_{mv,i+1}$ is

$$s^2_{mv,i+1} = \sum_{j=i-\tau+1}^{i} w_j^2 s_j^2$$

where $s_j^2$ is the sample variance of $y_j$. From our calibration studies, we have found that the logarithmic transformation stabilizes the variance, making all of the variances of $y_j$ approximately equal and the distribution of the $y_j$'s approximately normally distributed. We estimated that the stabilized variance is approx 0.125 log units squared, making the standard deviation approx 0.25 log units. However, the variance of $y_{i+1}$ is approximately $s_j^2$, making

$$t = \frac{y_{i+1} - \hat{y}_{mv,i+1}}{\sqrt{s_i^2 + s_{mv,i+1}^2}}$$

approximately distributed as the $t$-distribution with $\tau$ degrees of freedom. For the one-sided test to determine if $y_{i+1}$ is above $y_{mv,i+1}$, use the one-sided critical value of the t-distribution at significance $\alpha$. Thus, the alarm rule to signal a significant increase in $\log_{10}(BM - PCR)$ is as follows: If $t$ is greater than the one-sided critical value of the t-distribution with $\tau$ degrees of freedom, then there has been a significant increase in $\log_{10}(BM - PCR)$. One of the disadvantages of the method is that it works best in steady-state situations, where the mean of each $y_j$ is estimated by $y_{mv,i+1}$. If the weights are weighted toward the $i$th observation, the influence will be primarily that of the last observation, minimizing the effect of the whole series $\{y_j; j = 1, ..., i\}$. The other problem is that the moving-average method works most efficiently if the $\{t_j; j = 1, ..., i + 1\}$ are equally spaced, a situation often violated in clinical practice. The $\{w_j\}$ can be adjusted to account for unevenness.

## *Linear Regression Models*

An alternative to simple moving-average models is a moving linear regression. In this case, use the model

$$y_{i+1} = a + bt_{i+1}$$

where $a$ and $b$ are estimated using the model at time $i$ with $\tau$ data points minimizing the sum of squares

$$Q = \sum_{j=i-\tau+1}^{i} (y_j - (a + bt_j))^2$$

using the usual linear regression approach obtaining $\hat{a}$ and $\hat{b}$, respectively. Then, $y_{i+1}$ is estimated by

$$\hat{y}_{i+1} = \hat{a} + \hat{b}t_{i+1}$$

and compared to $y_{i+1}$ using

$$t = \frac{y_{i+1} - \hat{y}_{i+1}}{\sqrt{s_t^2 + s_{y,t}^2 \left( \left(\frac{1}{\tau}\right)^2 + \frac{(t_{i+1} - \hat{t_i})^2}{\sum (t_j - \hat{t_i})^2} \right)}}$$

where $s_{yt}^2$ is the error mean square of the linear regression and $\hat{t_i}$ is the mean of the $\tau$ times in the regression. The expression is approximately t-distributed with $\tau - 1$ degrees of freedom. The alarm rule for the autoregressive linear model is more complicated than the moving-average model. One such rule would have three possibilities. The first is if t is greater than the one-sided critical value with $\tau - 2$ degrees of freedom, then $y_{i+1}$ is significantly above the line. However, this is not necessarily a problem if the slope is significantly negative, so test if $b$ is significantly less than 0. If not, then $y_{i+1}$ could be significant or just leveling off (at minimum perhaps or other steady-state value and the data points on the line are still decreasing). A visual determination of which situation is the case or the use of the moving average as a secondary test is suggested.

Secondary, if t is not greater than the one-sided critical value, but the slope is significantly greater than 0, then the data points are still increasing and $y_{i+1}$ should be considered as significantly increased. The third possibility is if t is significantly below the negative one-sided critical value but the slope is significantly greater than 0, then $y_{i+1}$ is leveling off or decreasing, in which case $y_{i+1}$ should not be considered as increasing.

The principal advantage of the moving linear regressive model over the autoregressive model of the previous subsection is that the model accounts for simple trends in the $\log_{10}(BM - PCR)$ that are modeled by the slope. We have seen that the population of patients is very heterogeneous, especially those who eventually relapse. This model is an effort to individualize the prediction. The principal disadvantage is that we have to estimate the slope. This requires an additional degree of freedom. The minimum number of times $\tau$ that are needed for the model is three, as we must estimate the intercept and the slope and have at least one degree of freedom for the estimate of the error mean square (the residual variance $s_{yt}^2$). It would be much better for $\tau \geq 4$, so that the number of degrees of freedom in $s_{yt}^2$ is increased, reducing the critical values of the t-distribution and making the estimates more sensitive. The trade-off is that as the number of data points increases, the ability of a linear equation to fit the data decreases. Also, because the number of bone marrows before the model is usable increases, this implies that early relapses will not be predicted. In our preliminary tests, $\tau = 4$ worked better than $\tau = 3$ and fits the changes well enough.

## *Curvilinear Predictive Models*

Curvilinear predictive models use a polynomial,

$$y_j = a_0 + a_1 t_i + a_2 t_j^2 + \ldots + a_k t_j^k; \; j = 1, \ldots, i$$

to estimate $y_{i+1}$. As in the linear case, we wish to use the last $\tau$ times to produce a moving curvilinear model. The model to estimate the coefficients based on the last $\tau$ times is

$$
\begin{bmatrix} y_\tau \\ y_{\tau+1} \\ \vdots \\ y_i \end{bmatrix} =
\begin{bmatrix} 1 & t_\tau & \cdots & t_\tau^k \\ 1 & t_{\tau+1} & \cdots & t_{\tau+1}^k \\ \vdots & \vdots & \ddots & \vdots \\ 1 & t_i & \cdots & t_i^k \end{bmatrix}
\begin{bmatrix} a_0 \\ \vdots \\ a_k \end{bmatrix}
$$

$$Y_{\tau,i} = H_{\tau,i} A_{\tau,i}$$

where $Y_{\tau,i}$ is the vertical vector containing the $\log_{10}(\text{BM} - \text{PCR})$ data, $H_{\tau,i}$ is the corresponding $\tau \times k + 1$ design matrix of the times, and $A_{\tau,i}$ is the vertical vector of coefficients of the curvilinear model. To simplify the equations, the matrices will be written without the subscripts $\tau$ and, which will be assumed to be present. The least-squares solution is then the solution to the normal equations

$$\widehat{A} = (H^T H)^{-1} H^T Y$$

with the residual error being $s^2_{yt...k} = Y^T H (H^T H)^{-1} H^T Y$ and the variance–covariance of $\widehat{A}$ being $s^2_{yt...k} (H^T H)^{-1}$, where the superscripts $T$ and $-1$ denote matrix transpose and inverse, respectively *(17)*. The estimate of $y_{i+1}$ is

$$\widehat{y}_{i+1} = \widehat{a}_0 + \widehat{a}_1 t_{i+1} + \ldots + \widehat{a}_k t_{i+1}$$

and the one-sided test if $y_{i+1} > \widehat{y}_{i+1}$ is the one-sided t-test

$$t = \frac{y_{i+1} - \widehat{y}_{i+1}}{\sqrt{s^2_{yt..t_k} (1 + X^T (H^T H)^{-1} X)}}$$

$$X^T = (0, t_{i+1} - \overline{t}_i, \ldots, t_{i+1}^k - \overline{t}_i^k)$$

where the overbar denote the mean of the powers of $t$ from $\tau$ to $i$. The slope of the curvilinear model at $t_{i+1}$ is given as

$$\widehat{b}_{i+1} = \widehat{a}_1 + 2\widehat{a}_2 t_{i+1} + \ldots + k\widehat{a}_k t_{i+1}^{k-1}$$

A test of whether the slope is greater than zero is based on the one-sided t-test

$$t = \frac{\hat{b}_{i+1}}{\sqrt{s^2_{yt...k}(D^T(H^TH)^{-1}D)}}$$

$$D^T = (0, 1, 2(\bar{t}_{i+1} - \bar{t}_i), ..., k(t_{i+1}^{k-1} - t_i^{-k-1}))$$

## *Other Predictive Models*

Other predictive models may be used analogously to the others proposed in this section. The most promising is the use of cubic splines, which may be used as soon as the number of biopsies reaches seven. The theoretical framework for the method is complicated *(9,18–20)*. In a basic explanation, adapted from the work of Press et al. (9, pp. 94–98), the method is derived from the linear interpolation formula

$$y = ay_i + by_{i+1}$$

where

$$a = \frac{t_{i+1} - t}{t_{i+1} - t_i}$$

$$b = 1 - a = \frac{t - t_i}{t_{i+1} - t_i}$$

and $t_1 < t_2 < ... < t_n$ is the ordered sequence of times corresponding to the $\log_{10}(BM - PCR)$ values $y_1, y_2, ..., y_n$. The time at which the estimate is to be made is the next bone marrow time $t_{n+1}$. If linear interpolation were employed, the result would be a two-point linear model, similar to the mean method described above. The problem with linear interpolation is that the estimating line is a succession of broken lines, broken at the time-points. To smooth the line, the estimate is based on a smoother interpolation using the second derivatives of the predictor

$$y = ay_i + by_{i+1} + cy''_i + dy''_{i+1}$$

with

$$c = 1/6 \, (a^3 - a) \, (t_{i+1} - t_i)^2$$

$$d = 1/6 \, (b^3 - b) \, (t_{i+1} - t_i)^2$$

and requiring continuity of the predictor at the interior nodes $y_i$, $1 < i < n$, and choosing the values of the second derivatives at 1 and $n$. Because the prediction and error bounds at $t_{n+1}$ are desired, the specification of these end points strongly influence the prediction. The standard estimate for the second derivatives at the end points is to set them to zero. If this assumption is made, then the prediction at $t_{n+1}$ is

$$\hat{y}_{n+1} = y_n + (t_{n+1} - t_n)\acute{y}_n$$

where

$$\acute{y}_n = \frac{y_n - y_{n-1}}{t_n - t_{n-1}} + 1/6\,(t_n - t_{n-1})\ddot{y}_{n-1}$$

The problem arises in the estimate of the variance at $t_{n+1}$. The error variance can be estimated by using local differences (19)

$$\hat{\sigma}_R^2 = \frac{1}{2(n-1)} \sum_{i=2}^{n} (y_i - y_{i-1})^2$$

but the correction factor to extrapolate to $\hat{y}_{n+1}$ is not yet known. The form should be similar to

$$\hat{\sigma}_{\hat{y}_{n+1}}^2 = \sigma_R^2 \left( 1 + \frac{(t_{n+1} - \bar{t}_n)^2}{\sum\limits_{i=1}^{n}(t_i - \bar{t}_n)^2} \right)$$

but over a reduced set of $t$'s with the appropriate number of degrees of freedom. The ratio could use local differences instead of a mean. A similar expression is defined within the range of times (21, p. 15).

To predict an increasing $y_{n+1}$ in terms of $\hat{y}_{n+1}$ and the variance $\hat{\sigma}_{\hat{y}_{n+1}}^2$, test if

$$y_{n+1} > \hat{y}_{n+1} + t_{a,f}\hat{\sigma}_{\hat{y}_{n+1}}$$

and test the slope $y_n'$ for positivity following the rule given in an earlier subsection.

## Clinical Results of Predictive Models

In the event that $y_{i+1}$ is determined to be increasing, several clinical steps might be possible. The patient can be asked to return at a shorter interval based on the rate of increase to verify the increase and the prediction of relapse. We have observed a rapid increase in BM – PCR to eventual relapse. If nothing is done, it is probable that the patient will have continually increasing BM – PCR until relapse. An alternative therapy may be tried at the time of prediction. These approaches need to be tested in supervised clinical trials. More of this will be discussed in the next chapter.

## ACKNOWLEDGMENT

This work was supported, in part, by grant R21 CA68235 from the National Cancer Institute.

## REFERENCES

1. Fieller EC. *The Biological Standardization of Insulin, J. Roy. Statist. Soc.*, (**Suppl. 7**) (1940) 1–64.
2. Fieller EC. Some problems in interval estimation, *J. Roy. Statist. Soc. B* (1954) 175–185.
3. Box GEP and Jenkins GM. *Time Series Analysis Forecasting and Control.* San Francisco: Holden-Day, 1970.
4. Taswell C. Limiting dilution assays for the determination of immunocompetent frequencies, *J. Immunol.*, **126** (1981) 1614–1619.
5. Ouspenskaia MV, Johnston DA, Roberts WM, Estrov Z, and Zipf TF. Accurate quantitation of residual B-precursor acute lymphoblastic leukemia by limited dilution and a PCR-based detection system: a description of the method and the principles involved, *Leukemia*, **9** (1995) 321–328.
6. Creasy MA. Limits for the ratio of two means, *J. Roy. Statist. Soc. B* (1954) 186–194.
7. Finney DJ. *Statistical Methods in Biological Assay*, London: Griffin, 1971, 27–35.
8. Zar JH. *Biostatistical Analysis*, 4th ed. Upper Saddle River, NJ: Prentice-Hall, 1999.
9. Press WH, Flannery BP, Teukolsky SA, and Vetterling WT. *Numerical Recipes in C*, Cambridge: Cambridge University Press, 1998.
10. Johnson DE. *Applied Multivariate Methods for Data Analysts.* Pacific Grove, CA: Duxbury, 1998.
11. Roberts WM, Estrov Z, Ouspenskiai MV, Johnston DA, McClain KL, and Zipf TF. Measurement of residual leukemia during remission in childhood acute lymphoblastic leukemia, *N. Engl. J. Med.*, **336** (1997) 317–323.
12. Cavé H, van der Werff ten Bosch J, Suciu S, Guidal C, Waterkeyn C, Otten J, et al. Clinical significance of minimal residual disease in childhood acute lymphoblastic leukemia, *N. Engl. J. Med.*, **339** (1998) 591–598.
13. Nachman JB, Sather HN, Sensel MG, Trigg ME, Cherlow JM, Lukens JN, et al. Augmented post-induction therapy for children with high-risk acute lymphoblastic leukemia and a slow response to initial therapy, *N. Engl. J. Med.*, **338** (1998) 1663–1671.
14. van Dongen JJM, Seriu T, Panzer-Grumayer ER, Biondi A, Pongers-Willemse MJ, Corral L, et al. Prognostic value of minimal residual disease in childhood acute lymphoblastic leukemia, *Lancet*, **352** (1998) 1731–1738.
15. Feinstein AR. *Clinical Biostatistics.* St. Louis, MO: Mosby, 1977.
16. Manton KG, Woodbury MA, and Tolley HD. *Statistical Applications Using Fuzzy Sets.* New York: Wiley, 1994.
17. Draper NR and Smith H. *Applied Regression Models*, 3rd ed. New York: Wiley, 1998.
18. de Boor C. *A Practical Guide to Spline.* New York: Springer-Verlag, 1978.
19. Green PG and Silverman BW. *Nonparametric Regression and Generalized Linear Models.* Boca Raton, FL: Chapman & Hall/CRC, 1994.

20. Wahba G. *Spline Models for Observational Data*. Philadelphia: Society for Industrial and Applied Mathematics, 1990.
21. Silverman BW. Some aspects of the spline smoothing approach to non-parametric regression curve fitting, *J. Roy. Statist. Soc. B*, **47** (1985) 1–52.
22. Sykes PJ, Neoh SH, Brisco MJ, Hughes E, Condon J, and Morley AA. Quantitation of targets for PCR by use of limiting dilution, *BioTechniques*, **13** (1992) 444–449.

# 5

# The Application of Minimal Residual Disease Detection Methodology to the Clinical Decision-Making Process

*Theodore F. Zipf and Dennis A. Johnston*

## INTRODUCTION

Chapter 4 was devoted to a mathematically rigorous and comprehensive examination of some of the methods used to quantify and analyze residual disease measurements. This may not have been comprehensible to those investigators who do not have experience in either statistics or advanced mathematics. In this chapter, we will present a nonmathematical description of our view of the approach that will be required for minimal residual disease (MRD) measurements to achieve a significant role in the clinical decision-making process.

Now that submicroscopic detection of disease is possible, these methods must first undergo extensive testing to establish their reproducibility, sensitivity of detection, and specificity of the detection. In addition, the standard error that can be assigned to the individual measurements must be determined. This testing process must also include a careful examination of the quantification process. This examination must include a determination of the lower limit of detection. When all of this has been accomplished, it is then appropriate to inquire about the role of MRD measurements in clinical decision making.

First, the clinical problem that we would like to be resolved by this new technique must be defined. In our view, the majority would select the determination of treatment outcome as the prime target. Thus, the goal would be to predict either treatment failure or a successful treatment with long-term disease-free survival. Both of these outcomes must be predicted well in advance

From: *Leukemia and Lymphoma: Detection of Minimal Residual Disease*
Edited by: T. F. Zipf and D. A. Johnston © Humana Press Inc., Totowa, NJ

in order to both be of practical benefit to the patient and further our understanding of the mechanism of cure. For example, the prediction of treatment failure, or relapse, must occur at a time when the disease level is sufficiently low so that when an alternate therapy is initiated, it will be possible to determine, at the outset, whether it is effective against small amounts of disease. This statement assumes that the failure of a treatment regimen when the level of disease is low implies that a failure would also occur if the same treatment were initiated at high levels of disease. The converse of this statement may not necessarily be true. This is the reason for determining a relapse prediction signal at the lowest possible level consistent with the technology. Similarly, the identification of the patient destined for either long-term disease-free survival or cure must be made at the optimum time such that treatment-associated morbidity can be minimized.

## APPROACH TO EVALUATING
## THE DECISION-MAKING PROCESS

If the goals of the previous section are to be achieved, it is necessary to develop a method of analyzing the predictive capability of the MRD results obtained during a clinical trial. There will, inevitably, be a threshold of some quantity derived from the measurement(s) of disease level(s) that will be used to predict the outcome for a particular patient. The most straightforward way to evaluate the capability to predict either of the two outcomes (i.e., relapse or continued remission) is to determine the fraction of the particular outcome that was correctly predicted according to chosen criterion. This section will give a brief description of a way to accomplish this goal that can be used with little difficulty by all clinical investigators. This method of analyzing clinical data to determine the predictive reliability of an assay has been discussed in detail by Feinstein *(1)*. For the purposes of this discussion, an assay is defined as a method of using MRD data to predict clinical outcome.

In order to evaluate the predictive reliability of an assay, the types of failure must be identified. When we are concerned with a binary outcome (event/non-event), there are two types of prediction failure: the failure to predict the event and the false prediction of the event. In terms of the nonevent, these errors are identical and are the false prediction of the nonevent and the failure to predict the nonevent. In this case, the event may be *considered* to be relapse and the non-event to be continued remission, and the two types of prediction failure are the failure to predict relapse and the failure to predict continued remission.

The fraction of correctly predicted relapses is termed the *sensitivity* and is easily determined from the data from the clinical trial:

$$\text{Sensitivity} = \frac{\text{Correctly predicted relapses}}{\text{Actual relapses}}$$

Note that the term "actual relapses" contains the number of relapse prediction failures; that is, (Actual relapses – Relapse prediction failures) = Correctly predicted relapses; conversely, the fraction of assays that the assay failed to predict is 1 – Sensitivity.

The fraction of correctly predicted continued remissions, the alternate outcome, is determined from the clinical trial data in a similar manner. This fraction is termed the *specificity* of the assay and is

$$\text{Specificity} = \frac{\text{Correctly predicted continued remission}}{\text{Actual continued remissions}}$$

The fraction of continued remissions that were not correctly predicted is 1 – Specificity.

By defining the sensitivity and the specificity of an assay, we have two measures of the predictive capability of the assay. The statistical significance of the actual results is determined from the coefficients of variation (CVs) for the sensitivity and the specificity. The CV is a rough measure of the spread of the individual results and provides information on the extent that the results can deviate from their calculated value. It is

$$\text{CV Sensitivity (Specificity)} = \sqrt{\frac{1 - \text{Sensitivity (Specificity)}}{\text{Correctly predicted relapses (remissions)}}}$$

For most clinical tests that are considered to be predictive, or diagnostic, the CV must be less than or equal to 5%. It is apparent that an MRD assay that is to have useful predictive value will need a sensitivity and a specificity that both have values near 1 and the CV must be less than or equal to 5%. In the next section, we will choose one study from the literature and discuss the predictive reliability of the MRD data in terms of the methodology presented in the preceding paragraphs.

## AN ILLUSTRATIVE EXAMPLE
## OF DETERMINING THE PREDICTIVE CAPABILITY
## OF AN MRD-BASED ASSAY

The study of van Dongen et al. is one of several excellent clinical MRD studies that have appeared during the last 5 yr *(2)*. We have chosen to use it as an example because it presents results on a single group of 129 patients that had semi-quantitative estimates of MRD levels determined at two time-points during the first 12 wk of therapy, the first at 5 wk and the second at 12 wk since the start of treatment. At each time-point, the levels of MRD were assigned to one of four categories: $\geq 10^{-2}$, $10^{-3}$–$10^{-2}$, $10^{-4}$–$10^{-3}$, and negative (i.e., undetectable). These four categories of disease level make possible the assignment of three possible

Table 1
Separation of MRD Results at 5 and 12 wk
of Treatment from 129 Patients into Categories
Defined by Levels $>10^{-4}$ and $\leq10^{-4}$

| MRD at 12 wk | MRD at 5 wk | |
| --- | --- | --- |
| | $>10^{-4}$ | $\leq10^{-4}$ |
| $>10^{-4}$ | 19 (15) | 2 (0) |
| $\leq10^{-4}$ | 29 (5) | 79 (8) |

thresholds for predicting relapse. Because there were two time-points, this implies that there could be $4^2$ possible groupings of these data. The authors chose to reduce this number to a more manageable size and assigned the patients to three groups based on the relapse rates and disease levels from the two time-points. The first group represented about 43% of the total population; the patients were MRD negative at both time-points and they had a relapse rate of 2%. A second group of 55 patients had, at both time-points, MRD levels less than $10^{-3}$ and a relapse incidence of about 22%; the third group of 19 patients, or about 15% of the total, had 15 relapses or a rate of 79% and MRD levels in the greater than or equal to $10^{-3}$ category at both times. An analysis of these data using population-based statistics yielded a significant difference between each of the three groups ($p < 0.001$).

If these results are examined with the intent of creating a method of relapse prediction, the first decision that must be made is the assignment of a threshold for relapse. Levels of MRD that are above this threshold confer a prediction of relapse, whereas levels below it are predicted to remain in remission. These data are given in Table 1. For the purposes of this example, we arbitrarily choose less than or equal to $10^{-4}$ as the threshold for relapse. We examine the two time-points separately and then with the results combined using the $10^{-4}$ threshold. At time-point 1, the end of induction therapy, there were 81 patients with MRD levels less than or equal to $10^{-4}$ and, of these, 8 relapsed and 48 patients had values greater than $10^{-4}$. Thus, from a total of 28 relapses, 20 were predicted and the sensitivity equals 0.71 with a CV = 12%. At time-point 2, there were 108 patients with levels less than or equal to $10^{-4}$, and 13 of these ultimately relapsed. Among the remaining 21 patients with MRD levels greater than $10^{-4}$, there were 15 relapses. Because there were 28 total relapses and 15 of these were predicted by the data from time-point 2, this leads to a sensitivity of 0.53 (CV = 12%). The specificities at these two time-points were 0.72 (CV = 6%) and 0.94 (CV = 2.5%), respectively. Note that because the greater proportion of patients remain in remission, this specificity is easier to predict and the spread in the possible results is less. This effect becomes more evident as the time on treatment progresses. Finally, we will determine the sensitivity and the specificity for the combined results from both time-points. The threshold for relapse remains at less than or equal to $10^{-4}$ at both time-points. There were a total of 79 patients out of the 129 patients who had both MRD levels equal to or below $10^{-4}$, and within this group, there were 8 relapses. Because there were a total of 28 relapses in the entire 129 patients, this results in a sensitivity of 0.71 (CV = 12%) and a specificity of 0.70 (CV = 6.5%). These results are very similar to the results at time-point 1 and it appears that although the additional time-point has allowed the definition of additional groups of patients according to the paired results of MRD measurements, it does not necessarily improve the predictive capability when a single threshold is chosen for the entire population as the criterion for relapse.

The reason for the result obtained when the data from the two time-points are combined to calculate the sensitivity and specificity is that this determination ignores the data from those patients who moved from the greater than $10^{-4}$ group at the first time-point to the less than or equal to $10^{-4}$ group at the second time-point; that is, there was a group of patients that had a response to the second phase of treatment and were moved into the MRD-level category of patients who responded very well to the first phase of therapy. This movement is the result of the observed heterogeneity in the response to therapy that is known to be present in most disease entities. The most obvious demonstration of this heterogeneity is found in the results of a treatment protocol; that is, one fraction of the patients attain cure, whereas the remaining fraction do not, and the proportion often changes when a different treatment regimen consisting of other drugs, timing, or dosages is used. This heterogeneity in treatment response is apparent in the data presented in Table 1, where the outcome is mixed in the group of patients who had MRD levels less than $10^{-4}$ on both measurements and those who were initially greater than $10^{-4}$ and then less than $10^{-4}$ on the second measurement. This overlap of, or migration across, thresholds makes the assignment of a single threshold for relapse prediction based on MRD data taken at a particular time during treatment very problematic. In brief, it is very difficult to define a threshold for relapse prediction at an early time-point during therapy that separates those patients who will relapse and those who will remain in remission.

The question that faces the clinical investigator is whether a sensitivity that fails to predict the relapse of approx 30% of the actual relapses is satisfactory. The goal of early relapse prediction is to enable a switch to another type of therapy to control the malignant cells that are resistant to the present treatment regimen. Thus, the question becomes whether not being able to initiate early salvage therapy for 30% of the patients is appropriate. Early prediction for 70% of the patients who will relapse will improve the overall outcome if an effective augmented protocol is available, but a valid evaluation of its efficacy for all patients who relapse may not be possible. If the augmented therapy is as effective in patients in morphologic relapse as it is in patients predicted to relapse but still in morphologic remission, then there would be no advantage to effective relapse prediction. Conversely, if relapse is averted by initiating the salvage therapy during morphological remission for those patients predicted to relapse, then the effect of the alternate therapy administered at similar MRD levels to those patients destined to relapse but not identified by the relapse prediction assay would remain unknown.

A low sensitivity denies a group of patients an alternate therapy that could be beneficial to their long-term disease-free survival, but a low specificity has the effect of exposing patients, destined to remain in remission, to treatment that is both unnecessary and with associated morbidity. This strongly implies that an acceptable relapse prediction assay must have a specificity close to 1. The overall result of this brief discussion of the sensitivity and specificity is that it should be determined for the proposed relapse prediction assay before it is used in a clinical trial. These quantities have profound scientific, cost-effective, and ethical implications.

In a separate article, we have reviewed the problem of relapse prediction using treatment response measured by morphology, immunophenotype, or polymerase chain reaction (PCR) in childhood acute lymphoblastic leukemia (ALL) (3). This leukemia is one that is highly curable, with a cure rate greater than 70% and also one that has been prospectively studied by several MRD techniques (4–6). Heterogeneity in response has a very significant role in predicting overall outcome in this disease and the results shown here for the study of van Dongen et al. are also found in the other studies of treatment response.

We have concluded that a successful relapse-prediction methodology for childhood ALL must be one that follows the individual patient sequentially. In a previous study, we used a moving-line model that required three or more data points before predicting either relapse or continued remission (7). The prediction was based on the slope of the least-squares-fitted straight line and the associated confidence intervals. Over an extended period of time, the MRD data for a single patient will probably not be a straight line and it is likely that other, more sophisticated, models need to be developed. Before this can be accomplished, it will be necessary to conduct studies that collect sequential MRD results from a sizable cohort of patients throughout their course of treatment. We have estimated that with relapse rates of contemporary protocols, the size of the patient group will be about 250 patients. This is within the capability of the large cooperative groups and the time to complete the study would be slightly longer than 5 yr.

In closing, we urge that clinical investigators collaborate closely with statisticians to develop reliable methods to use MRD to make clinical decisions.

## ACKNOWLEDGMENT

This work was supported in part by grant R21 CA 68235 from the National Cancer Institute.

# REFERENCES

1. Feinstein AR. Clinical biostatistics—XXXI. On the sensitivity, specificity, and discrimination of diagnostic tests, *Clin. Pharmacol. Ther.*, **17** (1973) 104–117.
2. van Dongen JJM, Seriu T, Panzer-Grumayer ER, Biondi A, Pongers-Willemse MJ, Corral L, et al. Prognostic value of minimal residual disease in childhood acute lymphoblastic leukemia, *Lancet*, **352** (1998) 1731–1738.
3. Johnston DA and Zipf TF. Prediction of treatment outcome in a highly curable disease, childhood acute lymphoblastic leukemia, submitted.
4. Roberts WM, Estrov Z, Kitchingman GR, and Zipf TF. The clinical significance of residual disease in childhood acute lymphoblastic leukemia as detected by polymerase chain reaction amplification of antigen-receptor gene sequences, *Leuk. Lymphoma*, **20** (1995) 181–197.
5. Gaynon PS, Desai AA, Bostrom BC, Hutchinson RJ, Lange BJ, Nachman JB, et al. Early response to therapy and outcome in childhood acute lymphoblastic leukemia, *Cancer*, **80** (1997) 1717–1726.
6. Coustain-Smith E, Sancho J, Hancock ML, Boyett JM, Raimondi SC, Sandlund JT, et al. Clinical importance of minimal residual disease in childhood acute lymphoblastic leukemia, *Blood*, **96** (2000) 2691–2695.
7. Roberts WM, Estrov Z, Ouspenskia MV, Johnston DA, McClain KL, and Zipf TF. Measurement of residual leukemia during remission in childhood acute lymphoblastic leukemia, *N. Engl. J. Med.*, **336** (1997) 317–323.

# 6

# Measurement of Minimal Residual Disease in Children Undergoing Allogeneic Stem Cell Transplant for Acute Lymphoblastic Leukemia

*John Moppett, Amos Burke,*
*Christopher Knechtli, Anthony Oakhill,*
*Colin Steward, and Nicholas J. Goulden*

## INTRODUCTION

Allogeneic stem cell transplant (ASCT) is the most intensive therapy currently available to clinicians and, therefore, its use is limited to children deemed to be at an unacceptably high risk of relapse after chemotherapy alone. Although indications for ASCT vary between major treatment cooperatives, it is generally considered to be the treatment of choice for a minority of children with ALL in first remission and many of those who suffer a bone marrow relapse *(1)*.

## PRINCIPLES OF ASCT FOR ALL

Allogenic SCT effects cure of ALL by three major mechanisms. First, it allows dose intensification of chemoradiotherapy (conditioning). Second, it provides a "clean" source of stem cells to restore hemopoiesis. Third, some of the donor cells are immunocompetent and, therefore, may recognize and eliminate residual host malignant cells by a graft versus leukemia effect (GvL). The two major nonrelapse causes of treatment failure after allogeneic bone marrow transplantation (BMT) are rejection and graft versus host disease (GvHD). These are a product of confrontation between donor and recipient alloreactive cells, which recognize the proteins of the human leukocyte antigen (HLA) system. Having identified an appropriately HLA-matched donor, the alloreactive cells of the

From: *Leukemia and Lymphoma: Detection of Minimal Residual Disease*
Edited by: T. F. Zipf and D. A. Johnston © Humana Press Inc., Totowa, NJ

recipient immune system must be ablated to prevent rejection, a process known as conditioning. Conditioning therapy is also designed to treat residual disease and is therefore tailored to suit the potential side effects of previous treatment as well as the perceived risk of rejection. The most widely used protocols include cyclophosphamide and/or etoposide and total-body irradiation (TBI).

Immunocompetent donor cells recognize normal recipient cells as non-self and cause graft versus host disease. Their impact on the transplant course can be modified in a number of ways. Immunosuppressive drugs, commonly combinations of cyclosporin, steroids, and methotrexate, may be given to the recipient after transplant. Alternatively, various methods of reduction of the number of immunocompetent donor cells in the graft, known as T-cell depletion (TCD), can be employed. It is important to note that, at present, the effectors responsible for GvHD cannot be reliably differentiated from those leading to GvL Thus, any measure aimed at reducing GvHD may theoretically increase the risk of relapse.

The risk of rejection and GvHD is related to the degree of HLA matching between the donor and the recipient, which, in turn, governs the transplant protocol. If an HLA-matched sibling donor is available, the standard approach involves conditioning with TBI and either cyclophosphamide, etoposide, or cytosine arabinoside. This is followed by transplant of at least $3 \times 10^6$ CD34 positive stem cells per kilogram from a fully HLA-matched (MSD). If the graft is unmanipulated, approx $3 \times 10^8$ T-cells/kg are also infused. GvHD prophylaxis is provided by cyclosporin and methotrexate. Graft rejection occurs in less than 1% of children treated in this way. Severe (grades III–IV) acute GvHD occurs in 10% and extensive chronic GvH in 10% (2).

Only 25% of candidates for stem cell transplant (SCT) have a matched sibling donor. The 1990s saw a vast expansion in unrelated donor BMT, and, in our experience, if one accepts some degree of mismatch, it is now possible to offer an unradicated donor BMT (UDBMT) to 9 of every 10 children lacking a matched sibling (3). However, the increased alloreactivity of 10 antigen-matched unrelated grafts is such that 45% of children will develop severe acute (grades III–IV) GvHD and more than 31% extensive chronic GvHD in spite of prophylaxis with cyclosporin and methotrexate. In the mismatch group, as many as 60% suffer from severe acute grades III–IV GvHD. This contributes to a transplant-related mortality of 20–30% (4). Many groups believe that such a high incidence of GvHD is unacceptable and have resorted to T-cell depletion of unrelated grafts using either lympholytic antibodies or cell selection. This reduces the incidence of severe acute and extensive chronic GvHD to rates equivalent to that seen after MSD grafts (5). Although there is no evidence from controlled trials that TCD increases relapse in acute lymphoblastic leukemia (ALL), this remains a concern. Previous studies of sibling SCT reported that those with mild GvHD had a lower incidence of relapse when compared to those who did not develop GvHD. Two further concerns are the increased risk of rejection (up to 12% after mismatched UDBMT) and the poor immune reconstitution with such procedures. Taken together these complications result in a transplant-related mortality (TRM) after UDBMT of 10% (5).

A minority of candidates for ASCT lack either a matched sibling or suitable unrelated donor. In the last few years, it has become possible to offer these children effective haploidentical grafts. Traditionally, unmanipulated haploidentical grafts were associated with a high incidence of lethal GvHD. By contrast, TCD led to unacceptable risk of rejection (6). It is now possible to overcome these risks by the use of heavily T-cell-depleted (CD3 dose $<5 \times 10^4$/kg) peripheral blood stem cell transplants in which massively augmented stem cell doses (at least $10 \times 10^6$ CD34/kg) are used to overcome HLA disparity. This procedure is in its infancy and no reliable comment can be made about the risk of relapse. However, it is already clear that such profound TCD leads to a very high risk (20–40%) of severe viral infection and, at present, the TRM of this procedure is at best 20%.

## INDICATIONS FOR AND RESULTS OF ASCT FOR ALL

More than 80% of children with ALL can be cured without resorting to ASCT. SCT during first remission is reserved for $Ph^+$ and true hypodiploid ALL. A 50% 5-yr event-free survival (EFS) has been reported after ASCT for $Ph^+$ disease. This compares favorably with outcome after chemotherapy (7).

Treatment of relapsed ALL is the commonest indication for ASCT in childhood. Whereas precise indications for BMT in relapsed disease vary among the major treatment consortia, it is generally agreed that prognosis if chemotherapy alone is given after relapse is dependent on the duration of first remission and the site of relapse. This is exemplified by consideration of the results of the MRC UKALL R1 protocol (1). Here, the overall 5-yr EFS for children treated with chemotherapy was 42%; however, there were no survivors among those suffering a bone marrow relapse on therapy. This is in marked contrast to the 77% EFS seen in those children relapsing without bone marrow involvement (extramedullary relapse) more than 2.5 yr from diagnosis. An intermediate prognosis is seen in those suffering a bone marrow relapse following completion of therapy. In the United Kingdom this has led to the recommendation that BMT is reserved for those who relapse in the marrow within 2 yr of the completion of therapy (1).

## INCORPORATION OF MRD ANALYSIS
## INTO PROTOCOLS FOR ASCT IN ALL

Our unit has now performed more than 150 ASCT for relapsed ALL; the majority of these have TCD unradicated donor (UD) grafts. It is now clear that the major cause of death in these children is recurrent disease (5). We have examined whether analysis of MRD can highlight children at high risk of relapse so that they may be offered more effective therapy. Our initial studies involved measurement of MRD after ASCT; more recently, we have concentrated on the measure of tumor burden prior to the graft.

## MRD Post-ASCT

The last decade has seen a massive expansion in the use of cellular immunotherapy (donor lymphocyte infusions) to treat relapse after ASCT *(8)*. This strategy has been most successful in adult-type chronic myeloid leukemia (CML). It is now clear that in CML immunotherapy is most effective (and least toxic) when given at times of molecular relapse as defined by MRD analysis. It is reasonable to postulate that measurement of MRD in the early months post-ASCT for ALL may provide early warning of relapse and target children who may benefit from immunotherapy. This is particularly relevant to centers such as our own who perform T-cell-depleted ASCT for ALL in an attempt to reduce transplant-related mortality and morbidity resulting from GvHD.

## Methods of Measuring MRD

In a study published in 1998 we retrospectively analyzed the behavior of MRD *(9)*, as detected by antigen-receptor gene polymerase chain reaction (PCR), after allo-BMT in 71 children with ALL. The method employed four sets of primers that were designed to generate short products that could readily be resolved in polyacrylamide gel electrophoresis (PAGE) gels. Following sequencing, a clone-specific oligonucleotide was designed to match the junctional region of the rearrangement and this was used to detect MRD. One microgram of DNA from the marrow under analysis was amplified using IgH or TcR primers along with equivalent amounts of DNA from two normals, a non-DNA-containing control, and logarithmic dilutions of leukemic DNA into normal. The products were then subjected to PAGE and visualized after ethidium bromide staining.

Electroblotting of the gel on to a nylon membrane was then performed and the products were probed with a 20-base radiolabeled clone-specific oligonucleotide. It is important to note that electrophoretic resolution of PCR products generated from samples taken post-ASCT is vital if one is to avoid false-positive results *(11)*. The technique allows the study of 90% of all children with ALL and has a median sensitivity of $10^{-4}$. MRD was said to be present at high level (gel positivity) when a distinct clonal band of the same size as that seen at relapse prior to BMT was seen after PAGE. Probing and sequencing confirmed the identity of this band. Low-level or probe-positive disease was defined as hybridization stronger than that seen in the normal controls after autoradiography *(10)*.

In this study, 55 children received T-cell-depleted marrow unrelated donors and 16 unmanipulated grafts from related donors. All were conditioned with 120 mg/kg cyclophosphamide and 1440 Gy TBI in eight fractions. Patients receiving T-cell-depleted marrow also received further immunosuppression with Campath 1G. Cyclosporin ± methotrexate was used for GvHD prophylaxis posttransplant. More complete details of the transplant protocol can be found in ref. 5.

Minimal residual disease was measured in bone marrow taken at 1, 3, 6, 12, 18, and 24 mo after BMT. The correlation between MRD and clinical outcome is shown in Figs. 1 and 2. Three children were excluded from this analysis because of transplant-related mortality.

## RESULTS IN PATIENTS WHO REMAINED IN REMISSION

Thirty-six children (26 transplanted from unrelated donors, 10 from matched sibling donors) remain in continuing complete remission (CCR) with a median follow-up of 78.8 (range: 55–130) mo from BMT. In 28 of these children, MRD was not detected at any time post-BMT. In the remaining eight, at least one positive result was obtained. However, in each instance, disease was present at the lowest limits of detection of the technique. Moreover, evidence of MRD was confined to early time-points after BMT; in six of these cases, the positive sample was found solely within 3 mo of the BMT. All positive samples from this remission group have been followed by at least two negative samples with a minimum follow-up of 60 mo in the patients involved.

## RESULTS IN CHILDREN WHO RELAPSED

Thirty-two children (26 transplanted from unrelated donors, 6 from related donors) relapsed at a median of 5 mo after BMT (range: 2.4–64.9 mo). Of these, 16 were MRD positive at all times post-BMT and 12 were initially negative but became positive at a median of 3 mo (range: 1.5–11 mo) prior to relapse. The stability of clonal rearrangements amplified at relapse post-BMT was examined in 31 cases. In 24 cases, identical rearrangements were seen pre-BMT and post-BMT. Eleven rearrangements in seven patients were found to have changed from those seen prior to BMT: eight of the rearrangements were lost and three underwent a change to an unrelated sequence (complete clonal change). Another stable rearrangement was available for the reliable tracking of MRD in six of these seven patients. In the remaining child, no MRD was detected at any time post-BMT: a false-negative result consequent on complete clonal change.

No MRD was detected prior to relapse in four patients. The reasons for this failure bear further consideration. In one child, a single sample of poor quality was available for analysis; in a second child, marrow was available: Relapse occurred at 19 mo, but the last sample available for testing was taken 5 mo earlier. In the third case, isolated testicular relapse occurred 65 mo after ASCT and 41 mo since the last MRD analysis. In a single patient, a false-negative result was obtained because of complete clonal change (see above).

## STATISTICAL ANALYSIS OF TOTAL PATIENT POPULATION

At least one sample positive for MRD over the first 3 mo after ASCT was found in 7/36 (19%) of the patients in CCR compared with 18/26 (69%) of those

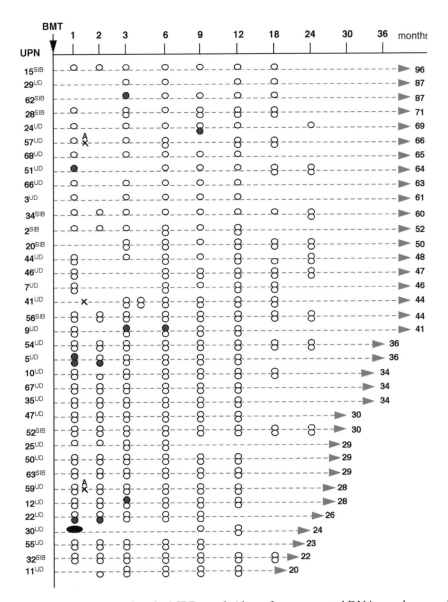

**Fig. 1.** Diagram representing the MRD result (those from extracted DNA are above and those from immunomagnetically selected cells are below each gray horizontal broken line) from individual patients with time for patients remaining in continuing complete remission (CCR). The unique patient number (UPN) for each patient is detailed on the left with the source of the donor in superscript (SIB = sibling, UD = unrelated donor, PAR = parent donor, and SYN = syngeneic twin donor) and the follow-up in patients in CCR is in months on the right. ○ = MRD negative; ⊕ = low-level MRD detected after PAGE and allele-specific oligoprobing; ● = high-level MRD evident after PAGE only; ℞ = overt hematological relapse; ▷ = continuing complete remission; X = failed to engraft; A = autologous marrow rescue; and ▮ = allogeneic peripheral blood progenitor cell infusion. [Reproduced from *Br. J. Haematol.* **102** (1998) 860–876 with permission].

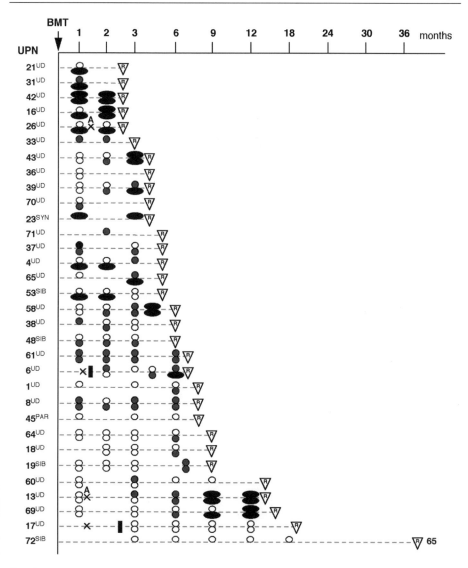

**Fig. 2.** Diagram representing the MRD results for patients who have relapsed. See legend to Fig. 1 for complete explanation. [Reproduced from *Br. J. Hematol.*, **102** (1998) 860–876 with permission.]

who relapsed at least 4 mo after BMT ($\chi^2 = 13.55$, [two-sided] $p = 0.0002$, odds ratio = 9.32, 95% confidence interval = 2.89–30.12). Of those who were investigated over the first 2 mo, 4/32 (13%) of the CCR group and 20/30 (67%) of the relapse group had at least one positive MRD result ($\chi^2 = 16.93$, [two-sided] $p < 0.0001$, odds ratio = 14.00, 95% confidence interval = 3.84–51.07).

CLINICAL VALUE OF MRD ANALYSIS POST-ASCT FOR ALL

Immunotherapy is of unproven value in ALL moreover it is associated with a high incidence of acute and chronic GvHD. Data from CML suggests that a minimum period of 2 mo is required to achieve cytoreduction by donor leukocyte infusion (DLI) *(8)*. Therefore, any strategy of targeted immunotherapy must fulfill two criteria. First, the risk of death from relapse in those patients who receive such therapy must be so great that the risk of added toxicity is justified. Second, DLI should be given as soon as possible after BMT to maximize efficacy. Unfortunately, we believe that in its current state, a positive MRD measurement fails to adequately provide a high-risk measure or early timing to permit an efficacious DLI.

In our study, a positive MRD result within the first 6 mo after the graft was not specific for relapse. Thus, if one chose to administer DLI on the basis of a positive MRD result within 2–3 mo of BMT, a significant minority of children would be unnecessarily exposed to potential toxicity. This obstacle could be overcome by targeting only those with high-level MRD, a finding universally correlated with relapse. However, the median time from obtaining such a result to eventual relapse was 2 mo and may be too short a time frame for successful immunotherapy.

## MRD PRE-ASCT FOR CHILDHOOD ALL

Allogeneic SCT for ALL is rarely, if ever, successful if performed when the marrow is not in hematological remission, suggesting that the leukemic burden must be adequately reduced to maximize the efficacy of conditioning and graft versus leukemia *(11)*. It is logical to use MRD measurements to attempt to correlate the submicroscopic tumor burden with transplant outcome.

### Methods

We therefore measured MRD in marrows taking a median of 13 days (range: 1–62) prior to conditioning for BMT in 64 children. MRD methodology and conditioning regimes were identical to those described earlier. Of those studied, 19 were in CR1, 39 in CR2, and 6 in CR3 or later *(12)*.

### Results

Results are shown in Table 1 and Fig. 3. The most notable single finding of this study is that the presence of high-level MRD immediately prior to conditioning for a TCD ASCT is universally associated with relapse. By contrast, 3-yr event-free survival for the MRD-negative group was 73%, and for those with low-level MRD positively was 36%. In univariate chi-square analysis, MRD status pre-BMT was significantly related to EFS ($p < 0.001$). However, when clinical risk factors are included in analysis, significant correlation is seen between the known

Table 1
Clinical Outcome According to MRD Status
Prior to BMT in 64 Children; $\chi^2$ for Trend = 21.16; $p < 0.0001$

|           | Negative | Low-level positive | High-level positive | Total |
|-----------|----------|--------------------|---------------------|-------|
| Remission | 30       | 4                  | 0                   | 34    |
| Relapse   | 8        | 5                  | 12                  | 25    |
| TRM       | 3        | 2                  | 0                   | 5     |
| Total     | 41       | 11                 | 12                  | 64    |

*Source*: Ref. *12*.

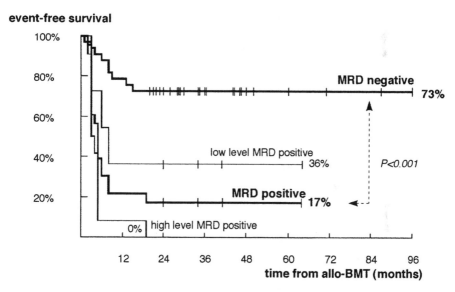

**Fig. 3.** Kaplan–Meier plot of outcome according to MRD status pre-BMT. (From ref. *12*; used by permission of the American Society of Hematology.)

clinical risk factors [Ph(1) disease, on treatment medullary relapse] and MRD detection pretransplant.

It is interesting to focus on patients transplanted in CR2, currently the most common indication for ASCT in ALL. Of 39 children, 9 had high-level MRD posttransplant, and of them, 7 had suffered an on-treatment bone marrow relapse. No patient who had high-level MRD had relapsed at more than 1 yr from the end of treatment. In a multivariate analysis of patients transplanted in CR2 following a medullary relapse, MRD lost statistical significance once adjustment was made for the duration of first remission. Nevertheless, analysis of MRD illustrates that

## Table 2
### Significance of Pre-BMT MRD Status in Univariate and Multivariate
### (Including Duration of CR1 and Site of Relapse) Analysis

|  | Univariate | | Multivariate | |
| --- | --- | --- | --- | --- |
|  | Hazard ratio | p-Value | Hazard ratio | p-Value |
| Negative | 1 |  | 1 |  |
| Low level | 3.79 |  | 3.41 |  |
| High level | 13.91 | <0.001 | 6.50 | 0.058 |

Source: Ref. 12.

the poor prognosis of children who suffer an medullary relapse on treatment relates to their failure to clear MRD, which, at least in part, reflects the resistance of their disease to chemotherapy (see Table 2).

Two subsequent studies have extended our knowledge of the relevance of MRD pre-ASCT for ALL. Bader et al. used identical techniques in a cohort of patients transplanted in Tubingen (14). The patient group ($n = 36$) was similar, with the exception that the majority (30/36) of transplants were T-cell replete. Seven patients were transplanted in CR1, 25 in CR2, and 4 in CR3 or more. Using the same definitions of MRD level as Knechtli et al., 14 were found to be high-level MRD[+], 7 low-level MRD[+], and in 11 no evidence of MRD could be found. The EFS for MRD negative, low-level, and high-level MRD[+] patients were 82%, 42%, and 21% respectively. These results concur with our own, confirming the excellent prognosis of MRD negative patients and the poor prognosis of high-level MRD[+] patients. However, there is one notable difference. High-level MRD pre-ASCT was not universally associated with relapse. In three cases (all had received T-cell-replete marrow), it appears that this high burden of MRD was overcome by either GvHD (two cases) or DLI (one case) or the patient responded to the conditioning regimen.

Further evidence of the potential for GvHD and by inference GvL to overcome a high tumor burden at the time of conditioning is drawn from Uzunel et al., who measured MRD by gene-rearrangement PCR immediately prior to conditioning in 30 patients (age and remission status unspecified) (15,16). MRD was present at a high level in 20 patients and at low level in 5 patients. Of these 25 MRD-positive patients, 11 developed GvHD, of whom 3 relapsed, whereas the risk of relapse was much higher (10 of 14) in those with no GvH.

### Clinical Value of MRD Analysis Pre-ASCT for ALL

Our large study of a homogeneously conditioned group of children undergoing ASCT for ALL in our unit revealed that the procedure is futile if conditioning begins at a time when high-level MRD is present in the marrow. However, other groups have shown that this is not a universal finding. In particular, it would seem that GvHD (as a surrogate for GvL) or the conditioning regimen may be able to overcome a high disease load prior to the conditioning regimen.

## BLUEPRINT FOR THE CLINICAL APPLICATION OF MRD MEASUREMENT DURING ASCT FOR ALL

Although ASCT in ALL is intensive, expensive, and toxic it is not a panacea. Attempts to define the place of the procedure in the treatment of relapse and to reduce the risk of treatment failure have been frustrated by the lack of large-scale randomized studies. MRD analysis offers physicians a unique opportunity to overcome this obstacle.

It is now clear that a simple measurement of MRD status prior to conditioning would allow clinicians to compare the success of different transplant protocols. We recommend that this should be come an integral part of all reports of ASCT in ALL. This must be allied with an examination of mechanisms by which disease persists and attempts to achieve better cytoreduction and augment the graft versus leukemia effect.

Currently, our data suggest that the measurement of residual disease after ASCT is not useful. However, this approach should be revisited when well-validated, rapid, truly quantitative techniques, which can measure MRD in peripheral blood, become the norm.

## ACKNOWLEDGMENTS

This work in Bristol has been supported by Leukaemia Research Fund of Great Britain and the Ben Drewer trust. As ever, we are indebted to clinical colleagues and research staff for their continued efforts.

## REFERENCES

1. Chessells JM. Relapsed lymphoblastic leukaemia in children: a continuing challenge, *Br. J. Haematol.*, **102** (1998) 423–438.
2. Barrett AJ. Bone marrow transplantation for acute lymphoblastic leukaemia, *Baillieres Clin. Haematol.*, **7** (1994) 377.
3. Heslop HE. Haemopoietic stem cell transplantation from unrelated donors, *Br. J. Haematol.*, **105** (1999) 2–6.
4. Woolfrey A, Frangoul H, Anasetti C, Storer B, Getzendaner L, Hansen J, et al. Unrelated transplants for children with acute lymphoblastic leukaemia, *Blood*, **94(1)** (1999) 712a (abstract).
5. Oakhill A, Pamphilon DH, Potter MN, Steward CG, Goodman S, Green A, et al. Unrelated donor bone marrow transplantation for children with relapsed acute lymphoblastic leukaemia in second complete remission, *Br. J. Haematol.*, **94** (1996) 574.
6. Aversa F, Tabilio A, Velardi F, Falzetti S, Ballanti A, Carotti F, et al. Advances in full haplotype mismatched transplants in acute leukaemia, *Blood*, **94(Suppl. 1)** (1999) 565a (abstract).

7. Marks D, Bird JM, Cornish JMM, Goulden NJ, Jones CG, Knechtli CJC, et al. Unrelated donor bone marrow transplantation for children and adolescents with Philadelphia positive acute lymphoblastic leukaemia, *J. Clin. Oncol.*, **16** (1998) 931–936.

8. Aricò M, Valsecchi MG, Camitta B, Schrappe M, Chessells J, Baruchel A, et al. Outcome of treatment in children with Philadelphia chromosome-positive acute lymphoblastic leukaemia, *N. Engl. J. Med.*, **342** (2000) 998–1006.

9. McKinnon S. Who may benefit from donor leucocyte infusions after allogeneic stem cell transplantation? *Br. J. Haematol.*, **110** (2000) 12–17.

10. Knechtli CJC, Goulden NJ, Hancock JP, Garland RJ, Jones CG, Grandage V, et al. Minimal residual status as a predictor of relapse after allogeneic bone marrow transplant for children with acute lymphoblastic leukaemia, *Br. J. Haematol.*, **102** (1998) 860–876.

11. Langlands K, Goulden NJ, Steward CG, Potter MN, Cornish JM, and Oakhill A. False positive residual disease assessment post-bone marrow transplant in acute lymphoblastic leukaemia, *Blood*, **84** (1994) 1352–1353.

12. Franklin IM. Consensus conference on unrelated-donor bone marrow transplantation, October 29 & 30, 1996: its use in leukemias and allied disorders. Royal College of Physicians of Edinburgh, *Transfusion*, **38** (1998) 100–101.

13. Knechtli CJC, Goulden NJ, Hancock JP, Garland RJ, Jones CG, Grandage V, et al. Minimal residual disease status prior to allogeneic bone marrow transplantation is an important determinant of successful outcome for children and adolescents with acute lymphoblastic leukaemia, *Blood*, **92** (1998) 4072–4079.

14. Bader P, Kreyenberg H, Beck J, Hancock J, Goulden N, Oakhill A, et al. Minimal residual disease in ALL prior to allogeneic stem cell transplantation, *Bone Marrow Transplant.*, **(Suppl. 1)** (2000) 149 (abstract).

15. Uzunel M, Mattson J, Matsche M, and Ringden O. High level MRD pre SCT is not necessarily associated with relapse in ALL, *Bone Marrow Transplant.*, **(Suppl. 1)** (2000) 146 (abstract).

16. Uzunel M, Matsson J, Jaksch M, Remberger M, and Ringden O. The significance of graft-versus-host disease and pretransplantation minimal residual disease status to outcome after allogeneic stem cell transplantation in patients with acute lymphoblastic leukaemia, *Blood*, **98** (2001) 2982–2984.

# 7

# Molecular Investigation of Minimal Residual Disease in Adult Acute Lymphoblastic Leukemia of B Lineage

*Letizia Foroni, Forida Y. Mortuza, and A. Victor Hoffbrand*

## INTRODUCTION

Although chemotherapy achieves clinical remission (CR) within 1 mo in the majority (≥80%) of adults with B-lineage acute lymphoblastic leukemia (ALL), less than 40% are considered to be cured at 5 yr *(1,2)*. Clinical relapses, following complete clinical remission (CCR) after induction therapy, indicate that leukemia cells, undetected by light microscopy (theoretically up to 1 in $10^{10}$ cells), expand at any time after achievement of remission until there is full-blown clinical relapse.

Consequently, the detection of residual disease at levels below 1 in $10^3$ leukemic cells among normal bone marrow (BM) cells has recently been explored using sensitive immunological and cytogenetic approaches. The use of leukemia-specific antigen profiles and four-color cell-sorting techniques *(3–5)* has improved the sensitivity and specificity of detecting leukemic cells. These techniques will be extensively described in a separate chapter of this volume.

Cytogenetic examination, even using the fluorescent *in situ* hybridization (FISH) technique, has, so far, failed to achieve the sensitivity required for the detection of residual disease in ALL, but it remains valuable for the identification of genetic changes in presentation material *(6,7)*. This allows the identification of chromosomal translocations, which are potentially valuable as clone-specific markers for tracking residual disease by molecular methods (see below). Molecular techniques have indeed had the greatest impact on the monitoring of

From: *Leukemia and Lymphoma: Detection of Minimal Residual Disease*
Edited by: T. F. Zipf and D. A. Johnston © Humana Press Inc., Totowa, NJ

residual disease in acute and chronic hematological malignancies. It is the scope of this chapter to describe their value in the MRD investigation focusing on adults with ALL and discussing data from our own laboratory and data presented in the literature.

## DEFINITION OF MINIMAL RESIDUAL DISEASE

Minimal residual disease (MRD) is defined as the "lowest level of disease detectable in patients in CR by the methods available." In order to detect MRD, it is necessary to identify leukemic-specific markers using sensitive detection techniques. In Table 1 *(8–16)*, we have listed some of the most frequent markers used in patients with ALL for the investigation of MRD.

## MRD ANALYSIS USING MOLECULAR MARKERS

Markers can be distinguished into (1) "clone-specific" and (2) "patient-specific" (*see* Table 1). The former are present in the leukemic but not normal background cells. All patients with that particular type of leukemia and abnormality show that molecular marker. This applies principally to markers linked to chromosomal translocations that create novel fusion genes. Among these, the first to be studied were the t(14;18) in non-Hodgkin's lymphoma (NHL) follicular lymphoma and the t(9;22) in chronic myeloid leukemia (CML) and ALL. Because the translocation is essentially the same in all patients, this facilitates its detection by common and widely applicable tests, irrespective of the age, gender, phenotype, and clinical features of the patient cohort. In adult ALL, the incidence of these abnormalities varies greatly. The t(9;22) is the most common abnormality (15–30%) and leads to the fusion of the BCR and ABL genes. Other translocations are more rarely detected in adult ALL. These include t(4;11) (5–10%) and t(1;19) (5%) *(17)*, which, like t(9;22), also carry a poor prognosis. Other translocations, such as t(12;21) (<1%) *(18)*, have limited relevance to the overall clinical outcome, as they are rare in adult ALL. Recent reviews of the cytogenetics and frequency of these abnormalities have been published in the past few years *(19–21)*. The use of these clone-specific markers for MRD investigation in adult ALL is described in Chapter 11.

## PATIENT-SPECIFIC MARKERS

These markers are almost exclusively the unique rearrangements that happen to the antigen-receptor genes, both immunoglobulin (Ig) and T-cell receptor (TCR) during leukemogenesis and subsequent clonal expansion. The unique type of DNA rearrangement associated with Ig and TCR production *(22,23)* involves deletion and rejoining of large stretches of DNA and insertion of novel nucleotides by the enzyme terminal deoxynucleotidyl transferase (TdT), which

Table 1

Markers Applied to the Investigation of MRD in Adult ALL Patients

| Markers | Incidence[a] | Sensitivity | Specificity[b] | Impact on survival | Ref. |
|---|---|---|---|---|---|
| Immunophenotype | 90–95% | $1:10–1:10^5$ | Clone-specific[c] | Based on phenotypes | 3 |
| WT1 | 5–10% | $>1:10^4$ | Clone-specific | NK[f] | 8, 9 |
| TAL-1 deletion | <5% of T | $>1:10^4$ | Patient-specific | NK | 10 |
| Cytogenetic abn. | >50% | $<1:10^2$ | Clone-specific | Depends on type | 7 |
| RT-PCR | ≥30% | $>1:10^4$ | Clone-specific | None[d] | 11 |
| Ag-receptor genes | >90% | $>1:10^4$ | Patient-specific | None[d] | 11 |
| MTHFR RFLP | 28% | NK | Clone-specific | Increased risk of ALL | 12 |
| ATM deletion | 10% | NK | Clone-specific | Good | 13 |
| del (13q14) | 51% | NK | Clone-specific | Poor | 14 |
| RB1[e] | 41% | NK | Clone-specific | Poor[e] | 15 |
| P16 (INK4A)[e] | 26% | NK | Clone-specific | Poor | 15 |
| p53[e] | 34% | NK | Clone-specific | Poor | 15 |
| Ikaros-6 isoforms | | NK | Clone-specific | NK | 16 |

[a]Incidence of some markers may vary depending on the marker.
[b]Specificity is defined as clone-specific when the same marker is present in different patients and it is indistinguishable from patient to patient by the method used; a marker is defined patient-specific when the method used identifies differences specific to each patient. The latter are the most sensitive methods.
[c]Some combination of surface markers can be patient-specific and therefore highly sensitive.
[d]The occurrence of these changes has no impact per se on survival.
[e]The combination of one or more of these defects is associated with worse outcome.
[f]NK, not known.

creates a gene sequence unique to each cell. During the normal course of early B-cell development, 1 each of 55 variable (VH), 30 diversity (D), and 6 joining (JH), segments are selected and undergo a somatic VH-(D)-JH recombination event *(22,23)*. This is associated with a change from the germ-line configuration of the IgH genes, which can be revealed by using Southern blotting and the polymerase chain reaction (PCR). Southern blotting is an easy and widely applicable technique, but it fails to provide the sensitivity required for MRD investigation, as it can only detect clonal cell populations at a sensitivity of 5–10%. The detection, however, of a clone by Southern blotting and PCR exploits the fact that following IgH rearrangement, the resultant complementarity-determining region 3 (CDR3) is unique (in size and sequence) to each B-cell and its clonal progeny. Therefore, the CDR3 sequence provides a leukemia-specific target for tracking MRD. PCR identification of leukemia-specific CDR3 is based on the principle that a monoclonal population of CDR3-bearing leukemic cells will exhibit amplification of one particular size of CDR3 at presentation (known as a fingerprint), compared to the heterogeneously sized CDR3-bearing B-cells seen in normal specimens *(24)*.

The combination of amplification using primers for the VH segments of the six major V families (VH1–VH6) and a JH primer yields a clonal IgH pattern that can be demonstrated following either separation on an agarose gel by electrophoresis and ethidium bromide staining or by separation of PCR products pulsed with a radiolabeled nucleotide ($\alpha$-$^{32}$P dCTP) (Fig. 1). The two methods have levels of sensitivity between one leukemic cell in $10^2$ to $10^3$, respectively. Primers can be designed for the framework (FR) 1, FR2 and FR3 regions and used in combination with the antisense JH primer.

The leukemic CDR3 region can be further analyzed for DNA sequence and an allele-specific oligonucleotide (ASO) can be generated. If this is used in combination with the forward FR1 primers a 10-fold higher sensitivity (>1–5 in $10^4$) can be obtained (Fig. 2).

Higher sensitivity of detection has been achieved in various laboratories by running 10 duplicate reactions for each sample (allowing analysis of increased DNA substrate), cellular enrichment of lymphoid cells, or in vitro culture prior to DNA amplification *(25)*. However, these more sensitive PCR-based assays have considerable implications in terms of cost, manpower, and time required. The different methods have recently been extensively reviewed *(11)*.

## MRD: THE TESTS

The Ig and TCR rearrangements are the most common markers used for the investigation of MRD in ALL, as they can be detected in most cases of B- and T-cell ALL, irrespective of age or of additional molecular or cytogenetics changes. They are by far more frequent than the most frequent chromosomal

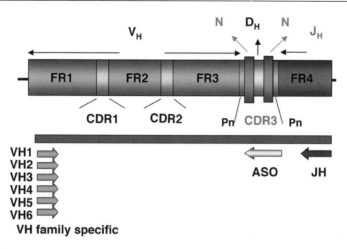

**Fig. 1.** IgH gene rearrangement. Each VH segment joins, by a random recombinatorial event, a D and JH segment to generate the VDJ segment encoding the "variable" part of the IgH molecule. In the joining process, random nucleotides (N) are added at the VD and DJ junction. Also, nucleotides complementary to trimmed basepairs (P nucleotides; Pn) are added to increase variability to the complementarity region 3. Abbreviations are as follows: V, variable; D, diversity: J, joining; CDR: complementarity-determining region; FR: framework region; ASO, allele-specific oligonucleotide.

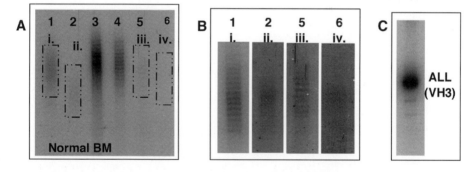

**Fig. 2.** Radiolabeled fingerprinting IgH gene analysis. PCR amplifications using VH family-specific forward primers and JH reverse primers were spiked with radiolabeled nucleotides and then separated on denaturing gel and autoradiographed. **(A)** PCR amplification using normal bone marrow; **(B)** prolonged exposure (5 d) of individual VH PCR amplifications as in (A); **(C)** autoradiograph of VH3 amplification of a VH3 clone in an adult ALL patient as a comparison.

abnormality and they allow monitoring of MRD in over 90–95% of cases of ALL. In Table 2, we compare the different approaches used for MRD investigation in relation to the amount of material required, level of sensitivity, speed, and cost.

Table 2
Technical Approaches to the Investigation of MRD in Adult ALL

| Methods | Required amount of material | Sensitivity[a] (%) | Time to result (d) | Cost-effectiveness[b] |
|---|---|---|---|---|
| Southern blotting | 10 µg | 5–10 | 4–10 | Low |
| Agarose gel PCR | 100–500 ng | 1–5 | 1 | Low |
| Heteroduplex | 100–500 ng | 1–5 | 1–2 | Medium |
| Gene scanning | 50–100 ng | 0.1–1 | 1–2 | High |
| Real-time PCR | 50–100 ng | 0.01–0.001 | 1 | High |

[a]The sensitivity increases using an allele-specific primer derived from the CDR3 region, which is patient-specific.
[b]Mainly the result of the high cost of the equipment required for these tests.

These techniques are also described more fully in other chapters of this volume. Some of the more recently introduced and widely used techniques are described next.

## REAL-TIME QUANTITATIVE PCR

This technology introduced by Heid and colleagues (26) promises to revolutionize the time and effort in using PCR for MRD investigation. In this system, the PCR reaction results in the displacement of a fluorogenic product-specific probe that is degraded while the PCR product is being generated and emits a detectable fluorescent signal (i.e., real-time detection). This amplification system results in a fivefold increase in sensitivity, eliminating the requirement for nested PCR amplification. In the few studies published to date, particularly using the breakpoint-specific fusion genes for the t(9;22) (27), (t(8;21) (28), and t(14;18) (29) translocations, have shown an excellent level of specificity and sensitivity ($10^{-5}$).

More recently, real-time quantitative (RQ)-PCR has been used for the amplification of IgH rearrangements in multiple myeloma (30,31) and ALL patients (30–33). Larger and more comparative studies are in progress to fully assess the impact of this new technique on MRD investigation in ALL, both using leukemia-specific breakpoints and antigen-receptor–specific rearrangements.

## MRD: USEFULNESS OF MONITORING ADULT ALL PATIENTS

At present, ALL patients are classified as standard (low or intermediate) and high risk based on clinical findings at presentation, such as age, sex, white blood count (WBC), immunophenotype, and cytogenetics. On these criteria, over 70–75% of adult ALL patients fall into the standard risk group and 20–25% into the particularly high-risk group. The latter predominantly include patients with t(9;22), T-ALL with high WBC and patients with t(4;11). Clinicians are still unable, however, to predict overall clinical response in the standard-risk group and identify, within the first 6 mo from presentation, those patients who may benefit from less intensive treatment because they are responding well to chemotherapy or to identify patients whose prognosis will improve by having more intensive treatment. Because postinduction clinical and morphological CR is achieved by over 85% of all adults treated with the UKALLXII protocol *(2)*, the use of molecular studies has been explored as possible means to separate high-risk from low- and intermediate-risk patients in remission within 1–3 mo from presentation.

Studies in children have shown that patients who have achieved morphological remission at the end of induction carry detectable residual disease (by molecular detection of leukemic-specific markers) in approx 30% of cases. Moreover, measurement of the level of leukemic cell infiltration in the BM has been shown to predict the relative risk of relapse. Conversely, approx 60–70% of children have been shown to achieve complete molecular remission by 1–3 mo, as revealed by failure of detection at a level of less than 1 leukemic cell in $10^5$ BM normal cells. In these patients, the prediction for continuous clinical remission (CCR) was far more accurate than using other standard criteria previously available, providing continuous monitoring for residual disease showed no re-emergence of the disease during the first 24 mo of therapy. These observations have prompted our and other laboratories to extend molecular monitoring to adult ALL patients. The principle information derived from this analysis will be summarized below.

## MRD: RELEVANT TECHNICAL AND BIOLOGICAL INFORMATION

### Clonality Assessment in Adult ALL

The most common combination of patient-specific markers for B-lineage adult ALL are the IgH and TCR-γ gene rearrangements (85–90%), followed by IgH and TCR-δ (in 50–60% of cases). Frequency of single-locus rearrangement (in our experience) in adults varies from 75% to 80% for the IgH, from 60% to 70% for TCR-γ and from 40% to 50% for TCR-δ. For the IgH rearrangement (the most common), efficiency of amplification using FR1 primers or leader sequence primers is successful in the identification of a clonal marker in 70–80% of patients. This frequency is only slightly lower than the frequency of the same type of rearrangement in childhood ALL (80–90%). Therefore, IgH remains the first choice of marker for MRD studies in ALL. Two events decrease the efficiency of detection of the marker: (1) somatic mutations within the V and J coding regions at sequences where primers are conventionally designed for amplification and (2) incomplete VDJ rearrangements. Somatic mutations, restricted to the IgH genes, introduce sequence changes resulting in poor annealing of the primers and poor amplification efficiency. To avoid this problem, several laboratories use mRNA and real-time (RQ) PCR for amplification of the rearranged alleles encompassing the variable to constant region. This is, however, more successful in chronic lymphoid malignancies, where the rearranged allele is transcribed and results in a surface immunoglobulin. In the acute leukemias, only pre-B-ALL (cytoplasmic IgM positive) and mature B-ALL are amenable to such investigation. Both null and common (CD10+) ALL have no detectable cytoplasmic Ig heavy chains.

In addition, the lower efficiency of amplification in adult compared to childhood ALL has been explained by the presence of more immature IgH rearrangements with DJ rearrangements in approx 10–15% of adult cases. We have analyzed 110 diagnostic BM DNA samples from adult B-lineage ALL patients and found PCR amplifiable rearrangements in 85 (77%), in agreement with other reports (34–36).

## Oligoclonality

Investigation of VH rearrangement in ALL has also revealed the frequent occurrence of oligoclonality. Oligoclonality is defined as the expansion of subclones from the primary leukemic cell. It leads to the generation of as many as five to six different subclones in the same patient and is detected in 20–30% of cases of adult and childhood ALL with little difference between the two age groups. In our study, the majority of the cases carried 1 clone (59%), 18 had 2 clones (21%), and 17 had 3 or more clones (20%). It is important to identify cases with oligoclonality to allow the monitoring of all subclones. We have recently shown that the rates of proliferation of different clones vary greatly because subclones can acquire additional molecular changes with different growth potential and resistance to therapy (37,38).

## VH Gene Usage

Analysis of IgH rearrangement of 245 alleles in adult ALL has confirmed that the clonal cells in adult ALL are derived from a relatively more immature B-cell than in chronic B-cell malignancies such as chronic lymphocytic leukemia (CLL) and non-Hodgkin's lymphoma (39). VH6, the most JH proximal VH gene, is used in a statistically higher proportion of ALL patients than expected. With the exclusion of VH6 and genes within the JH proximal region (within 150–200 kilobases [kb] from JH), there is no other preferential usage of individual VH genes (39).

## MRD MONITORING AND CLINICAL OUTCOME

Although the value of MRD in predicting outcome has been extensively evaluated in childhood ALL (4,5,40,41), little is known of its value in adult ALL (34,42,43). We have analyzed adult ALL patients using BM aspirate specimens taken postinduction (between 28 and 35 d) and at three later time-points (3–5 mo, 6–9 mo, and 10–24 mo) during the first 24 mo of treatment. No Philadelphia-positive patient or patients with T-ALL were included. ALL patients were between 15 and 55 yr of age and treated according to the UKALLXII trial protocol. For patients with an IgH rearrangement (77% of all cases investigated), their MRD status was monitored while in clinical CR at available time-points. End points were latest CCR recording, relapse event, or death (in CR).

In agreement with Brisco's study *(42)*, approx 50% of patients showed residual disease at the end of induction (1 mo). With the exception of one patient, a level of disease of $1:10^2-10^3$ was identified. As time progressed, a reduction in level of residual disease was observed among patients who remained in CCR compared to patients who later relapsed.

Brisco and colleagues *(42)* showed that a test between d 28 and d 42 postinduction could correlate with outcome if accurate quantification was conducted. They showed that the incidence of relapse was greater with increased level of disease at time of assessment *(42)*. Our results *(44)* demonstrate how, among Philadelphia (Ph)-negative B-lineage ALL patients, subgroups with different outcomes can be identified depending on the MRD pattern during the first 6 mo of treatment. Among 49 patients who had been tested at least twice in the first 6 mo of treatment, the following four patterns emerged: (1) only positive MRD tests were recorded; (2) a positive test was followed by conversion to negative test; (3) conversion from negative to positive was observed; (4) all tests were negative. Our data indicate that patients with patterns (1) and (3) have the worst outcome (77% and 71.5% incidence of relapse, respectively) and can therefore be pooled into a high-risk group, whereas patients with pattern (2) or (4) had the greatest chance of CCR (16% and 22%, respectively) and were entered into the low-risk group (*see* Table 3). The individual subgroups will be discussed next.

## *High-Risk Group*

Two consecutive positive tests were detected in 18 patients; 7 patients converted from a negative to a positive test during the period of observation (1–6 mo from induction). We investigated the correlation between these patterns and outcome, and the impact of chemotherapy (CHT), autologous stem cell transplant (SCT) (ASCT), or allogeneic SCT (allo-SCT) treatment on overall outcome. All patients were in CR at time of SCT. Among patients with pattern 1 or 4, the incidence of relapse was comparable (14 [77%] of 18 patients and 5 [71.5%] of 7 patients), indicating the association between positive MRD tests and conversion to positive MRD and high relapse rate.

Only 2 of 15 patients in this high-risk group treated with CHT remained in CCR. All four patients, who received ASCT relapsed. In all four patients, BM harvests pre-BMT were found to contain more than $1:10^3$ leukemic cells. By contrast, four of five patients who received allo-SCT have remained in CCR.

Table 3
MRD Patterns and Association with Outcome

| MRD pattern | Total no. | CHT | ASCT | Allo-SCT | Predictive value[a] |
|---|---|---|---|---|---|
| (1) +/+ | 18 | 9 | 4 | 5 | |
| | Relapses (14) | 9 | 4 | 1 | **PPV: 77%** |
| | CCR (4) | 0 | 0 | 4 | NPV: 22% |
| | % of relapses | 100% | 100% | 20% | |
| (2) +/– | 6 | 3 | 1 | 2 | |
| | Relapses (1) | 0 | 0 | 1 | PPV: 16% |
| | CCR (5) | 3 | 1 | 1 | **NPV: 83%** |
| | % of relapses | 0% | 0% | 50% | |
| (3) –/+ | 7 | 6 | 1 | 0 | |
| | Relapses (5) | 4 | 1 | 0 | **PPV: 71.5%** |
| | CCR (2) | 2 | 0 | 0 | NPV: 28.5% |
| | % of relapses | 71.5% | 100% | NA | |
| (4) –/– | 18 | 11 | 4 | 3 | |
| | Relapses (4) | 3 | 0 | 1 | PPV: 22% |
| | CCR (14) | 8 | 4 | 2 | **NPV: 77%** |
| | % of relapses | 27% | 0% | 33% | |

Abbreviations: +/+, only positive MRD tests during the first 6 mo postinduction; +/–, MRD positive conversion to negative during the first 6 mo; –/+, a conversion from negative to positive tests; –/– only negative tests recorded during the first 6 mo post-induction.

[a]As a whole group. The PPV and NPV are provided. NA: not available; PPV: positive predictive value; NPV: negative predictive value.

Relapse occurred in only one patient who received allo-SCT, but this patient had failed to clear residual disease 2 mo posttransplant and progressed rapidly (within 1 mo) to a clinical relapse.

These data indicate that allo-SCT appears to be the only procedure with an impact on outcome in this high-risk group. Consequently, if we exclude patients who received allo-SCT, relapse was then observed in 18 (90%) of 20 patients with patterns 1 and 4. CHT and ASCT appeared to have little or no effect in preventing relapse in these patients.

### Low-Risk Group

Six patients showed conversion from a positive to a negative test (pattern 2) during the first 6 mo of treatment. All patients remained in CCR. Three had received CHT, one had ASCT, and two had allo-SCT, suggesting a favorable outcome irrespective of treatment.

Two consecutive negative tests during the first 6 mo of observation (pattern 4) were recorded in 18 patients. Except for four patients, all remained in CCR. Three of the relapsed patients received CHT and one received allo-SCT. Four patients receiving ASCT and two patients receiving allo-SCT remained in CCR.

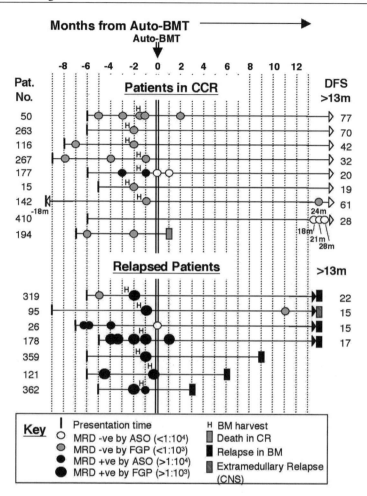

**Fig. 3.** Autologous-BMT patient time lines, showing MRD status at various times from presentation. The time in months has been shown relative to the point at which transplantation took place. The patients have been divided according to clinical outcome.

In this group, analysis of MRD pattern and outcome showed that a negative test is associated with CCR in 77% of cases investigated.

## ASCT Patients

No information is yet available in adult ALL patients in complete remission undergoing ASCT relating level of residual disease in the bone marrow samples to clinical outcome. We were able to collect data on a limited cohort of patients and the findings are described in this subsection.

We observed that patients who receive ASCT showed a striking concordance between MRD results at the time of transplant and clinical outcome (Fig. 3).

Apart from one patient (patient 142), all transplantation procedures took place 5–9 mo from presentation. Almost all samples from patients in long-term CCR were MRD negative (21 of 23; 91.3%) at time-points mainly prior to SCT, and none were positive after SCT. The only patient to remain in CCR with a positive test prior to SCT (patient 177) converted to MRD negativity immediately after SCT.

The opposite is true for those patients who relapsed, with all but one patient (six of seven; 85.7%) testing MRD positive prior to SCT. Interestingly, one patient (patient 95) who was positive at 1 mo prior to SCT (at level greater than 1 in $10^3$) became negative at 10 mo post-SCT, but then had an extramedullary relapse at 15 mo. There was good concordance between the MRD status of the harvested BM sample (usually taken at between 1 and 2 mo prior to ASCT) and clinical outcome of the SCT, with all six MRD-negative harvests being associated with subsequent CCR and six of seven (85.7%) MRD-positive harvest being associated with relapse. Fisher's exact test revealed the relationship to be highly significant ($p = 0.005$).

## Allogeneic SCT Patients

Similar to the autologous SCT, BM assessment in patients undergoing allogeneic bone marrow transplantation showed features important in planning future studies (Fig. 4). Apart from one patient (patient 289), all transplantation procedures took place 5–8 mo from presentation. In contrast to autologous SCT, there was no correlation between MRD result prior to allo-SCT and clinical outcome (Fig. 4). Among 14 patients who remained in CCR, 8 (57%) were MRD positive and 6 (43%) were MRD negative prior to SCT. Among three patients who relapsed (or died with residual disease) after transplantation, only one was MRD positive and two were MRD negative prior to SCT.

By contrast, there was good correlation between the MRD test post-SCT and clinical outcome. Patients in long-term CCR showed no MRD after SCT, and the two patients who were MRD positive either relapsed or died with detectable MRD soon after SCT.

However, because of the low number of relapse patients tested and treated, these results should be considered as very preliminary and suggestive for further testing.

## RELAPSES AND MRD TESTS

The value of MRD tests is also judged by their ability to predict relapse within a specified lapse of time. This is still under investigation in several studies. We applied this analysis to 37 patients in a homogeneous cohort of *de novo* ALL patients. In 26 (70%), relapse was preceded by a positive MRD test, indicating the strong ability of MRD assessment to predict impending relapse. However, in 11 (30%), the last test prior to relapse showed no evidence of MRD. There are

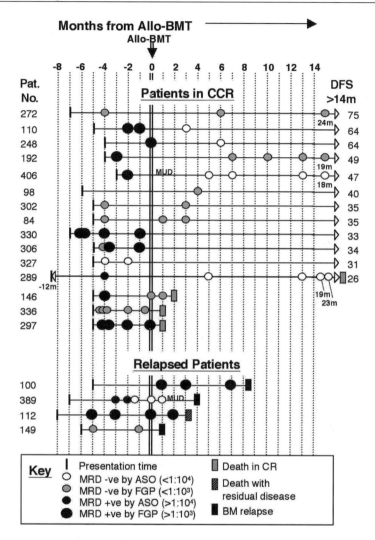

**Fig. 4.** Allogeneic-BMT patient time lines, showing MRD status at various times from presentation. In this group of patients (19 patients in total), follow-up (in months) has been shown relative to the point at which transplantation took place. The patients have been divided according to clinical outcome.

a number of possible explanations for this discrepancy: (1) It could be a consequence of extramedullary relapse with no evidence of BM involvement (in two patients) or (2) prolonged interval (longer than 5 mo) between the last MRD test and relapse (in four patients). Sensitivity of the test may also be relevant. Tests should guarantee level of detection $\geq 1:10^4$ to avoid false-negative tests. Four relapses occurred in patients where no allele-specific oligonucleotide (ASO) was available. Only one patient relapsed within 3 mo after a test, with sensitivity of $1:10^4$ showing no evidence of residual disease. The patient had received a matched-unrelated donor (MUD) transplant 4 mo prior to relapse. The rapid rise of residual disease in transplant patients has been previously recorded both in Ph-positive and Ph-negative patients *(45)*.

The results in our group of patients suggest that (1) monitoring for MRD should be done at regular intervals; we suggest 3 monthly testing. As several patients carry multiple IgH clones (oligoclonality), efforts should be made to follow all available clones. Markers for the TCR-δ and TCR-γ rearrangements should be followed in parallel. In our experience, however, the IgH genes are, by far, the most reliable markers in B-lineage ALL as clonal TCR-δ rearrangement in particular can be lost during the follow-up period preceding relapse.

## MRD TESTS AS INDEPENDENT PREDICTOR OF OUTCOME

The Cox regression multivariant model was used to determine the most significant independent prognostic variable comparing age, sex, WBC, and days to first remission. This analysis made use of information collected from the cohorts of patients discussed above and another 40 patients who had been tested at different times during the first 24 mo of treatment *(44)*. As our study excluded Ph+ ALL, cytogenetics were not taken into account, as other cytogenetics subgroups [e.g., t(4;11) and t(1;19)] were too small to have an impact. We therefore compared MRD status at each time period with age, WBC, count at presentation, and time to first CR for effects on disease-free state (DFS) rates. The only covariable to have any significant independent effects on DFS was MRD.

## MRD IN ADULT ALL:
## COMPARISON WITH CHILDHOOD ALL STUDIES

Comparison between MRD data in childhood and adult ALL highlights differences between responses in the two age groups but similarity in the predictive value of MRD detection. Data for comparison have been derived from recent studies in childhood ALL *(4,5,40,41)*.

### *Differences*

1. Effect of induction therapy. Children show a better response rate to induction therapy than adults, in that a larger proportion reach molecular remission as well as morphological remission (75%) compared to adults (50%) by the end of induction therapy.
2. Less effective response to treatment in adult versus children. The prolonged persistence of residual disease in adults indicates comparative resistance to therapy because they are treated at least as aggressively as children. In our cohort of patients, over 50% of patients still had detectable disease between 3 and 5 mo and this was strongly associated with a high relapse rate (70%).

3. Bone marrow transplant and outcome. The MRD status prior to allo-SCT appears to be the most important indicator of outcome in children *(46,47)*. On the other hand, in adults, we have found that the presence or absence of MRD prior to allogeneic transplant carries little or no impact on outcome. The reason for this difference is not apparent, but it is possible that children selected for allo-SCT have more resistant disease than adults (all in first CR in our study). In children, allogeneic transplants are T-cell depleted (a procedure not applied to adults), removing the antileukemic effect. As there are no large-scale reports in autologous SCT, the data we have collected suggest that all harvested BM should be tested for residual disease, which is the most important factor in predicting outcome in the autologous procedures.

## *Similarities*

1. MRD is a valid parameter for measuring therapy response. In both adult and childhood ALL, MRD is the most important prognostic factor in measuring outcome and it is independent of total WBC, gender, immunophenotype, and age. In children, this has been strongly corroborated by the publication of two large European studies that reported MRD investigation in a total of 178 and 240 childhood ALL patients, respectively *(4,40,41)*. These data have now been corroborated among adult ALL through our study.
2. There is direct correlation between level of disease and incidence of later relapse *(42)* when measuring MRD postinduction, as previously demonstrated in children *(4,40,41)*.

# MRD ANALYSIS: IMPORTANT CRITERIA

## *Peripheral Blood Versus Bone Marrow*

There is strong agreement that peripheral blood (PB) is about 1 log less sensitive than BM for detection of MRD *(45,48,49)*. TCR-$\gamma$ is the least sensitive of markers used *(50)*. Molecular remission in the PB is therefore compatible with residual disease in the BM. Consequently, marrow is preferable for analysis. Most reports have utilized mononuclear cell preparations from fresh marrow samples. If not available, DNA can be obtained from archival glass slides, but the DNA is frequently of inferior quality, which may compromise the sensitivity of the test. There are now several kits that facilitate the preparation of DNA or RNA for analysis. No study has extensively compared the use of RT-PCR versus DNA analysis for antigen-receptor genes in ALL and, therefore, DNA remains the preferred material for analysis.

## *Timing of Testing*

Although testing for MRD at only one time-point may provide informative results, most investigators advocate testing on two or more occasions (e.g., immediately postinduction and at 3–5 mo and 6–9 mo of therapy). More frequent testing may be desirable, particularly if MRD is being assessed by a more sensitive and quantitative technique to detect an emerging clone of proliferating cells. However, the practicality and ethics of this need to be considered carefully.

## BM Testing for Extramedullary Relapse

We have limited information on the efficiency of MRD analysis using BM for prediction of extramedullary relapse. In children, several studies have shown that BM testing is not yet sufficiently sensitive to predict extramedullary relapse (central nervous system, testis, and skin) in all cases *(40,41,51,52)*. There are too few cases of extramedullary relapses in our study to reach any meaningful conclusion. It is only noteworthy that two of three extramedullary relapses were preceded by negative tests. Larger studies and more regular monitoring are required in the future.

At the time of extramedullary relapse, the bone marrow in children almost invariably contains low-level MRD *(41,53)*. This observation explains why there is a high incidence of subsequent marrow relapse in such patients and provides a rationale for systemic treatment, in addition to site-directed treatment.

## MRD in Harvested Bone Marrow Specimens

Minimal residual disease analysis has been useful in the assessment of residual disease both prior to or after purging in BM harvested for ASCT. A direct relationship between PCR-positive BM and incidence of relapse following ASCT has been described in patients with non-Hodgkin's lymphoma *(54,55)*, CLL *(56)*, and ALL *(44,57)*. Whether relapse originates from residual disease in the BM graft or from persisting medullary disease that survives the effect of high-dose therapy is unknown. Relapse derived from the grafted cells has occurred in AML *(58)*. Purging studies with MRD monitoring may help to resolve this issue in cases of ALL.

## CONCLUDING REMARKS

The evaluation of MRD following chemotherapy or bone marrow transplantation has progressed in the past 10–15 yr from morphological assessment of BM aspirates to the use of immunological and cytogenetic tests. The application of molecular techniques, including PCR, has enabled us to detect MRD to levels of sensitivity of $10^{-5}$–$10^{-4}$. We now have the ability to trace leukemic cells among normal counterparts using both clonal changes in antigen-receptor genes (IgH and TCR) and leukemic-specific changes (translocations, point mutations). These tests have been used, to date, to study more than 900 patients with ALL, predominantly children. In at least three large prospective studies that together evaluated over 500 childhood ALL patients *(4,40,41)*, this predictive value has been found to be independent of other risk factors such as age, sex, and presenting leukocyte count. Quantitative and semiquantitative assessment of MRD is becoming important with three of these large studies defining relapse risk as a function of MRD level immediately postinduction and at later time-points.

We have now been able to evaluate the same parameters in adult ALL and show that MRD detection has similar predictive value *(44)*. Both for children and adults, the challenge is to incorporate routine, regular MRD analysis into prognostic indices for testing in large randomized trials. The potential benefit would seem to be largest in "standard-risk" ALL as judged by conventional criteria (age, sex, presenting leukocyte count, chromosomal translocations). In this, the largest category of patients, overall benefit has been obtained by treatment intensification, but this is at the expense of overtreating a substantial number of patients (who may be cured with less intensive protocols), especially in children. In adults, a large number of patients appear to be cured by standard chemotherapy and could be spared invasive SCT procedures. The corollary to this is the potential for detecting a new group of high-risk patients, both adults and children on the basis of slow MRD clearance or rapid rise following negative MRD. These could be candidates for further treatment intensification including the possibility of SCT in first CR or alternative, more aggressive treatments.

For such decisions to be made, there will need to be a high level of confidence in interpreting MRD results. As we have described, these results can be affected by the technique used and a host of other potential pitfalls. The availability of several different markers helps to rule out false-positive or false-negative tests but increases the total labor and costs substantially. The current technology is labor intensive, but improvements including kits for DNA/RNA extraction, automated sequencing, fluorescent-based methodology, and, more recently, real-time PCR may lead to a more widespread availability of MRD testing.

We hope that within the next 5 yr MRD analysis will be used routinely and prospectively to assess treatment response in all patients with ALL treated on major national and international protocols. The challenge will be how to incorporate the information learned into new studies for the overall benefit of the patients.

## ACKNOWLEDGMENTS

The Kay Kendall Leukemia Research Fund (KK98) and Leukemia Research Fund, UK (Grant 91-75 and 95-03) supported our study. We would like to thank the research team in the Laboratory of Molecular Genetics at the Royal Free and University College (Dr. James Chim, Dr. Luke A. Coyle, Dr. Mary Papaioannou, Dr. Ilidia Moreira, Dr. Giulio L. Palmisano, Dr. Paola Carrara, and Paula Gameiro) for their continuous effort in analyzing material. We would like to thank the clinical colleagues at the Royal Free Hospital and all participating centers that have supplied material for MRD investigation.

# REFERENCES

1. Hoelzer D and Gokbuget N. Recent approaches in acute lymphoblastic leukemia in adults, *Crit. Rev. Oncol. Hematol, * **36** (2000) 49–58.
2. Durrant IJ, Richards SM, Prentice HG, and Goldstone AH. The Medical Research Council trials in adult acute lymphocytic leukemia, *Hematol. Oncol. Clin. North Am.*, **14** (2000) 1327–1352.
3. Campana D and Behm FG. Immunophenotyping of leukemia, *J. Immunol. Methods*, **243** (2000) 59–75.
4. Coustan-Smith E, Behm FG, Sanchez J, Boyett JM, Hancock ML, Raimondi SC, et al., Immunological detection of minimal residual disease in children with acute lymphoblastic leukemia, *Lancet*, **351** (1998) 550–554.
5. Coustan-Smith E, Sancho J, Hancock ML, Boyett JM, Behm FG, Raimondi SC, et al., Clinical importance of minimal residual disease in childhood acute lymphoblastic leukemia, *Blood*, **96** (2000) 2691–2696.
6. Harrison CJ. The genetics of childhood acute lymphoblastic leukemia, *Bailliere's Best Pract. Res. Clin. Haematol.*, **13** (2000) 427–439.
7. Harrison CJ. The management of patients with leukemia: the role of cytogenetics in this molecular era [review], *Br. J. Haematol.*, **108** (2000) 19–30.
8. Inoue K, Sugiyama H, Ogawa H, Nakagawa M, Yamagami T, Miwa H, et al. WT1 as a new prognostic factor and a new marker for the detection of minimal residual disease in acute leukemia, *Blood*, **84** (1994) 3071–3079.
9. Im HJ, Kong G, and Lee H. Expression of Wilms tumor gene (WT1) in children with acute leukemia, *Pediatr. Hematol. Oncol.*, **16** (1999) 109–118.
10. Stock W, Westbrook CA, Sher DA, Dodge R, Sobol RE, Wurster-Hill D, et al. Low incidence of TAL1 gene rearrangements in adult acute lymphoblastic leukemia: a cancer and leukemia group B study (8762), *Clin. Cancer Res.*, **1** (1995) 459–463.
11. Foroni L, Harrison CJ, Hoffbrand AV, and Potter M. Investigation of minimal residual disease in childhood and adult lymphoblastic leukemia by molecular analysis, *Br. J. Haematol.*, **105** (1999) 7–24.
12. Skibola CF, Smith MT, Kane E, Roman E, Rollinson S, Cartwright RA, et al. Polymorphisms in the methylenetetrahydrofolate reductase gene are associated with susceptibility to acute leukemia in adults, *Proc. Natl. Acad. Sci. USA*, **96** (1999) 12,810–12,815.
13. Haidar MA, Kantarjian H, Manshouri T, Chang CY, O'Brien S, Freireich E, et al. ATM gene deletion in patients with adult acute lymphoblastic leukemia, *Cancer*, **88** (2000) 1057–1062.
14. Chung CY, Kantarjian H, Haidar M, Starostik P, Manshouri T, Gidel C, et al. Deletions in the 13q14 locus in adult lymphoblastic leukemia: rate of incidence and relevance, *Cancer*, **88** (2000) 1359–1364.
15. Stock W, Tsai T, Golden C, Rankin C, Sher D, Slovak ML, et al. Cell cycle regulatory gene abnormalities are important determinants of leukemogenesis and disease biology in adult acute lymphoblastic leukemia, *Blood*, **95** (2000) 2364–2371.
16. Nakase K, Ishimaru F, Avitahl N, Dansako H, Matsuo K, Fujii K, et al. Dominant negative isoform of the Ikaros gene in patients with adult B-cell acute lymphoblastic leukemia, *Cancer Res.*, **60** (2000) 4062–4065.
17. Rambaldi A, Attuati V, Bassan R, Neonato MG, Viero P, Battista R, et al. Molecular diagnosis and clinical relevance of t(9;22), t(4;11) and t(1;19) chromosome abnormalities in a consecutive group of 141 adult patients with acute lymphoblastic leukemia, *Leuk. Lymphoma*, **21** (1996) 457–466.
18. Aguiar RC, Sohal J, van Rhee F, Carapeti M, Franklin IM, Goldstone AH, et al. TEL-AML1 fusion in acute lymphoblastic leukemia of adults. M.R.C. Adult Leukemia Working Party, *Br. J. Haematol.*, **9** (1996) 673–677.

19. Rabbitts TH. Chromosomal translocations in human cancer [review], *Nature*, **372(10)** (1994) 143–149.
20. Rabbitts TH. Perspective: chromosomal translocations can affect genes controlling gene expression and differentiation—why are these functions targeted? [review], *J. Pathol.*, **187** (1999) 39–42.
21. Look AT. Oncogenic transcription factors in the human acute leukemias [review], *Science*, **278** (1997) 1059–1064.
22. Tonegawa S. Somatic generation of antibody diversity, *Nature*, **302** (1983) 575–581.
23. Alt FW, Blackwell TK, and Yancopoulos GD. Development of the primary antibody repertoire, *Science*, **238** (1987) 1079–1087.
24. Chim JC, Coyle L, Yaxley JC, Cole Sinclair MF, Cannell PK, Hoffbrand AV, et al. The use of IgH fingerprinting and ASO-dependent PCR for the investigation of residual disease (MRD) in ALL, *Br. J. Haematol.*, **92** (1996) 104–115.
25. Roberts WM, Estrov Z, Ouspenskaia MV, Johnston DA, McClain KL, and Zipf TF. Measurement of residual leukemia during remission in childhood acute lymphoblastic leukemia, *N. Engl. J. Med.*, **30** (1997) 317–323.
26. Heid CA, Stevens J, Livak KJ, and Williams PM. Real time quantitative PCR, *Genome Res.*, **6** (1996) 986–994.
27. Mensink E, van de Locht A, Schattenberg A, Linders E, Schaap N, Geurts van Kessel A, et al. Quantitation of minimal residual disease in Philadelphia chromosome positive chronic myeloid leukaemia patients using real-time quantitative RT-PCR, *Br. J. Haematol.*, **102** (1998) 768–774.
28. Marcucci G, Livak KJ, Bi W, Strout MP, Bloomfield CD, and Caligiuri MA. Detection of minimal residual disease in patients with AML1/ETO-associated acute myeloid leukemia using a novel quantitative reverse transcription polymerase chain reaction assay, *Leukemia*, **12** (1998) 1482–1489.
29. Luthra R, McBride JA, Cabanillas F, and Sarris A. Novel 5' exonuclease-based real-time PCR assay for the detection of t(14;18)(q32;q21) in patients with follicular lymphoma, *Am. J. Pathol.*, **153** (1998) 63–68.
30. Gerard CJ, Olsson K, Ramanathan R, Reading C, and Hanania EG. Improved quantitation of minimal residual disease in multiple myeloma using real-time polymerase chain reaction and plasmid-DNA complementarity determining region III standards, *Cancer Res.*, **58** (1998) 3957–3964.
31. Ladetto M, Donovan JW, Harig S, Trojan A, Poor C, Schlossnan R, et al. Real-time polymerase chain reaction of immunoglobulin rearrangements for quantitative evaluation of minimal residual disease in multiple myeloma, *Biol. Blood Marrow Transplant.*, **6** (2000) 241–253.
32. Verhagen OJ, Willemse MJ, Breunis WB, Wijkhuijs AJ, Jacobs DC, Joosten SA, et al. Application of germline IGH probes in real-time quantitative PCR for the detection of minimal residual disease in acute lymphoblastic leukemia, *Leukemia*, **14** (2000) 1426–1435.
33. Pongers-Willemse MJ, Verhagen OJ, Tibbe GJ, Wijkhuijs AJ, de Haas V, Roovers E, et al. Real-time quantitative PCR for the detection of minimal residual disease in acute lymphoblastic leukemia using junctional region specific TaqMan probes, *Leukemia*, **12** (1998) 2006–2014.
34. Salo A, Pakkala S, Jansson S-E, et al. Monitoring of adult B-cell lineage acute lymphoblastic leukemia: validation of a simple method for detecting immunoglobulin heavy chain gene clonality, *Leukemia*, **7** (1993) 1459–1468.
35. Coyle LA, Papaioannou M, Yaxley JC, Chim JS, Attard M, Hoffbrand AV, et al. Molecular analysis of the leukaemic B cell in adult and childhood acute lymphoblastic leukaemia, *Br. J. Haematol.*, **94** (1996) 685–693.
36. Li AH, Rosenquist R, Forestier E, Holmberg D, Lindh J, Lofvenberg E, et al. Clonal rearrangements in childhood and adult precursor B acute lymphoblastic leukemia: a comparative poly-

merase chain reaction study using multiple sets of primers, *Eur. J. Haematol.*, **63** (1999) 211–218.

37. Zhu Y-M, Foroni L, McQuaker IG, Papaioannou M, Haynes A, and Russell N. Mechanisms of relapse in acute lymphoblastic leukemia: involvement of p53 mutated subclones in disease progression, *Br. J. Cancer*, **79** (1999) 1151–1157.

38. Moreira I, Papaioannou M, Mortuza F, et al. Oligoclonality: an insight into the biology of acute lymphoblastic leukaemia. *Leukemia* **15** (2001) 1527–1530.

39. Mortuza FY, Moreira IM, Papaioannou M, Coyle LA, Yaxley JC, Gricks CS, et al. Immunoglobulin heavy-chain gene rearrangement in adult acute lymphoblastic leukemia reveals preferential usage of J(H)-proximal variable gene segments, *Blood*, **97** (2001) 2716–2726.

40. Cavé H, van der Werff ten Bosch J, Suciu S, Guidal C, Waterkeyn C, Otten J, et al. Clinical significance of minimal residual disease in childhood acute lymphoblastic leukemia, *N. Engl. J. Med.*, **339** (1998) 591–598.

41. Van Dongen JJM, Seriu T, Panzer-Grümayer ER, Biondi A, Pongers-Willemse MJ, Corral L, et al. Prognostic value of minimal residual disease in acute lymphoblastic leukemia in children, *Lancet*, **352** (1998) 1731–1738.

42. Brisco J, Hughes E, Neoh SH, Sykes PJ, Bradstock K, Enno A, Szer J, et al. Relationship between minimal residual disease and outcome in adult acute lymphoblastic leukemia, *Blood*, **87** (1996) 5251–5256.

43. Foroni L, Coyle LA, Papaioannou M, Yaxley JC, Cole Sinclair MF, Chim JS, et al. Molecular detection of minimal residual disease in adult and childhood Acute lymphoblastic leukaemia reveals differences in treatment response, *Leukemia*, **11** (1997) 1732–1741.

44. Mortuza FY, Papaioannou M, Moreira IM, Coyle LA, Gameiro P, Gandini D, et al. Minimal residual disease tests provide an independent predictor of clinical outcome in adult acute lymphoblastic leukemia, *J. Clin. Oncol.*, **20** (2002) 1094–1104.

45. van Rhee F, Hochhaus A, Lin F, Cross NCP, and Goldman JM. High *BCR-ABL* transcript levels precede haematological relapse in Philadelphia positive acute leukemia [Abstract], *Exp. Haematol.*, **23** (1995) 922.

46. Knechtli CJC, Goulden NJ, Hancock JP, Grandage VLG, Harris EL, Garland R, et al. Minimal residual disease status before allogeneic bone marrow transplantation is an important determinant of successful outcome for children and adolescents with acute lymphoblastic leukemia, *Blood*, **92** (1998) 4072–4079.

47. Goulden NJ, Knechtli CJC, Garland RJ, Langlands K, Hancock JP, Potter MN, et al. Minimal residual disease analysis for the prediction of relapse in children with standard-risk acute lymphoblastic leukemia, *Br. J. Haematol.*, **100** (1998) 235–244.

48. Gribben JG, Neuberg D, Barber M, Moore J, Pesek KW, Freedman AS, et al. Detection of residual lymphoma cells by polymerase chain reaction in peripheral blood is significantly less predictive for relapse than detection in bone marrow, *Blood*, **83** (1984) 3800–3807.

49. Brisco MJ, Sykes PJ, Hughes E, Dolman G, Neoh SH, Peng LM, et al. Monitoring minimal residual disease in peripheral blood in B-lineage acute lymphoblastic leukaemia, *Br. J. Haematol.*, **99** (1997) 314–319.

50. Sykes PJ, Snell LE, Brisco MJ, Neoh SH, Hughes E, Dolman G, et al. The use of monoclonal gene rearrangement for detection of minimal residual disease in acute lymphoblastic leukemia of childhood, *Leukemia*, **11** (1997) 153–158.

51. Cave' H, Guidal C, Rohrlich P, Delfau MH, Broyart A, Lescoeur B, et al. Prospective monitoring and quantification of residual blasts in childhood acute lymphoblastic leukemia by polymerase chain reaction study of the δ and γ T-cell receptor genes, *Blood*, **83** (1994) 1892–1902.

52. Seriu T, Yokota S, Nakao M, Misawa S, Takaue Y, Koizumi S, et al. Prospective monitoring of minimal residual disease during the course of chemotherapy in patients with acute lymphoblastic leukemia, and detection of contaminating tumour cells in peripheral blood stem cells for autotransplantation, *Leukemia*, **9** (1995) 615–623.

53. Goulden N, Langlands K, Steward C, Katz F, Potter M, Chessells J, et al. PCR assessment of bone marrow status in "isolated" extramedullary relapse of childhood B-precursor acute lymphoblastic leukaemia, *Br. J. Haematol.*, **87** (1994) 282–285.
54. Gribben JG, Freedman AS, Neuberg D, Roy DC, Blake KW, Woo SD, et al. Immunologic purging of marrow assessed by PCR before autologous bone marrow transplantation for B-cell lymphoma, *N. Engl. J. Med.*, **325** (1991) 1525–1533.
55. Zwicky CS, Maddocks AB, Andersen N, and Gribben JG. Eradication of polymerase chain reaction detectable immunoglobulin gene rearrangement in non-Hodgkin's lymphoma is associated with decreased relapse after autologous bone marrow transplantation, *Blood*, **88** (1996) 3314–3322.
56. Provan D, Bartlett-Pandite L, Zwicky C, Neuberg D, Maddocks A, Corradini P, et al. Eradication of polymerase chain reaction-detectable chronic lymphocytic leukemia cells is associated with improved outcome after bone marrow transplantation, *Blood*, **88** (1996) 2228–2235.
57. Atta J, Martin H, Bruecher J, Elsner S, Wassmann B, Rode C, et al. Residual leukemia and immunomagnetic bead purging in patients with BCR-ABL-positive acute lymphoblastic leukemia, *Bone Marrow Transplant.*, **18** (1996) 541–548.
58. Brenner MK, Rill DR, Moen RC, Krance RA, Mirro J Jr, Anderson WF, et al. Gene-marking to trace origin of relapse after autologous bone-marrow transplantation, *Lancet*, **341** (1993) 85–86.

# 8 Investigation of Minimal Residual Disease in Acute Myeloid Leukemia by Immunophenotyping

*Jesús F. San Miguel, María B. Vidriales, and Alberto Orfao*

## INTRODUCTION

Current treatment strategies for patients with acute myeloid leukemia (AML) result in a high complete remission (CR) rate (60–80%). However, relapses due to the persistence of low numbers of residual neoplastic cells which are undetectable by conventional morphological techniques (minimal residual disease [MRD]), still occur in most patients; in fact, only around one-third of patients with AML are leukemia-free at 5 yr. Owing to this, patients are indiscriminately subjected to consolidation treatments, including conventional chemotherapy and autologous and allogeneic stem cell transplantation, in order to eradicate possible MRD. Therefore, more sensitive techniques are needed to lay the foundations for the design of patient-adapted consolidation therapies that would reduce the risk of both: toxic deaths resulting from overtreatment in patients that could be cured with conventional chemotherapy and relapses resulting from insufficiently intensive consolidation treatment in patients at high risk of relapse because of persistence of residual leukemic cells. In addition, such sensitive methods for MRD detection can contribute to the assessment of the efficacy of ex vivo purging protocols for autologous stem cells prior to reinfusion and to a more precise evaluation of the effectiveness of new treatment strategies.

A detailed analysis of the literature shows that different methodological approaches have been used for the detection of MRD *(1–17)*. The efficacy and applicability of the different methodological approaches that are available for the detection of MRD depend on three main features: (1) *specificity*: discrimination between malignant and normal cells, without false-negative and false-positive

From: *Leukemia and Lymphoma: Detection of Minimal Residual Disease*
Edited by: T. F. Zipf and D. A. Johnston © Humana Press Inc., Totowa, NJ

results; (2) *sensitivity*: leukemic cells are undetectable by morphology when their number falls below 1–5% of the total bone marrow (BM) nucleated cells, and, consequently, the detection limit of an MRD technique must be at least $10^{-3}$ (i.e., discrimination of 1 leukemic cell among 1000 normal cells); and (3) *clinical applicability*: the technique should allow for easy standardization and rapid collection of results for their clinical application.

In general, the strategies that are currently used for the detection of MRD in hematological malignancies are based on the identification at diagnosis of uniquely characteristic features of the leukemic cells, which would be used later to distinguish them from a major population of normal cells in samples in which neoplastic cells are not detected by conventional morphology *(1,2,6,8,12,15–29)*. On the basis of these leukemia-associated features, one or several patient-specific probes can be built at diagnosis to be used later during the follow-up of patients who achieved morphologic complete remission for MRD detection. According to the cell characteristics explored, MRD techniques are classically grouped into: (1) cell culture techniques; (2) cytogenetic approaches based on conventional karyotyping, fluorescence *in situ* hybridization (FISH), or chromosome analysis by flow cytometry; (3) flow-cytometric analysis of total cell DNA contents; (4) molecular biology, mainly based on polymerase chain reaction (PCR) techniques, and (5) immunophenotyping using multiple stainings analyzed by flow cytometry *(1–4,6–9,11,12,29)*. Based on the relative sensitivity and applicability of the different techniques, the two most commonly used methods for detection of MRD are the multiparametric immunophenotypic flow-cytometry studies and PCR analysis.

It should be noted that these techniques cannot be indiscriminately used for all types of leukemia, but they should be adapted to each individual case, depending on the markers (cytogenetic, immunologic, molecular, etc.) that best characterize the malignant clone. Thus, immunophenotyping is ideal for T-ALL, whereas PCR analysis is the method of choice for chronic myeloid leukemia (CML). Ideally, at present it is recommended that two or more techniques should be simultaneously explored in each patient, in order to define the best approach for investigation of MRD. In this chapter, we review the use of flow-cytometry immunophenotyping for the investigation of MRD in patients with AML. First, we will focus on technical-related aspects and then we will comment on the information that is currently available regarding the clinical utility of MRD studies using immunophenotyping.

## IMMUNOPHENOTYPIC DETECTION OF MRD: METHODOLOGICAL APPROACH

Immunophenotypic analysis of leukemic cells has proved to be an attractive approach for MRD investigation, owing to its relative simplicity and speed

*(8,9,11,12,26,30–32)*. Moreover, the combination of multiple antigen stainings and flow cytometry has increased the sensitivity and reproducibility of the method by providing the possibility to (1) simultaneously analyze several parameters on a single-cell basis, (2) allow the study of high numbers of cells within a relatively short period, at the same time it permits storage of the information for latter analysis, (3) quantitatively evaluate antigen expression, and (4) combine the detection of surface and intracellular antigens.

In spite of these advantages, flow-cytometry immunophenotypic detection of MRD has, at least from the theoretical point of view, two major disadvantages that would hamper the specificity and applicability of immunophenotype for MRD detection *(33,34)*: (1) At present we should consider that, in most cases, leukemic cells do not express well-characterized leukemia-specific antigens; in addition, although there are some proteins resulting from fusion genes, such as BCR/ABL or PML/RARα, that would represent true specific leukemic markers, no reliable monoclonal antibody (MoAb) for their routine detection are available, and (2) several groups have reported on the existence of phenotypic changes at relapse and this may lead to an increased proportion of false-negative results *(23,35–41)*. Although the first disadvantage poses the question as to whether leukemia-associated phenotypes exist and could overcome the lack of leukemia-specific antigens, the second points out the need to ensure that the abnormal phenotypic characteristics detected at diagnosis remain stable during follow-up evaluation. Accordingly, two key prerequisites for the immunophenotypical investigation of MRD are the demonstration that leukemic cells display singular antigenic profiles that allow their distinction from normal hemopoietic cells even when present at very low frequencies and the demonstration that such antigenic characteristics remain stable during the course of the disease; in other words, that immunophenotypic probes are reliable markers for the identification of residual leukemic cells.

## Characterization and Incidence
## of Leukemia-Associated Phenotypes

Precise identification of leukemia cells is essentially based on the ability to clearly distinguish them from the normal cells present in the specimen. Accordingly, phenotypic patterns of not only leukemic cells but also normal cells, present in all types of sample used for the diagnosis of hematological malignances, must be well established in advance. Traditionally, it has been considered that leukemic cells reflect the immunophenotypic characteristics of normal cells blocked at a certain differentiation stage. However, the combined use of multiparametric flow cytometry and large panels of fluorochrome-conjugated MoAb reagents have shown that leukemic cells frequently display either aberrant or uncommon phenotypic features that allow their distinction from normal cells *(13,16,17, 22,24,28,42–56)*. Accordingly, those phenotypes that go undetected in normal hematopoiesis, either because they do not exist or they are present at very low frequencies, could be considered as leukemia-associated phenotypes (LAPs). These unusual or aberrant phenotypes generally result from (1) cross-lineage antigen expression (i.e., expression of lymphoid-associated markers in myeloid blast cells), (2) asynchronous antigen expression (i.e., coexpression in neoplastic cells of antigenic characteristics that correspond to different maturational stages in normal hematopoiesis), (3) antigen overexpression (i.e., presence of an antigen in leukemic cells at abnormally high amounts), (4) ectopic antigen expression (i.e., presence of a marker outside of its normal homing area [i.e., presence of TdT+ cells in the spinal fluid], and (5) the existence of abnormal light-scatter patterns (i.e., lymphoid cells displaying high forward scatter [FSS] and side scatter [SSC] features) *(19,22,24,44,46,47,52,56–59)*. The detection of these aberrancies at diagnosis represents a prerequisite for the investigation of MRD during follow-up evaluation once morphologic CR has been attained. Together with these phenotypic aberrancies, there are other situations that may herald the presence of leukemic hematopoiesis. The most relevant one is the detection of an increased proportion of immature cell populations with abnormal maturation patterns *(60)*. Accordingly, it has been suggested that an abnormally high ratio between CD34+ myeloid and CD34+ lymphoid progenitors after intensification treatment could reflect the existence of MRD in AML patients *(60)*.

From the clinical point of view, the applicability of the use of immunophenotyping for the investigation of MRD is directly dependent not only on the existence of these abnormal phenotypes but also on the frequency at which they are detected. In this sense, careful analysis of the literature shows the existence of disturbing levels of variability in the incidence of LAP in AML as well as in other hematologic malignancies *(19,22,24,28,42–54,59)*. Such discrepancies are probably related to technical pitfalls, including the use of different fluorochrome-conjugated reagents, monoclonal antibody clones, single- versus multiple-staining combinations, different gating strategies, the methods used to assess fluorescence expression, sample preparation protocols, and the use of distinct control samples to establish normal phenotypes *(57,61)*. In any case, it may be stated that the frequency at which LAPs are detected has increased during the last years in parallel to the technical improvements and the availability of new analytical capabilities *(16,17,19,22,24,45–47)*. At present, the incidence of aberrant or LAP in AML ranges from 30% to 85%, depending on the criteria used for their definition and the panel of MoAbs employed. In our experience, 70% of AML patients display aberrant phenotypes, two or more aberrancies coexisting in more than a half of them (56%) *(22,27,62)*. Therefore, according to these results, immunophenotypic detection of MRD is feasible in around three-quarters of AML patients. Below, we will discuss how the most relevant antigenic aberrancies present in AML.

## ASYNCHRONOUS ANTIGEN EXPRESSION

The most common type of LAP found in AML is the presence of asynchronous antigen expression (60% of cases), usually caused either by the coexistence of two antigens in the same cell that are not simultaneously expressed in the normal myeloid differentiation or by the lack of reactivity for one of two myeloid-associated antigens that are coexpressed on normal cells (i.e., CD13 and CD33). During normal maturation of hematopoietic cells, expression of surface and intracellular antigens is finally controlled in such a way that downregulation of certain antigens precedes the expression of other molecules and vice versa. Therefore, antigens exist whose expression is characteristic of specific maturational stages within an hematopoietic cell lineage *(16,17,26,63,64)*. The use of multiple stainings analyzed by flow cytometry in which two or more antigens are simultaneously explored has shown that leukemic cells frequently display asynchronous antigen expression *(15,22–24,41,45,62,64)*. This implies the need for detailed knowledge on the sequence of antigen expression during normal differentiation, because some phenotypes that may appear to be asynchronous may actually either exist at low frequencies or they might be restricted to a specific myeloid lineage usually with a low representation (i.e., mast cells, dendritic cells).

In our experience the overall incidence of asynchronous antigen expression among AML is around 80%. The most representative examples of this aberrancy are illustrated in Table 1 and include CD33++DR–CD34–CD15–CD14– (17% of cases), CD33–CD13+ (14%), CD117+CD33+DR– (11%), CD34+DR– CD33+ (9%), CD34+CD56+ (8%); CD33+CD13– (7%), CD117+CD34–CD15– (6%), CD117+CD11B+ (5%), and CD34+CD11B++ (5%).

## CROSS-LINEAGE ANTIGEN EXPRESSION

Although several leukocyte antigens have long been associated with the lymphoid cell lineage either because they are absent or present at very low frequencies and/or intensity in myeloid cells, it was already observed in the late 1970s and early 1980s that some AML-expressed lymphoid-related markers and vice versa. Since then, a large number of reports have analyzed the incidence of expression of lymphoid-associated markers in blast cells from AML; the incidence ranges from 4% to 60%, with CD2 and CD7 being the markers most frequently found in neoplastic myeloblasts *(8,12,19,56,65,66)*. In our experience the overall incidence of cross-lineage aberrancies in AML is 29%, and the individual expression of CD2, CD7, and CD19 is 21%, 9%, and 2% respectively *(22,62)* (*see* Table 2). It is possible that upon using fluorochromes that have a high resolution (i.e., phycoerythrin), this incidence may even increase; nevertheless, the expression detected with sensitive fluorochromes may be so dim that it would limit their value during follow-up for the specific identification of MRD.

Table 1
Incidence of Aberrant Phenotypes in AML (I)

| | | |
|---|---|---|
| CD34+DR−CD33+ | 11 | 9% |
| CD34+CD56+ | 10 | 8% |
| CD34+CD11b+ | 6 | 5% |
| CD34+CD33++ | 4 | 3% |
| CD34+CD14+ | 4 | 3% |
| CD34+CD117+DR− | 3 | 2.3% |
| CD34+CD117−CD15+ | 3 | 2.3% |
| CD34+CD33−CD13+DR+ | 2 | 1.5% |
| CD34+CD33−CD13+DR− | 1 | 0.8% |
| CD34+CD33−CD117+DR+ | 1 | 0.8% |
| CD117+CD33+DR− | 14 | 11% |
| CD117+CD34−CD15−[a] | 8 | 6% |
| CD117+CD11b+ | 7 | 5.5% |
| CD117+CD33+CD34−CD15+ | 5 | 4% |
| CD117+DR−CD15+ | 3 | 2.3% |
| CD117+DR−CD15−[a] | 2 | 2.3% |
| CD117+DR+CD33+CD34− | 1 | 0.8% |
| CD33++DR−CD34−CD15−CD14− | 22 | 17% |
| CD33−CD13+ | 18 | 14% |
| CD33+CD13− | 9 | 7% |
| CD33+DR+CD4+CD45dim | 1 | 0.8% |
| CD33++DR+CD15−CD14−[b] | 1 | 0.8% |
| CD33+CD45d CD34−CD15−[c] | 1 | 0.8% |
| CD33+DR+CD56+CD13+ | 1 | 0.8% |

[a]Mast cells express this phenotype, but with higher expression of CD117.
[b]Minor phenotypes (dendritic cells).
[c]Minor phenotypes (basophilic lineage).

## ANTIGEN OVEREXPRESSION

Multiparametric flow cytometry allows not only the qualitative evaluation of antigen expression (presence vs absence) but also the assessment of quantitative expression on a single-cell basis. It has frequently been observed that leukemic blasts may express antigens that, in spite of being present in normal cells, are also observed at significantly higher amounts (intensity levels) in the malignant counterpart (antigen overexpression). The overall incidence of this aberrancy in AML is low (21%) and the antigens more frequently involved are CD33 (11%), CD34 (9%), and CD13 (2%) (*see* Table 2).

## ABNORMAL LIGHT-SCATTER PATTERNS

Flow-cytometry immunophenotyping combines the measurement of cell antigen-associated fluorescence with that of the light-scatter properties of the

Table 2
Incidence of Aberrant Phenotypes in AML (II)

| Cross-lineage infidelity | | Antigen overexpression | | Abnormal light-scatter pattern | |
|---|---|---|---|---|---|
| 37/126 | 29% | 26/126 | 21% | 22/126 | 17% |
| CD2 | 26 (21%) | CD33+++ | 14 (11%) | High FSC/SSC | |
| CD7 | 11 (9%) | CD34 | 11 (9%) | CD2 | 4 (2.6%) |
| CD19 | 3 (2%) | CD13 | 3 (2%) | CD34 | 4 (2.6%) |
| CD20 | 1 (0.8%) | CD117 | 1 (0.8%) | CD7 | 4 (2.6%) |
| CD5 | 1 (0.8%) | CD15[a] | 1 (0.8%) | CD117 | 2 (1.5%) |
| | | HLA DR | 1 (0.8%) | CD19 | 2 (1.5%) |
| | | | | CD20 | 1 (0.8%) |
| | | | | Low FSC/SSC | |
| | | | | CD13[b] | 3 (2%) |
| | | | | CD33[b] | 1 (0.8%) |
| | | | | CD15 | 1 (0.8%) |

[a]Overexpression of CD15 in nongranulocytic lineage.
[b]Minor phenotypes (basophilic lineage).

individual cells under study. These latter parameters include the light scattered at (1) low angles (forward light scatter, or FSC) and (2) angles of 90° (sideward scatter, or SSC). The amount of FSC is directly dependent on the size and the refractory index of the cell. In turn, SSC mainly reflects the relative homogeneity/heterogeneity of intracellular components that reflect the laser light such as cytoplasmic granules and cell membranes (55). Along the maturation process of normal hematopoietic precursors, cells gradually change their light-scatter properties, specific FSC/SSC patterns being associated with each maturational step within an individual hematopoietic cell lineage. Leukemic cells from AML patients usually display a relatively high FSC/SSC and the presence of cells expressing lymphoid-associated antigens in this area should be considered as aberrant. In our experience, this occurs in around 2% of AML cases for CD19 and 3% for CD2. It should be noted that this specific aberrancy parallels that of cross-lineage antigen expression. In normal differentiation, the expression of stem cell markers (CD34 and CD117) is associated with relatively low/intermediate FSC/SSC values; however, in approx 3% and 2% of all AML cases, these markers are present on cells with abnormally high FSC/SSC. Finally, myeloid markers can be observed on myeloid blast cells that resemble lymphoblasts as a result of a very small FSC/SSC. This aberrant expression involved CD13 in 2% of our AML cases and CD33, and CD15 in around 1% of the cases each (see Table 2). Overall, abnormal FSC/SSC patterns aberrancies occurred in 17% of our AML patients (62).

## Phenotypic Changes

Because the strategy for the immunophenotypical detection of MRD relies mainly on the identification of residual cells with the same phenotypic aberrancies detected at diagnosis, a possible major limitation for this type of approach is the existence of phenotypic switches during the evolution of the disease. In this sense, several groups, including our own *(23,35–41)* have suggested that phenotypic changes may occur with a relatively high frequency. However, few studies have been specifically devoted to the analysis of the frequency at which these phenotypic switches affect the aberrant criteria that could, in principle, be used for the investigation of MRD during follow-up evaluation. It has been reported that a high incidence of phenotypic changes (20–70%) *(23,35–41)* can be detected in AML when large panels of monoclonal antibodies are used to compare the antigenic expression of blast cells at diagnosis and at relapse. In our AML series, the incidence of changes in individual antigens was 62% *(23)*. However, most of these phenotypic switches involve individual differentiation-associated markers (CD15, CD14, CD11b, HLA-DR), whereas changes affecting aberrant phenotypes were much less frequent, only 16% of the cases in our series *(23)*, and at least one of the aberrancies detected at diagnosis remained stable at relapse *(23)*. These findings point out the need to use not only one but all phenotypic aberrancies detected at diagnosis for the follow-up of MRD, in order to avoid false-negative results.

Two major factors may account for the variability observed in the literature with regard to the incidence of phenotypic changes in AML: (1) technical pitfalls and (2) the presence of two or more phenotypically different blast cell subpopulations at diagnosis. Regarding the first factor, the use at relapse of different reagents (i.e., new monoclonal antibodies, clones, and fluorochrome conjugates) than those employed initially at diagnosis, may generate apparent, but not real, antigenic changes. The second possible pitfall derives from the presence of more than one cell subset at diagnosis. Until now, in most reports the immunophenotypic detection of MRD has been based on the antigenic characteristics of the predominant blast cell population at diagnosis *(1,2,9,10,19,31,36–38,44,45, 52,66)*. However, it is well known that in AML, several leukemic subpopulations with different phenotypic characteristics may be present at diagnosis *(24,56)*, and perhaps a minor one may be the resistant clone that is the responsible for the relapse. In our experience, around 60% of all AML patients have two or more cell populations, at diagnosis at least one of them being small in size (<10% of all blast cells) *(24)*. These subpopulations frequently correspond to different stages of maturation of the neoplastic clone. According to this observation, the investigation of MRD should be based on the phenotypic characteristics of each subpopulation even if it was present at low frequencies at diagnosis. It is important to note that many of these cell subsets share the same phenotypic aberrancy, which would eventually facilitate MRD follow-up. In fact, in our experience in most AML cases, MRD can be investigated with just two triple-antigen staining, this usually covers the leukemic-associated phenotypes present in all different cell subpopulations identified at diagnosis.

### Sensitivity of Flow-Cytometry Immunophenotyping for MRD Detection

Flow cytometry is a well-suited technology for the identification, enumeration, and characterization of rare cells. As a matter of fact, among other applications, flow cytometry is currently used as the preferred method for the enumeration of CD34+ hematopoietic progenitor cells *(67)*, dendritic cells, and mast cells *(68,69)* in both bone marrow and peripheral-blood-derived samples. Most of the information on the sensitivity of the flow-cytometric approach used for the immunophenotypic detection of MRD has been obtained through either dilutional experiments or the capacity to identify, in patients in morphological complete remission, residual cells with the same phenotype as that displayed by the blast cells at diagnosis *(1–3,5–12,27,59,70)*. Accordingly, experiments in which leukemic cells are progressively diluted in normal peripheral blood and bone marrow samples have shown that flow cytometry is able to reliably detect cells displaying aberrant phenotypes at frequencies ranging from $10^{-5}$ to $10^{-3}$ (*see* Fig. 1). Nevertheless, it should be noted that the level of sensitivity clearly varies depending on the type of phenotypic aberrancy, the combination of monoclonal antibody reagents used for their detection, and the sample under study.

### CLINICAL VALUE OF THE IMMUNOPHENOTYPIC INVESTIGATION OF MRD IN AML

Although the information available so far on the clinical value of the immunophenotypic detection of MRD in AML is still scanty, most preliminary studies suggest that it may contribute to predict relapse and to define different patient risk-group categories at specific time-points during follow-up. Figure 2 shows an example of follow-up of MRD in an AML patient. Initial studies were based not on a three- and four-color multiparametric flow-cytometry strategy, but simply on double-marker combinations analyzed by fluorescence microscopy. Accordingly, Adriaansen et al. *(31)* and Campana et al. *(1)* investigated MRD in AML patients, based on the aberrant coexpression of terminal deoxynucleotidyl transferase (TdT) and myeloid markers (CD13/33) (cross-lineage marker expression). The criteria used to define TdT positivity at diagnosis was different in both studies, as Adriaansen et al. *(31)* included all cases that displayed more than 1% TdT$^+$ myeloid leukemic cells, but the cutoff value was much higher in the study of Campana et al. *(1)*. In this latter series, from the seven

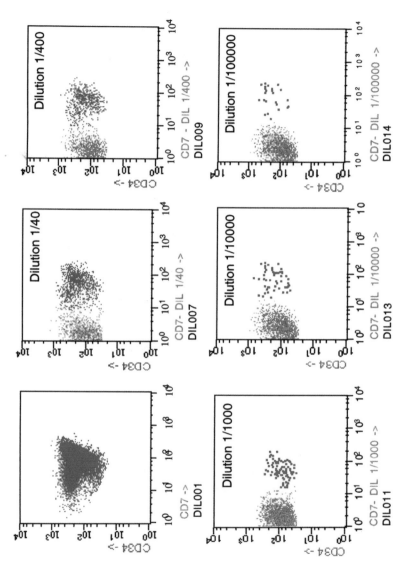

**Fig. 1.** Sensitivity of immunophenotyping for MRD detection. Serial dilutional experiments of leukemic cells (CD34+DR+) with normal BM cells were performed. The detection limit reached was 1 leukemic cell among $10^5$ normal cells ($10^{-5}$). The first plot corresponds to whole BM sample and the remaining plots correspond to CD34+-gated cells. The three plots on the bottom are shown in the highlight mode (Paint-A-Gate software program, Becton Dickinson).

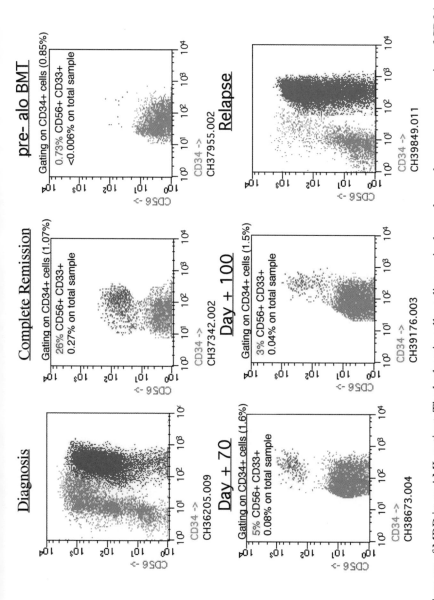

**Fig. 2.** Follow-up of MRD in an AML patient. The leukemic cells at diagnosis showed asynchronous coexpression of CD34 and CD56. A small number of residual leukemic cells were detectable during follow-up, even after allo-BMT (d +70 and +100), and the patient relapsed.

129

patients included, residual disease persisted during follow-up in four cases, all of whom subsequently relapsed; by contrast, only one of the three negative cases relapsed. In the Adriaansen et al. *(31)* series, 9 of the 10 relapses observed were preceded, over a period of 14–38 wk, by a gradual increase in the number of TdT/ CD13+ residual cells. In five additional patients who remained in continuous CR, TdT+ CD13+ blast cells were detected, but their number did not increase during follow-up. It should be noted that it has been shown that early lymphoid progenitors may coexpress the myeloid-related CD13 and CD33 markers, which could at least partially explain these latter findings *(71,72)*. In spite of this latter observation, both studies suggest that this phenotypic combination (TdT/myeloid antigen) may be very useful to predict relapse with very few false-positive results. Drach et al. *(44)* have followed three patients who also displayed cross-lineage antigen expression (CD13+CD7+) and in whom the persistence of these cells was predictive of relapse. More recently, Campana and Pui *(8)*, using multiparametric flow cytometry, have studied 13 children in CR after BMT. In four patients, residual leukemic cells were observed, and all relapsed within 2 mo after the phenotypical detection of MRD. In the remaining nine patients, leukemic cells were not detected, and seven of them remained in CR with a median follow-up of over 1 yr after transplant. The other two patients relapsed, and, according to the authors, should be considered as false-negative cases. Other reports have focused not on sequential follow-up studies, but on the analysis of the potential prognostic value of the levels of MRD detected at specific time-points of the treatment scheme, such as at the end of induction and intensification therapy. Thus, Reading et al. *(19)* have studied 16 AML patients in morphological CR using three-color stainings analyzed by flow cytometry: Six patients had more than 0.2% phenotypically aberrant cells in the first remission BM aspirate obtained following induction therapy, and all relapsed between 1 and 7 mo latter. Conversely, in the 10 patients with less than 0.2% aberrant cells, only 1 relapsed during the follow-up period. These findings are consistent with those of Wörman et al. *(45)*, who have also quantitated the number of residual cells in a series of 45 adult AML patients. In two-thirds of these cases, more than 0.5% phenotypically aberrant cells were detected in the first CR bone marrow sample, and half of these patients relapsed within 1 yr. As far as our own experience is concerned, we initially reported on a series of 53 AML patients who entered into morphological complete remission (mCR) following induction therapy and displayed an aberrant phenotype at diagnosis, allowing for MRD follow-up *(27)*. In this study, we observed that patients with $\geq 5 \times 10^{-3}$ residual cells with a leukemic-associated phenotype (LAP+) in the BM sample in mCR obtained after induction therapy showed a significant higher relapse rate (67% vs 20% for patients with less than $5 \times 10^{-3}$ LAP+ cells; $p = 0.002$) and a lower median relapse-free survival (17 mo vs not reached; $p = 0,01$). At the end of intensification therapy, the number of residual LAP+ cells slightly decreased, and, accordingly, a reduced cutoff value of LAP+ cells was used ($2 \times 10^{-3}$ cells) for the discrimination of the two AML risk groups with relapse rates of 69% versus 32%, respectively ($p = 0.02$). Interestingly, we also analyzed which one of the two time-points explored (BM after induction or after intensification therapy) was more informative in terms of relapse prediction. Our results show a high degree of concordance once the MRD levels at both time-points are compared, because all except two patients with high and low MRD levels after intensification therapy corresponded to the same cases identified as high and low risk in the postinduction BM. Accordingly, the analysis of the first BM in mCR immediately after induction therapy should be the first choice in terms of clinical applicability, because it already allows the discrimination of different patient risk groups, which could contribute either to individualize or to stratify postinduction treatment in AML patients. Furthermore, we explored whether residual disease was related with the functional expression of multidrug resistance (MDR-1) at diagnosis. Patients with high rhodamine-123 efflux displayed significantly higher levels of residual leukemic cells, probably reflecting that immunophenotypical detection of MRD represents an "ex vivo" test for drug resistance.

More recently, we have expanded the investigation of MRD to a series of 126 consecutive AML patients who displayed aberrant phenotypes at diagnosis and achieved mCR with induction therapy *(62)*. Current results confirm the clinical value of these immunophenotypical studies. Accordingly, four different risk group categories can be established based on the level of MRD found in the BM in morphological CR obtained after induction therapy: patients at very low risk of relapse ($<10^{-4}$ LAP+ cells), at low risk ($10^{-4}$–$10^{-3}$ LAP+ cells), at intermediate risk ($10^{-3}$–$10^{-2}$ LAP+ cells), and at high risk ($>10^{-2}$ LAP+ cells) with a cumulative incidence of relapses at 3 yr of 0%, 14%, 50%, and 84%, respectively. It should be mentioned that the adverse prognostic influence of having high levels of MRD after induction therapy was also observed when M3 and non-M3 leukemias were analyzed separately. Moreover, high levels of MRD were associated with some of the most relevant prognostic factors identified in AML, such as adverse cytogenetics subtypes, the need for two or more cycles of chemotherapy to achieve mCR, and both high white blood cell (WBC) and blast cell counts at diagnosis. In spite of these associations, multivariate analysis showed that the level of MRD detected by immunophenotypic flow-cytometry techniques was the most powerful independent prognostic factor for predicting both disease-free survival and overall survival in AML *(62)*. This finding is of particular interest for clinical practice because, at present, the only relevant factors for risk stratification of AML are cytogenetics and morphologic evaluation of response to induction therapy. However, this latter parameter is of limited value because it only identifies a subgroup of patients with a very bad prognosis: those who fail to achieve morphological CR; by contrast, information provided by morphology within those patients who enter into mCR is not really relevant, because although some of these patients will remain in continuous CR, many others will relapse. Therefore, more sensitive techniques for a more precise assessment of the magnitude of the response to induction therapy are needed and, according to our results, multiparametric immunophenotypic investigation of MRD by flow cytometry could represent a very useful tool for the management of AML patients who achieve mCR after induction therapy.

## REFERENCES

1. Campana D, Coustan-Smith E, and Janossy G. The immunologic detection of minimal residual disease in acute leukemia, *Blood*, **76** (1990) 163–174.
2. van Dongen JJM, Breit TM, Adriaansen HJ, Boishuizen A, and Hooijkaas H. Detection of minimal residual disease in acute leukemia by immunological marker analysis and polymerase chain reaction, *Leukemia*, **6(Suppl. 1)** (1992) 47–59.
3. van Dongen JJM and San Miguel JF. Techniques for detection of minimal residual disease in leukaemia patients, in *Meet the Expert Sessions of the Second EHA*, Oxford: Blackwell Science, 1996, pp. 39–46.
4. Lo Coco C, Divorsio D, Pandolfi PD, et al. Molecular evaluation of residual disease as a predictor of relapse in acute promyelocytic leukemia, *Lancet*, **340** (1992) 1437–1438.
5. Campana D, Otubo Freitas R, and Coustan-Smith E. Detection of residual leukemia with immunologic methods: Technical developments and clinical implications, *Leuk. Lymphoma*, **13(Suppl. 1)** (1994) 31–34.
6. Orfao A, Ciudad J, Lopez-Berges MC, Lopez A, Vidriales B, Caballero MD, et al. Acute lymphoblastic leukemia (ALL): detection of minimal residual disease (MRD) at flow cytometry, *Leuk. Lymphoma.*, **13(Suppl. 1)** (1994) 87–90.
7. Nowak R, Oelschlaegel U, Schuler U, Zengler H, Hofmann R, Ehninger G, et al. Sensitivity of combined DNA/immunophenotype flow cytometry for the detection of low levels of aneuploid lymphoblastic leukemia cells in bone marrow, *Cytometry*, **30** (1997) 47–53.
8. Campana D and Pui CH. Detection of minimal residual disease in acute leukemia: methodologic advances and clinical significance, *Blood*, **85** (1995) 1416–1434.
9. Sievers EL, Lange BJ, Buckley JD, Smith FO, Wells DA, Daigneault-Creech CA, et al. Prediction of relapse of pediatric acute myeloid leukemia by use of multidimensional flow cytometry, *J. Natl. Cancer Inst.*, **88** (1996) 1483–1488.
10. Sievers EL and Loken M. Detection of minimal residual disease in acute myelogenous leukemia, *J. Pediatr. Hematol. Oncol.*, **17** (1995) 123–133.
11. Van Dongen JJM and San Miguel JF. Methods of detection of minimal residual disease, in *Acute Leukemias VI Prognostic Factors and Treatment Strategies*. Büchner T, Hiddenmann W, Wörman B, et al. (eds). Berlin: Springer-Verlag, 1997, pp. 307–312.
12. Campana D and Coustan-Smith E. Detection of minimal residual disease in acute leukemia by flow cytometry, *Cytometry*, **38(4)** (1999) 139–152.
13. Ciudad J, San Miguel JF, Lopez-Berges MC, Garcia Marcos MA, Gonzalez M, Vazquez L, et al. Detection of abnormalities in B-cell differentiation pattern is a useful tool to predict relapse in precursor-B-ALL, *Br. J. Haematol.*, **104** (1999) 695–705.
14. Ciudad J, San Miguel JF, López-Berges MC, Valverde B, Vidriales B, López A, et al. Immunophenotypic detection of minimal residual disease (MDR) in acute lymphoblastic leukaemia (ALL), in *Acute Leukemias VI: Prognostic Factors and Treatment Strategies*. Büchner T, Hiddenmann W, Wörman B, et al. (eds). Berlin: Springer-Verlag, 1997, pp. 321–327.
15. Weir EG, Cowan K, LeBeau P, and Borowitz MJ. A limited antibody panel can distinguish B-precursor acute lymphoblastic leukemia from normal B precursors with four color flow cytometry: implications for residual disease detection, *Leukemia*, **13** (1999) 558–567.

16. Lucio P, Parreira A, van den Beemd MW, van Lochem EG, van Wering ER, Baars E, et al. Flow cytometric analysis of normal B cell differentiation: a frame of reference for the detection of minimal residual disease in precursor-B-ALL, *Leukemia*, **13** (1999) 419–427.
17. Porwit-MacDonald A, Bjorklund E, Lucio P, van Lochem EG, Mazur J, Parreira A, et al. BIOMED-1 concerted action report: flow cytometric characterization of CD7+ cell subsets in normal bone marrow as a basis for the diagnosis and follow-up of T cell acute lymphoblastic leukemia (T-ALL), *Leukemia*, **14** (2000) 816–825.
18. Ross CW, Stoolman LM, Schnitzer B, Schlegelmilch JA, and Hanson CA. Immunophenotypic aberrancy in adult acute lymphoblastic leukemia, *Am. J. Clin. Pathol.*, **94** (1990) 590–599.
19. Reading CL, Estey EH, Huh YO, Claxton DF, Sánchez G, Terstappen LWMM, et al. Expression of unusual immunophenotype combinations in acute myelogenous leukemia, *Blood*, **81** (1993) 3083–3090.
20. Harada N, Kawano MM, Huang N, Harada Y, Iwato K, Tanabe O, et al. Phenotypic differences of normal plasma cells from mature myeloma cells, *Blood*, **81** (1993) 2658–2663.
21. Campana D and Coustan-Smith E. The use of flow cytometry to detect minimal residual disease in acute leukemia, *Eur. J. Histochem.*, **40(Suppl. 1)** (1996) 39–42.
22. Macedo A, Orfao A, Vidriales MB, Lopez-Berges C, Valverde B, González M, et al. Characterization of aberrant phenotypes in acute myeloblastic leukemia, *Ann. Hematol.*, **70** (1995) 189–194.
23. Macedo A, San Miguel JF, Vidriales MB, Lopez-Berges C, García Marcos MA, González M, et al. Phenotypic changes in acute myeloid leukaemia: implications in the detection of minimal residual disease, *J. Clin. Pathol.*, **49** (1996) 15–18.
24. Macedo A, Orfao A, Gonzalez M, Vidriales MB, López-Berges MC, Martínez A, et al. Immunological detection of blast cell subpopulations in acute myeloblastic leukemia at diagnosis: implications for minimal residual disease studies, *Leukemia*, **9** (1995) 993–998.
25. Macedo A, Orfao A, Martinez A, Vidriales MB, Valverde B, Lopez-Berges MC, et al. Immunophenotype of c-kit cells in normal human bone marrow: implications for the detection of minimal residual disease in AML, *Br. J. Haematol.*, **89** (1995) 338–341.
26. Ciudad J, Orfao A, Vidriales B, Macedo A, Martinez A, Gonzalez M, et al. Immunophenotypic analysis of CD19+ precursors in normal human adult bone marrow: implications for minimal residual disease detection, *Haematologica*, **83** (1998) 1069–1075.
27. San Miguel JF, Martínez A, Macedo A, Vidriales MB, López-Berges C, González M, et al. Immunophenotyping investigation of MRD is a useful approach for predicting relapse in AML patients, *Blood*, **90** (1997) 2465–2470.
28. Coustan-Smith E, Behm FG, Hurwitz CA, Rivera GK, and Campana D. N-CAM (CD56) expression by CD34+ malignant myeloblasts has implications for minimal residual disease detection in acute myeloid leukemia, *Leukemia*, **7** (1993) 853–858.
29. Yin L. Detection of minimal residual disease in acute myeloid leukemia: methodologies, clinical and biological significance, *Br. J. Haematol.*, **106** (1999) 578–590.
30. Gore SD, Kastan MB, Goodman SN, and Civin CI. Detection of minimal residual T cell acute lymphoblastic leukemia by flow cytometry, *J. Immunol. Methods*, **132(2)** (1990) 275–286.
31. Adriaansen HJ, Jacobs BC, Kappers-Klunne MC, Hählen K, Hooijkaas H, and van Dongen JJM. Detection of residual disease in AML patients by use of double immunological marker analysis for terminal deoxynucleotidyl transferase and myeloid markers, *Leukemia*, **7** (1993) 472–481.
32. Coustan-Smith E, Behm FG, Sanchez J, Boyett JM, Hancock ML, Raimondi SC, et al. Immunological detection of minimal residual disease in children with acute lymphoblastic leukaemia, *Lancet*, **351** (1998) 550–554.
33. Behm FG, Smith FO, Raimondi SC, Pui CH, and Bernstein ID. Human homologue of the rat chondroitin sulfate proteoglycan, NG2, detected by monoclonal antibody 7.1, identifies childhood acute lymphoblastic leukemias with t(4;11)(q21;q23) or t(11;19)(q23;p13) and MLL gene rearrangements, *Blood*, **87** (1996) 1134–1139.

34. Smith FO, Rauch C, Williams DE, March CJ, Arthur D, Hilden J, et al. The human homologue of rat NG2, a chondroitin sulfate proteoglycan, is not expressed on the cell surface of normal hematopoietic cells but is expressed by acute myeloid leukemia blasts from poor-prognosis patients with abnormalities of chromosome band 11q23, *Blood*, **87** (1996) 1123–1133.

35. Abshire TC, Buchanan GR, Jackson JF, Shuster JJ, Brock B, Head D, et al. Morphologic, immunologic and cytogenetic studies in children with acute lymphoblastic leukemia at diagnosis and relapse: a Pediatric Oncology Group study, *Leukemia*, **6** (1992) 357–362.

36. Thomas X, Campos L, Archimbaud E, Shi ZH, Treille-Ritouet D, Anglaret B, et al. Surface marker expression in acute myeloid leukaemia at first relapse, *Br. J. Haematol.*, **81** (1992) 40–44.

37. Peters RE, Janossy G, Ivory K, Al-Ismail S, and Mercolino T. Leukemia associated changes identified by quantitative flow cytometry. III. B-cell gating in CD37/kappa/lambda clonality test, *Leukemia*, **8** (1994) 1864–1870.

38. Lavabre-Bertrand T, Janossy G, Ivory K, Peters R, Secker-Walkers L, and Porwith-MacDonald A. Leukemia associated changes identified by quantitative flow cytometry. I CD10 expression, *Cytometry*, **18** (1994) 209–217.

39. Chucrallah AE, Stass SA, Huh YO, Albitar M, and Kantarjian HM. Adults acute lymphoblastic Leukemia at relapse. Cytogenetic, immunophenotypic, and molecular changes, *Cancer*, **76** (1995) 985–991.

40. van Wering ER, Beishuizen A, Roeffen ET, van der Linden-Schrever BE, Verhoeven MA, Hahlen K, et al. Immunophenotypic changes between diagnosis and relapse in childhood acute lymphoblastic leukemia, *Leukemia*, **9** (1995) 1523–1533.

41. Guglielmi C, Cordone I, Boecklin F, Masi S, Valentini T, Vegna ML, et al. Immunophenotype of adult and childhood acute lymphoblastic leukemia: changes at first relapse and clinicoprognostic implications, *Leukemia*, **11(9)** (1997) 1501–1507.

42. Drexler HG, Thield E, and Ludwig WD. Review of the incidence and clinical relevance of myeloid antigen-positive acute lymphoblastic leukemia, *Leukemia*, **5** (1991) 637–645.

43. Kurec AS, Bealir P, Stefanu C, Barret DM, Dubowy RL, and Davey FR. Significance of aberrant immunophenotypes in childhood acute lymphoid leukemia, *Cancer*, **67** (1991) 3081–3086.

44. Drach J, Drach D, Glassl H, Gattringer C, and Huber H. Flow cytometric determination of atypical antigen expression in acute leukemia for the study of minimal residual disease, *Cytometry*, **13** (1992) 893–901.

45. Wörman B, Griesinger F, Innig G, et al. Detection of residual leukemic cells in patients with acute myeloid leukemia based on cell surface antigen expression, *Sangre*, **37(Suppl. 3)** (1992) 133–135.

46. Lauria F, Raspadori D, Martinelli G, Rondelli D, Ventura MA, Farabegoli P, et al. Increased expression of myeloid antigen markers in adult acute lymphoblastic leukaemia patients: diagnostic and prognostic implications, *Br. J. Haematol.*, **87** (1994) 286–292.

47. Lamkin T, Brooks J, Annett G, Roberts W, and Weinberg K. Immunophenotypic differences between putative hematopoietic stem cells and childhood B-cell precursor acute lymphoblastic leukemia cells, *Leukemia*, **8** (1994) 1871–1878.

48. Ludwig WD, Reiter A, Loffler H, Gokbuget Hoelzer D, Riehm H, and Thiel E. Immunophenotypic features of childhood and adult acute lymphoblastic leukemia (ALL): experience of the German Multicentre Trials ALL-BFM and GMALL, *Leuk. Lymphoma*, **13(Suppl. 1)** (1994) 71–76.

49. Boldt DH, Kopecky KJ, Head D, Gehly G, Radich JP, and Appelbaum FR. Expression of myeloid antigens by blast cells in acute lymphoblastic leukemia of adults. The Southwest Oncology Group experience, *Leukemia*, **8** (1994) 2118–2126.

50. Preti HA, Huh YO, O'Brien SM, Andreeff M, Pierce ST, Keating M, et al. Myeloid markers in adult acute lymphocytic leukemia. Correlations with patient and disease characteristics and with prognosis, *Cancer*, **76** (1995) 1564–1570.

51. Borowitz MJ, Shuster J, Carroll AJ, Nash M, Look AT, Camitta B, et al. Prognostic signifi-cance of fluorescence intensity of surface marker expression in childhood B-precursor acute lymphoblastic leukemia. A Pediatric Oncology Group Study, *Blood*, **89** (1997) 3960–3966.
52. Casasnovas RO, Campos L, Mugneret F, Charrin C, Bene MC, Garand R, et al. Immuno-phenotypic patterns and cytogenetic anomalies in acute non-lymphoblastic leukemia sub-types: a prospective study of 432 patients, *Leukemia*, **12** (1998) 34–43.
53. Orfao A, Almeida J, Sánchez ML, Sánchez-Guijo FM, Vallejo C, López-Berges MC, et al. Incidence of aberrant phenotypes in a large series of B-cell chronic lymphoproliferative dis-orders: Implications for minimal residual disease, *Cytometry*, **(Suppl. 9)** (1998) 53 (abstract).
54. Ocqueteau M, Orfão A, Almeida J, Bladé J, González M, García-Sanz R, et al. Immuno-phenotypic characterization of plasma cells from monoclonal gammopathy of undetermined significance (MGUS) patients. Implications for the differential diagnosis between MGUS and multiple myeloma, *Am. J. Pathol.*, **152** (1998) 1655–1665.
55. Terstappen LW, Mickaels RA, Dost R, and Loken MR. Increased light scattering resolution facilitates multidimensional flow cytometry analysis, *Cytometry*, **11** (1990) 506.
56. Terstappen LWMM, Safford M, Konemann S, et al. Flow cytometric characterization of acute myeloid leukemia. Part II. Phenotypic heterogeneity at diagnosis, *Leukemia*, **5** (1992) 757–767.
57. Orfao A, Schmitz G, Brando B, Ruiz-Arguelles A, Basso G, Braylan R, et al. For the standard-ization committee on clinical flow cytometry of the internal federation of clinical chemistry. Clinically useful information provided by the flow cytometric immunophenotyping of hemato-logical malignancies: current status and future directions, *Clin. Chem.*, **45** (1999) 1708–1717.
58. San Miguel JF, González M, and Orfao A. Minimal residual disease in myeloid malignancies, in *Textbook of Malignant Haematology*. Linch LH and Löwenberg B (eds). London: Martin Dunitz, 1999, pp. 871–891.
59. San Miguel JF, Almeida J, Ocqueteau M, Mateo G, Caballero MD, García-Sanz R, et al. Immunophenotyping and DNA ploidy analysis for detection of minimal residual disease in MM, *Cancer Res. Ther. Control*, **6** (1998) 299–302.
60. Martinez A, San Miguel JF, Vidriales B, Ciudad J, Caballero MD, López-Berges MC, et al. An abnormal CD34+ myeloid/ CD34+ lymphoid ratio at the end of chemotherapy predict relapse in patients with acute myeloid leukemia, *Cytometry*, **38** (1998) 70–75.
61. Howard MR and Reid MM. Expression of myeloid antigens in acute lymphoblastic leukaemia, *Br. J. Haematol.*, **88** (1994) 897–898.
62. San Miguel JF, Vidriales MB, López-Berges MC, Díaz-Mediavilla J, Gutiérrez N, Cañizo C, et al. Early immunophenotypical evaluation of minimal residual disease (MRD) in AML identifies different patient risk-groups and may contribute to post-induction treatment strati-fication, *Blood*, **98** (2001) 1746–1751.
63. Loken MR, Shah VO, Dattilio KL, and Civin CI. Flow cytometric analysis of human bone marrow. II. Normal B lymphocyte development, *Blood*, **70** (1987) 1316–1324.
64. Terstappen LW, Safford M, Unterhalt M, Konemann S, Zurlutter K, Piechotka K, et al. Flow cytometric characterization of acute myeloid leukemia: IV. Comparison to the differentiation pathway of normal hematopoietic progenitor cells, *Leukemia*, **6** (1992) 993–1000.
65. Del Vecchio L, Finizio O, Lo Pardo C, Pane N, Schiavone EM, Vacca C, et al. Co-ordinate expression of T-cell antigens on acute myelogenous leukemia and of myeloid antigens on T-acute lymphoblastic leukemia. Speculation on a highly balanced bilinearity), *Leukemia*, **5** (1991) 815–818.
66. Drexler HG, Thield E, and Ludwing WD. Acute myeloid leukemias expressing lymphoid-associated antigens: diagnostic incidence and prognostic significance, *Leukemia*, **7** (1993) 489–498.
67. Gratama JW, Orfao A, Barnett D, Brando B, Huber A, Janossy G, et al. Flow cytometric enumeration of CD34+ hematopoietic stem and progenitor cells. European Working Group on Clinical Cell Analysis, *Cytometry*, **34** (1998) 128–142.

68. Almeida J, Bueno C, Alguero MC, Sanchez ML, Canizo MC, Fernandez ME, et al. Extensive characterization of the immunophenotype and pattern of cytokine production by distinct subpopulations of normal human peripheral blood MHC II+/lineage-cells, *Clin. Exp. Immunol.*, **118** (1999) 392–401.

69. Escribano L, Orfao A, Villarrubia J, Diaz-Agustin B, Cervero C, Rios A, et al. Immunophenotypic characterization of human bone marrow mast cells. A flow cytometric study of normal and pathological bone marrow samples, *Anal. Cell Pathol.*, **16(3)** (1998) 151–159.

70. San Miguel JF, Ciudad J, Vidriales MB, Orfao A, Lucio P, Porwith MacDonald A, et al. Immunophenotypical detection of minimal residual disease in acute leukemia, *Crit. Rev. Oncol. Hematol.*, **32** (1999) 175–185.

71. Uckun FM. Regulation of normal B-cell ontogeny, *Blood*, **76** (1990) 1908–1923.

72. Tjonnfjord GE, Steen R, Veiby OP, Morkrid L, and Egeland T. Haematopoietic progenitor cell differentiation: flow cytometric assessment in bone marrow and tymus, *Br. J. Haematol.*, **91** (1995) 1006–1016.

# 9

# Minimal Residual Disease in Acute Myeloid Leukemia

*RT-PCR–Based Studies of Fusion Transcripts*

## Guido Marcucci and Michael A. Caligiuri

## INTRODUCTION

Acute myeloid leukemia (AML) is a biologically heterogeneous disease of the hematopoietic system characterized by a clonal accumulation of immature myeloid cells in the bone marrow. The management of this disease is clinically complex, with only approx 40% of the patients treated with conventional or high-dose chemotherapy reaching a long-term complete remission (CR). Nonrandom chromosomal abnormalities are identified at the cytogenetic level in approx 55% of all adult primary or *de novo* AML patients and have long been recognized as important independent prognostic indicators for the achievement of CR, duration of first CR, and survival following intensive chemotherapy treatment *(1,2)*. Among these recurrent aberrations, chromosome translocations and inversions often result in genomic structural rearrangements leading to the creation of chimeric fusion genes that, in turn, encode fusion transcripts readily detected in bone marrow (BM) and blood by highly sensitive molecular techniques such as the reverse transcription–polymerase chain reaction (RT-PCR). Because the fusion transcripts are thought to be specific to the leukemic cells, their detection in BM or blood from AML patients who achieve CR following intensive treatment has been used as a surrogate marker for minimal residual disease (MRD) *(3–5)*. It was anticipated that those patients with a positive assay would inevitably relapse as a consequence of the treatment failure to completely eradicate the leukemogenic clone, whereas those patients with a negative RT-PCR status would remain in continuous CR (CCR). Although this strategy has been relatively successful in predicting clinical outcome in chronic myeloid leukemia (CML) and acute promyelocytic leukemia (APL), its prognostic use in other

From: *Leukemia and Lymphoma: Detection of Minimal Residual Disease*
Edited by: T. F. Zipf and D. A. Johnston © Humana Press Inc., Totowa, NJ

types of myeloid leukemia has yet to prove useful *(6,7)*. In some cases, in fact, detection of minimal residual disease (MRD) during CR is not indicative of impending relapse, and chimeric transcripts have been found in patients with long-term clinical remission and in normal healthy individuals *(8,9)*. Similarly, a BM or blood sample deemed negative for MRD on the basis of an undetectable fusion transcript invariably has not been predictive of long-term remission. These data support the notion that different molecular subgroups of AML may have a diversified biology, and in some cases, persistence of chimeric clones following aggressive treatment is compatible with normal hematopoiesis. At the same time, it is important to underscore that a positive or negative result by RT-PCR in remission samples may not be the mere reflection of the presence or absence, respectively, of a target transcript, but may also depend on the experimental conditions used to develop the assay. Thus, the use of a very sensitive RT-PCR capable of detecting 1 leukemic cell in $10^5$–$10^6$ normal cells demands several precautions to avoid the potentials for cross-contamination, leading to false-positive results. On the other hand, an RT-PCR assay with an inferior level of sensitivity may fail to detect a small but potentially important residual tumor burden, leading to false-negative results. In this chapter, we discuss the applicability of MRD analysis by RT-PCR to the clinical management of AML patients in remission, exemplifying advantages and limitations of this strategy in the context of specific molecular subgroups of AML.

## CORE-BINDING FACTOR AML

Translocation (8;21)(q22;q22) and inversion or translocation of chromosome 16 [inv(16)(p13q22) or t(16;16)(p13;q22)] are among the most common cytogenetic aberrations found in patients with AML and are generally associated with the most favorable prognosis *(10)*. These abnormalities result in the disruption of genes encoding subunits of the core-binding factor (CBF), an heterodimeric transcriptional factor involved in the regulation of normal hematopoiesis. In almost all studies of adult primary AML, t(8;21) and inv(16) or t(16;16), here referred to as CBF AML, have been associated with the highest CR rate (approx 90%) and the longest disease-free survival (DFS) at 5 yr (approx 60%) *(1,10)*. These favorable results could be achieved with incorporation of high-dose ARA-C (HiDAC) into the consolidation treatment, as shown in a recent CALGB analysis (CALGB study 8695) *(11)*. In this study, patients with t(8;21) or abnormalities of chromosome 16 treated with HiDAC therapy showed a better DFS and overall survival (OS) when compared to patients with the same cytogenetic abnormalities but treated with lower doses of ARA-C, or compared to patients with no or other cytogenetic abnormalities. A similar favorable impact of the CBF gene rearrangements on clinical outcome was also found in the setting of bone marrow transplantation (BMT) *(11a)*. Despite these favorable treatment results, however, a subgroup of patients with CBF AML are destined to relapse, and implementation of strategies that have the potential to predict clinical outcome during remission are highly desirable.

## MRD STUDIES IN t(8;21) AML

The t(8;21)(q22;q22) is a balanced translocation between chromosomes 8 and 21. At the molecular level, this genomic abnormality results in the fusion of the *AML1* gene on chromosome 21q22 with the *ETO* gene on chromosome 8q22 *(12)*. A novel chimeric gene, *AML1/ETO*, created on the derivative chromosome 8, encodes the *AML1/ETO* fusion transcript that is readily amplified by RT-PCR *(13)*. Detection of the *AML1/ETO* fusion transcript in remission samples has been used in several studies to define the risk for relapse and the probability to continue in CR.

Using a highly sensitive RT-PCR assay with the ability to detect 1 malignant cell in $10^5$–$10^6$ normal cells, several groups have reported detection of the *AML1/ETO* fusion transcript in patients in early or long-term CR. Nucifora et al., for example, analyzed six t(8;21) AML patients by RT-PCR during various stages of their disease *(14)*. Three patients in early CR (1–4 mo) were found positive for the *AML1/ETO* fusion transcript. Two of these patients subsequently relapsed, whereas the third patient was alive and in CCR at 70 mo from remission. The *AML1/ETO* fusion transcript was also detected in blood samples from three additional patients in CCR for 83–94 mo. Chang et al. described three patients in CR with blood and BM samples positive for the *AML1/ETO* fusion transcript at 1–5 yr from diagnosis, and other authors have also reported patients in CR with positive RT-PCR following high-dose chemotherapy and autologous BMT (ABMT) *(15,16)*. Finally, the inability to completely eradicate the *AML1/ETO*-positive clone despite a successful treatment was also demonstrated in the setting of allogeneic BMT (alloBMT). We reported on 10 patients with t(8;21) AML who received alloBMT in either first or second remission or first or second relapse *(8)*. A variety of myeloablative regimens were used. Five patients developed acute and/or chronic graft versus host disease (GvHD). The furthest remission time-points analyzed for the *AML1/ETO* fusion transcript in these 10 patients ranged from 7.5 to 83.0 mo after alloBMT. The *AML1/ETO* fusion transcript was detected by RT-PCR in 9 of the 10 patients: 8 were positive in BM and 1 was negative in BM, but positive in blood. The *AML1/ETO* fusion transcript could not be detected in a BM sample from the remaining patient at 7.5 mo after alloBMT, but the amount of RNA available for analysis was deemed suboptimal. Similarly, Sanders et al. described a patient with t(8;21) AML who was found positive for the *AML1/ETO* fusion transcript in BM and blood at 18 mo following alloBMT performed in first CR (CR1) *(17)*.

In contrast with these data, other groups have reported patients who achieved RT-PCR-negative status following conventional chemotherapy or alloBMT. Sataka et al., for example, reported an undetectable *AML1/ETO* fusion transcript during remission in five patients at 52–198 mo following chemotherapy and in 1 patient at 61 mo following alloBMT *(18)*. Miyamoto et al. found that, although the *AML1/ETO* fusion transcript was detectable by RT-PCR in remission BM or blood from 18 patients treated with conventional chemotherapy, it was undetectable in 4 patients in CCR following alloBMT *(19)*. More recently, Elmaacagli et al. reported a series of patients with t(8;21) AML who underwent alloBMT *(20)*. Three of the five patients who were initially positive for the *AML1/ETO* fusion transcript by RT-PCR converted to negative test at 6, 9, and 30 mo following alloBMT and continued in CR. Two patients who were repeatedly positive for the *AML1/ETO* transcript instead relapsed. Finally, Morschhauser reported a retrospective analysis of five patients treated with alloBMT *(21)*. Three patients were transplanted in CR1 and two in second CR (CR2). All of these patients tested negative for the *AML1/ETO* fusion transcript in both BM and blood between 38 and 120 mo during remission. These same authors also prospectively studied eight additional t(8;21) AML patients who received alloBMT in CR1. Of the eight patients, three relapsed and five continued in CR. All three patients who relapsed remained positive for the *AML1/ETO* fusion transcript between 3 and 12 mo after transplantation. The five CCR patients instead tested negative between 6 and 50 mo after transplantation. Among patients transplanted in CR2, one was positive at 8 mo and relapsed, whereas three with positive BM samples died with no evidence of disease (NED) as a consequence of therapy-related toxicity. Only one patient continued in CR despite testing positive in BM at 12 mo; in this patient, the *AML1/ETO* fusion transcript became undetectable in blood at 15 mo following transplantation.

In the same study, the authors evaluated the predictive value of a negative or positive RT-PCR result in a total of 51 patients with t(8;21) AML by using two different assays, a nested RT-PCR with a sensitivity of $10^{-6}$ and a one-step RT-PCR with a sensitivity of $10^{-5}$ *(21)*. Patients who converted to RT-PCR negativity by the one-step assay (60%) or by both assays (48%) after treatment had a longer CR duration than those with a persistently positive RT-PCR status (two-sided log-rank test, $p = 0.0001$). Patients who became RT-PCR negative by the one-step assay before intensive consolidation (23%) had a lower relapse rate (11% vs 72%) and a longer CR duration than those who remained persistently RT-PCR positive at the same time-points (two-sided log-rank test, $p = 0.0015$). The authors concluded that in patients with t(8;21) AML, RT-PCR negativity can be achieved. Moreover, a negative RT-PCR result correlated well with decreased risk for disease relapse. Early conversion to a negative result before consolidation treatment seemed to carry an especially good prognosis, suggesting that RT-PCR analysis could be helpful in assessing therapy response and stratify patients to a different type of consolidation strategy according to the risk for relapse. However, it is to be noted that a negative result was more likely to be achieved with the one-step assay and a positive result with the nested RT-PCR. This disparity was likely to be related to the one-order difference in the sensitivity between the two assays. Furthermore, despite achieving RT-PCR negativity, a significant number of patients eventually relapsed, underscoring how a negative result does not necessarily mean eradication of the leukemogenic clone, but simply indicates a residual blast population below the detectable limit of the assay utilized. Nevertheless, the data reported by Morschhauser et al. suggest a very good correlation between molecular status and clinical outcome using the less sensitive one-step RT-PCR, which may be preferable to the nested RT-PCR because of its simplicity, a lower risk of contamination, and a lower cost. Interestingly, these results are similar to those obtained in other molecular subgroups of AML, such as the *PML/RARα* acute promyelocytic leukemia. In this context, a positive or negative result in remission sample by an RT-PCR assay with a sensitivity of $10^{-4}$ correlated well with risk of relapse or probability to remain in CCR, respectively *(22)*. In contrast, the presence or absence of a positive RT-PCR loses its clinical usefulness when an assay with a higher level of sensitivity is used, as suggested by Tobal et al., who detected the *PML/RARα* fusion transcript or its reciprocal *RARα/PML* in patients in long-term CR *(23)*.

Although a reduced sensitivity may improve the clinical usefulness of the MRD analysis by RT-PCR, it is also necessary to underscore the potential risks for false-negative results that occur in this context. Variation in the sensitivity of the RT-PCR assay or in the amount and the source of the starting material (i.e., BM vs blood) was shown to have a profound impact on the probability of obtaining a positive result. In our hands, for example, the sensitivity for a nested RT-PCR assay changed with individual reactions on the basis of the amount of RNA used in the reverse-transcription step *(8)*. Using 0.5 μg of total cellular RNA isolated from a *AML1/ETO*-positive Kasumi-1 cell line:*AML1/ETO*-negative K562 cell line dilutions of $1:10^5$ or $1:10^6$, the *AML1/ETO* fusion transcript could be detected in 89% or 29% of the RT-PCR amplifications, respectively. However, if the RNA amount isolated from $1:10^6$ Kasumi-1:K562 dilution was increased from 0.5 to 1.0. μg, a positive result was obtained in 78% of the RT-PCR amplifications, suggesting that detection of the *AML1/ETO* fusion transcript depends not only on the presence of MRD but also on the absolute number of transcript copies in the sample analyzed. In light of these results, we have, therefore, proposed that the following conditions should be applied to the analysis of remission samples from patients with t(8;21)AML: (1) three independent PCR amplifications using 2.0 μg of total cellular RNA per reaction, (2) coamplification of a housekeeping gene used as an internal control for each reaction; (3) a sensitivity for detection of the *AML1/ETO* transcript of at least $10^{-5}$ performed simultaneously in all three independent PCR amplifications, and (4) PCR amplification to be performed on both blood and BM. Using these criteria uniformly, it would be possible on the basis of a negative RT-PCR assay to score a remission sample as "truly" negative.

Finally, with regard to a persistent RT-PCR positivity in patients in long-term remission, more recent studies appear to support the inability of the currently available treatments to eradicate residual *AML1/ETO*-positive clones. Saunders et al., for instance, were able to demonstrate by RT-PCR that the *AML1/ETO* fusion gene is expressed in colony-forming cells of granulocyte–macrophage originated from remission BM samples of patients with t(8;21) AML in long-term CR after chemotherapy or BMT *(24)*. These results were confirmed by Miaymoto et al., who demonstrated that *AML1/ETO* fusion transcripts were present in a fraction of stem cells, monocytes, and B-cells from BM of t(8;21) AML patients in remission *(25)*. The *AML1/ETO* fusion transcripts were also detected in a fraction of colony-forming cells of erythroid, granulocyte–macrophage, and/or megakaryocyte lineages originated from the same samples. Both of these studies, therefore, strongly suggest that persistence of residual *AML1/ETO*-positive stem cells in BM is compatible with long-term CR. It is unlikely, however, that these precursors have the ability to produce a leukemic phenotype without the occurrence of additional genomic mutations, as supported by recent studies in *AML1/ETO* transgenic mice, where malignant growth resembling granulocytic sarcoma develops only when the animals are treated with additional mutagenic agents *(26)*.

## QUANTITATIVE RT-PCR FOR t(8;21) AML

Based on the current data, it is becoming clear that the use of MRD detection by RT-PCR to predict clinical outcome in t(8;21) AML is not straightforward and that, ultimately, it may be difficult to assign broad criteria to predict relapse or cure only on the basis of a positive or negative result in this group of patients. Therefore, we and others have recently tested the hypothesis that quantification of the *AML1/ETO* fusion transcripts during CR could be more useful than a qualitative assay to estimate the burden of the residual clonal cell population and, ultimately, to identify a critical level of MRD predictive of cure or relapse *(27–29)*. In the initial studies that used this strategy, calculation of levels of chimeric fusion transcripts was performed by quantitative competitive RT-PCR (QcRT-PCR) *(28,30)*. This is a method that uses a known amount of competitor cDNA, slightly different in size from the target cDNA but with a presumed equivalent efficiency of PCR amplification. A known amount of competitive cDNA is serially diluted into tubes containing equivalent but unknown amounts of cDNA from a patient sample. The equivalence point of target-to-competitor product ratio at the end of the PCR is used to calculate the starting amount of cDNA in the unknown patient samples. The dynamic range of target cDNA quantification is two to three logs, with the best accuracy in estimating the amount of target cDNA given by a target-to-product ratio 1:1, visualized after loading the amplification products on an ethidium-bromide-stained gel. Using this strategy, Muto et al. quantified the *AML1/ETO* fusion transcript in eight t(8;21) AML patients at diagnosis and thereafter *(28)*. Four of the eight patients had relapsed (time to relapse: 2–22 mo), and four were in CCR (follow-up duration: 4–43 mo). In all patients, the *AML1/ETO* fusion transcript decreased and, in some cases, became undetectable over time following induction and consolidation chemotherapy. In the four CCR patients, the level of the *AML1/ETO* fusion transcript was always <0.1 fg of the competitor dose throughout their courses. In contrast, in the four relapsed patients, the level of the *AML1/ETO* fusion transcript increased to >0.1 fg of the competitor dose before relapse. Similar results were recently reported by Tobal et al. BM and blood samples from 25 patients with t(8;21) AML were evaluated for levels of the *AML1/ETO* fusion transcript at different time-points during the course of their disease *(30)*. A considerable variation in the level of the *AML1/ETO* fusion transcripts was shown in diagnostic BM (range: $2.27 \times 10^6$ to $2.27 \times 10^7$ molecules/µg of RNA) or blood (range $0.71 \times 10^5$ to $2.27 \times 10^6$ molecules/µg of RNA) samples, with at least a one log-fold difference in the fusion transcript copies between BM and blood. A two to six log-fold reduction in the level of the *AML1/ETO* fusion transcript was detected over time, following induction and consolidation chemotherapy. There were no differences in the kinetics of molecular response between patients who received different chemotherapy regimens. Most of the patients evaluated, however, continued to be positive for the *AML1/ETO* fusion transcript during remission. Among these patients, those who continued in CR had a level of the *AML1/ETO* fusion transcript consistently $<10^3$ molecules/µg of RNA in BM and $<10^2$ molecules/µg of RNA in blood. In contrast, five patients who relapsed had a significant increase in the *AML1/ETO* fusion transcript level in BM (range: $0.71 \times 10^5$ to $2.27 \times 10^5$ molecules/µg of RNA) or blood (range: $2.27 \times 10^3$ to $2.27 \times 10^4$ molecules/µg of RNA) within 3–6 mo before onset of hematologic relapse.

Although these data support the concept that in t(8;21) AML, it may be ultimately possible to establish a threshold of MRD above which relapse can be predicted, the quantification methodology used in these studies was laborious and relatively inefficient to be applied to large patient populations. The introduction of an automated system called real-time (or Taqman) PCR has simplified the detection of the absolute amount of an amplified target by eliminating many of the extra steps necessary in the previous quantitative RT-PCR techniques *(31–33)*. In this system, a probe labeled with a reporter fluorescent dye at the 5' end and a quencher fluorescent dye at the 3' end is designed to hybridize to a target sequence (*see* Fig. 1). During the extension phase of the PCR cycle, the 5' nuclease activity of *Taq* DNA polymerase cleaves the probe from the target and releases the reporter dye from the proximity of the quencher dye, resulting in an increase of the target-specific fluorescent signal. The increase in reporter fluorescent dye emission is monitored in real time (i.e., during PCR amplification) using a

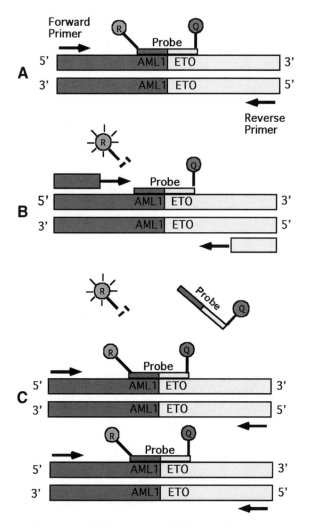

**Fig. 1.** A schematic illustration of the real-time PCR. (**A**) A detection probe labeled with a reporter fluorescent dye (R) at the 5' end and a fluorescence dye quencher (Q) at the 3' end specifically hybridizes to the *AML1/ETO* fusion cDNA. (**B**) During the extension phase of the PCR, the *Taq* DNA polymerase cleaves the probe from the target. The reporter fluorescent dye is released from the dye quencher and produces a specific fluorescence signal. (**C**) The fluorescence signal increases with each amplification cycle proportionally to the starting amount of the *AML1/ETO* fusion transcript present in a given sample. A charge-coupled device (CCD) camera measures the fluorescence signal emission spectra in real time, approximately every 7 s, allowing quantitation of the *AML1/ETO* fusion transcript during the PCR amplification (not shown). An excess of labeled probe is available for hybridization as the amount of amplicon increases during the PCR amplification.

144

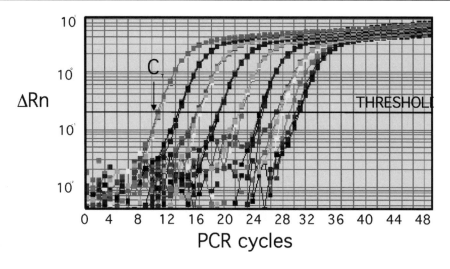

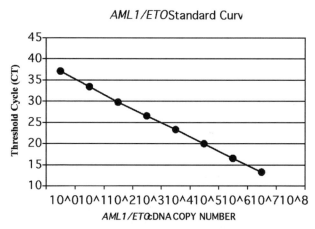

**Fig. 2.** The *AML1/ETO* cDNA standard curve for real-time RT-PCR. The $C_T$ decreases linearly with increasing copy numbers of the *AML1/ETO* cDNA. The standard curve can then be used to calculate the absolute *AML1/ETO* fusion transcript copy number present in an unknown patient sample, following reverse transcription and determination of the relative $C_T$ value during the real-time PCR amplification.

sequence detector system, the 7700 Sequence Detector (Applied Biosystems). The higher the starting copy of the nucleic acid target, the sooner a significant increase in fluorescence is observed. The parameter $C_T$ (threshold cycle) is defined as the PCR cycle number at which the reporter fluorescence generated by the cleavage of the probe passes a fixed threshold above the baseline. Because a plot of the log of initial target copy number for a set of standards versus $C_T$ is a straight line, it is possible to construct a standard curve (*see* Fig. 2). Quantifi-

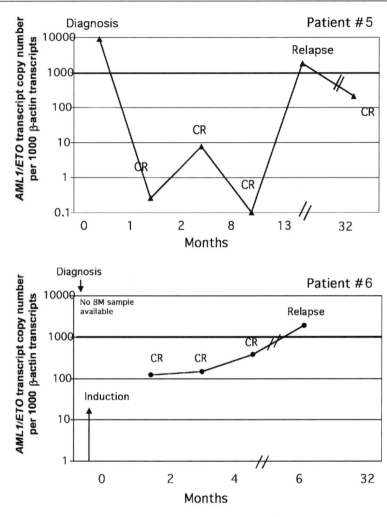

**Fig. 3.** Examples of serial quantification of the *AML1/ETO* fusion transcript by real-time RT-PCR at diagnosis, during remission and relapse. On the *y*-axis, the *AML1/ETO* fusion transcript copy number normalized to a housekeeping gene (i.e., *b-actin*), on the *x*-axis (time in months). (From ref. *33*.)

cation of the amount of target in unknown samples is accomplished by measuring $C_T$ and comparing this value with the standard curve. The entire process of calculating $C_T$, preparing the standard curve, and determining starting copy number for unknowns is performed by the software of the 7700 system.

We have applied the above principles to quantification of the *AML1/ETO* fusion transcript at diagnosis, during remission, and at relapse in patients with t(8;21) AML *(27)* (*see* Fig. 3). Using a limiting dilution of a known quantity of an *AML1/ETO* cDNA standard synthesized in our laboratory, we have constructed a standard curve to quantify the *AML1/ETO* fusion transcript in patient samples. In order to minimize variability in the results resulting from differences in the reverse-transcription efficiency and/or RNA integrity among the unknown patient samples, the absolute *AML1/ETO* fusion transcript copy number was then normalized to transcript copies of an internal housekeeping gene (i.e., β-*actin* or *GAPDH*). Six patients with t(8;21)(q22;q22) AML who achieved CR were studied by real-time RT-PCR at different time intervals following diagnosis. Different levels of *AML1/ETO* fusion transcript could be measured at diagnosis, but a direct correlation between number of blasts and *AML1/ETO* fusion transcript copy number could not be established. Each patient showed a two- to four-log decrease in the level of the *AML1/ETO* fusion transcript following successful induction chemotherapy. In one patient, relapse was preceded by an increase in *AML1/ETO* copy number. In another case, however, relapse occurred despite a stable copy number from the remission value. This could be merely the result of a technical error or illustrate the limits of the methodology. In fact, RNA-based MRD detection, as expression of a chimeric transcript in the leukemic clone, may vary dramatically from patient to patient, if not from leukemic cell to leukemic cell in the same patient. Thus, low fusion transcript copy numbers detected during remission may be either truly reflective of a low number of residual blasts or only indicative of a low expression of the fusion gene and not indicative of the number of blast cells or in the leukemic clone. In the latter case, the predictive value of a MRD level deemed "low" would be incorrectly estimated if a relatively high number of resistant leukemic cells with reduced fusion gene expression but high potential for reexpressing the leukemic phenotype is still present after treatment.

Other authors have since replicated our results *(34,35)*. Sugimoto et al., for instance, analyzed BM samples from seven AML patients with t(8;21) at different time points during the clinical courses of their disease by real-time RT-PCR and found levels of *AML1/ETO* expression quantitatively increased before relapse and decreased following reinduction chemotherapy or donor lymphocyte *(35)*. Krauter et al. quantified the *AML1/ETO* fusion transcript relative to the expression of the *GAPDH* housekeeping gene by real-time RT-PCR in 22 patients with t(8;21) AML at initial diagnosis and thereafter. The quantitative expression of the *AML1/ETO* fusion transcript varied considerably at diagnosis, with achievement of a marked decline in the levels of fusion transcript during remission *(34)*.

The collective analysis of these data demonstrated that quantification of levels of *AML1/ETO* fusion transcript by both QcRT-PCR and real-time RT-PCR is feasible and has a good correspondence with disease status. It is possible that the use of these strategies applied to larger *AML1/ETO*-positive patient populations would allow us to identify the threshold of MRD predictive of clinical outcome and to tailor therapeutic strategies during remission accordingly. Both methodologies appear comparable for sensitivity, linearity, and reproducibility, as recently reported by Wattjes et al. *(36)*. The real-time RT-PCR offers, however, some technical advantages by providing absolute quantification of the target sequence, expanding the dynamic range of quantification to over six orders of magnitude, eliminating the post-PCR processing, and reducing labor and carryover contamination, which make this technique a more attractive method to be applied in future studies.

## MRD STUDIES IN inv(16)(Q13Q22) AML

At the molecular level, inv(16)(p13q22) results in the fusion of the *CBF*β gene from chromosome 16q22 with the *MYH11* gene from chromosome 16p13 *(37)*. The *CBF*β gene encodes the β subunit of CBF. The *CBF*β fusion partner, the *MYH11* gene, encodes a smooth-muscle form of the myosin heavy chain. Several studies have demonstrated that the genomic breakpoints within *CBF*β and *MYH11* are extremely variable, resulting in the production of *CBF*β*/MYH11* fusion transcripts of different sizes. At least eight different types of *CBF*β*/MYH11* fusion transcripts have been identified by RT-PCR *(38)*. The most common one is referred to as type A and has been detected in approx 85% of patients with AML and inv(16)(p13q22). Identical *CBF*β*/MYH11* fusion transcripts are detected in patients with t(16;16)(p13;q22), indicating that the genes involved in the translocation are the same as those involved in the inversion. Whether the different fusion transcripts have any clinical or biological significance is currently unknown, but there is preliminary evidence that rare *CBF*β*/MYH11* fusion transcripts (i.e., type B-H) are found more commonly than *CBF*β*/MYH11* type A in therapy-related inv(16)(p13q22) AML *(39)*.

Amplification of *CBF*β*/MYH11* fusion transcripts in patients with inv(16) (p13q22) AML using a qualitative RT-PCR assay in BM and blood samples has been used to detect MRD and assess the risk of relapse simply on the basis of a positive or negative result. Similar to t(8;21) AML, however, this strategy has produced conflicting results *(40)*. Several studies, for example, have reported patients who tested negative by RT-PCR, and although most of them continued in CR, others have relapsed. Claxton et al. reported the first two patients with inv(16) AML who were studied for MRD during remission *(41)*. Both patients in CR for more than 1 yr had a negative RT-PCR assay. Similarly, we have reported three patients in long-term remission *(40)*. Of the three patients, two were RT-PCR negative at 36 mo during CR1 following chemotherapy and one was RT-PCR negative at 12 mo during CR2 following alloBMT. Of these three patients, two continued in CR1 at 40 and 55 mo, respectively, and the remaining patient has died of infection with NED at 15 mo after alloBMT. In contrast, Martinelli et al. reported two patients who relapsed following ABMT, despite a negative RT-PCR assay for the *CBFβ/MYH11* fusion transcript at 8 and 12 mo before disease recurrence *(42)*. In the same study, however, seven additional patients, three of whom treated with alloBMT, continued in CR with a negative RT-PCR assay. Although it is possible that at the sampling time-points, fusion transcript levels in the relapsed patients were indeed below the detection threshold, it cannot be excluded that these negative results are related to a relatively low sensitivity level of the RT-PCR assay utilized. The results from this study, therefore, underscore the need for a standardized methodology that could efficiently elucidate the potential clinical significance of a fusion transcript deemed undetectable by nested RT-PCR. We have recently proposed that, as a minimum definition, the criteria that we used for the *AML1/ETO* AML to score a patient positive or negative for MRD should also be adopted for *CBFβ/MYH11* AML *(33)*.

Similarly unresolved is the prognostic value of a detectable *CBFβ/MYH11* transcript, because some studies have reported patients who continued in remission despite a positive RT-PCR status. Poirel et al. reported three patients in remission who were positive at 1, 3, and 6 mo from diagnosis *(43)*. Four additional patients in CR were found positive by Herbert et al. between 4 and 22 mo from diagnosis *(44)*. Costello et al. has proposed that although a positive RT-PCR assay can be found during remission, conversion from a positive to a negative status usually occurs in those patients destined to CCR *(45)*. These authors reported on 10 patients with inv(16) AML treated with alloBMT (*n* = 1), ABMT (*n* = 5), or chemotherapy (*n* = 4). Of the 10 patients, 5 were found positive at 2 mo from diagnosis. This early positivity, however, was not predictive of impending relapse, and only three patients who remained positive beyond 8 mo from diagnosis relapsed. In a larger study, Martin et al. reported 15 patients in first CR following treatment with chemotherapy (*n* = 8), ASCT (*n* = 6), or alloBMT (*n* = 1) *(46)*. All 15 tested positive at least once during remission. Of the 15 patients, 7 (chemotherapy = 3; ASCT= 3; alloBMT=1) remained in CCR after a median follow-up of 48 mo (range: 31–79 mo). These patients tested positive for the *CBFβ/MYH11* fusion transcript up to 24 mo from diagnosis (median: 7.5; range: 1–24 mo) before converting to a negative RT-PCR status. The remaining eight patients (chemotherapy = 5; ASCT = 3) tested positive for the chimeric transcript at a median time of 10.5 mo from diagnosis (range: 5 to 19 mo). These patients never converted to a negative RT-PCR status and eventually all relapsed. From the analysis of these data, it emerges that, although conversion from a positive to a negative test may be a necessary condition to achieve long-term remission, the prognostic value of a positive RT-PCR continues to remain uncertain. In fact, in both groups, patients destined to relapse and patients who continued in CR tested positive at the same time-points during remission. In the series from Martin et al., the last conversion from a positive to a negative status among CCR patients occurred at 24 mo. This was 5 mo beyond the longest time-point during remission at which the last of the patients destined to relapse tested positive before disease recurrence. In addition, Tobal et al. have recently reported two patients post-alloBMT and postchemotherapy who were positive at 30 and 108 mo from achievement of CR, respectively, supporting the notion that even a persistent positive RT-PCR assay may be compatible with long-term remission *(47)*.

Finally, it is possible that the intensity of the treatment received has a significant impact on the probability of converting from a positive to a negative RT-PCR status during remission. Elmaagacli et al. evaluated by nested RT-PCR a patient population with inv(16) AML undergoing high-dose chemotherapy with allogeneic or autologous BMT or peripheral stem cell transplantation (PSCT) *(48)*. Two patients who received ABMT and were positive for the *CBFβ/MYH11* fusion transcript at 3 mo following therapy eventually relapsed. The remaining eight patients underwent allogeneic BMT/PSCT in CR1 ($n = 7$) or CR2 ($n = 1$). At 3 mo following transplant, six of these eight patients were negative for the *CBFβ/MYH11* fusion transcript by RT-PCR and continued in remission. Of the two remaining patients, one continued to test positive at 6 mo following transplantation and eventually relapsed, whereas the other patients converted to a negative status and continued in CR. These data together with the results of other different studies indicated that, in contrast to t(8;21) AML, patients with inv(16) AML undergoing alloBMT are likely to achieve molecular remission. To date, of 15 patients who underwent alloBMT, only two tested positive for the *CBFβ/MYH11* fusion transcript during remission; 1 relapsed and 1 continued in long-term CR. Of the remaining 13 patients, all achieved RT-PCR negativity and continued in CR or died as consequence of therapy-related toxicity with NED. In contrast, of 21 reported patients who underwent ABMT or APSCT, 9 (43%) have relapsed, 7 with a positive RT-PCR during remission, and 2 with a negative RT-PCR during remission *(42,45,46,48)*. Whether contamination of the leukapheresis products by leukemic cells plays an important role in determining disease relapse remains unknown. Costello et al., however, studied four patients with inv(16) AML who underwent APSCT *(45)*. Three of these four patients who were reinfused with leukapheresis products negative for the *CBFβ/MYH11* fusion transcript by RT-PCR remained in CCR at 18–24 mo after therapy. In contrast, one patient who was reinfused with a *CBFβ/MYH11*-positive leukaphersis product experienced early relapsed. In contrast, Testoni et al. reported two patients who underwent APSCT with a negative leukapheresis product; one relapsed and one continued in CR.

## QUANTITATIVE ANALYSIS OF MRD IN inv(16) OR t(16;16) AML

Based on the current data, it continues to be difficult to stratify inv(16) or t(16;16) AML patients for risk of disease relapse only on the basis of the presence or absence of the *CBFβ/MYH11* fusion transcript by RT-PCR. Conversion from a positive to a negative RT-PCR status following treatment can occur and is potentially predictive of long-term CR, but conversions during long-term remission are not uncommon. Thus, in the case of a positive result, it remains difficult to determine whether a patient will become negative for the fusion transcript and continue in CR or, instead, will relapse. Two recent small retrospective studies have suggested that a quantitative RT-PCR methodology that detects residual levels of *CBFβ/MYH11* fusion transcripts in inv(16) AML during CR may prove more useful to assess treatment response and predict clinical outcome than a simple qualitative assay *(49,50)*. Utilizing QcRT-PCR, both of these studies found that the decline in the amount of fusion transcript following treatment occurs over a variable length of time and suggested that the degree of log-fold reduction in the level of the *CBFβ/MYH11* fusion transcript is predictive of patients' outcome. In neither study, however, was it possible to identify, during CR, an absolute threshold of fusion transcripts above which relapse occurs and below which cure is likely. Moreover, limitations such as the small number of patients analyzed in the two studies ($n = 7$ and $n = 5$, respectively), the variety of treatments used, and the narrow dynamic range of quantification of the technique utilized in both studies prevent any firm conclusion from being drawn. As discussed for the t(8;21) AML, the recent introduction of the real-time RT-PCR appears promising for resolving some of the technical limitations intrinsic in these initial quantitative analyses. We have recently reported on 16 uniformly treated patients with inv(16) AML *(51)*. The preliminary data from this study suggested that a high *CBFβ/MYH11* transcript copy number during remission correlated with risk of relapse and CR duration. Future large prospective studies that analyze cohorts of uniformly treated patients and utilize BM and/or blood samples collected at the same specific time-points are, however, necessary to establish the predictive value of *CBFβ/MYH11* fusion transcript quantification in order to provide useful information for the clinical management of patients with inv(16) or t(16;16) AML during remission.

## MLL-ASSOCIATED AML

Rearrangements of the *MLL* (*ALL1*, *HRX*, *Htrx-1*) gene, located on chromosome band 11q23, characterize 5–10% of adult and pediatric *de novo* acute leukemias and more than 50% of secondary AML following treatment with inhibitors of topoisomerase II *(2,52)*. The majority of these cases present with reciprocal translocations involving at least 25 other chromosomes, most commonly t(4;11)(q21;q23), t(6;11)(q27;q23), t(9;11)(p22;q23), and t(11;19) (q23;p13). In addition, a self-rearrangement of *MLL* was described in the absence of fusion with any other chromosome partner *(53,54)*. In most instances, abnormalities involving *MLL* are associated with a poor clinical outcome *(55)*.

To date, only a few studies have addressed the prognostic value of detection of fusion transcripts by RT-PCR in *MLL* AML, and it remains unknown whether molecular remission is a necessary condition for achievement of prolonged CR in this group of patients. In a recent study, 27 out of 210 patients (13%) were found with rearranged *MLL* genes by Southern blot analysis *(56)*. Of the 27, the *MLL/AF6* fusion transcript was detected in 6 patients by RT-PCR. Sequence analysis showed that in these patients different types of *MLL/AF6* fusion transcripts involving *MLL* exons 5, 6, or 7 and *AF6* exon 2 could be detected. *MLL/AF6*-positive patients were monitored by RT-PCR for a period of 6–33 mo following achievement CR *(56)*. Five of the six patients had *MLL/AF6* fusion transcripts detectable in every sample tested during remission and eventually relapsed (CR duration range: 2.6–8.3 mo). The remaining patient, who achieved molecular remission, remained in CR 33 mo after diagnosis. In a second study, four patients with t(9;11) AML were serially monitored by RT-PCR for the MLL/AF9 fusion transcript for a period of 4–23 mo during CR *(57)*. Two patients became RT-PCR negative in BM and blood after one cycle of induction chemotherapy and remained in CR at 15 and 22 mo from diagnosis, respectively. Two additional patients who initially achieved CR failed to become RT-PCR negative for the *MLL/AF9* fusion transcripts. One of these patients relapsed 5 mo after achieving CR, whereas the other received alloBMT in CR1 and became RT-PCR negative. Unfortunately, because of the small number of patients analyzed, it is difficult to draw a definite conclusion from these studies. However, it appears that in AML patients presenting with t(6;11) or t(9;11), the use of a qualitative RT-PCR in AML may be more applicable than in other subgroups of AML, and achievement of molecular remission can predict a favorable outcome.

In contrast with these results, for patients who present with a self-rearrangement of *MLL* in the absence of fusion with any other chromosome partner, analysis of MRD may not be so straightforward. This genomic abnormality results in a partial tandem duplication (PTD) of an internal portion of *MLL* that creates within the *MLL* gene transcript a unique fusion of exons in which the open reading frame (ORF) is always maintained. Since its initial discovery, the PTD of *MLL* has been found to be present in the majority of primary AML patients with trisomy 11 as a sole abnormality and in a fraction of primary AML patients with trisomy 11 accompanied by additional cytogenetic abnormalities *(58)*. Recently, we and others have reported that the PTD of *MLL* can also be found in 5–10% of adult patients with AML and normal cytogenetics *(59)*. It was anticipated that monitoring for evidence of MRD by RT-PCR in this patient population could be important for assessing treatment response and in a timely prediction of disease relapse. Therefore, we completed a study to determine if BM or blood from normal donors express the fusion transcripts that result from the PTD of *MLL* or whether these transcripts are instead restricted to leukemic blasts *(9)*. The ultimate goal of this study was to determine the specificity of fusion transcript amplification by RT-PCR to detect MRD in AML patients with the PTD of *MLL*. We analyzed 60 healthy normal donors for the PTD of *MLL* by nested RT-PCR and found that in 10 of the 60 samples (16%), it was possible to amplify a unique transcript showing an abnormal fusion of *MLL* exons. Marked differences, however, were observed between the *MLL* fusion transcripts detected in normal donors and those detected in leukemic patients with a PTD of *MLL* documented at the genomic level. First, the transcripts detected in normal individuals were not of similar size or composition compared to those described in AML patients. Second, fusion transcripts resulting from the PTD of *MLL* in AML have all been in-frame and found in the polyA+ fraction of the RNA, with the PTD of *MLL* that is always demonstrated at the genomic level as well. In contrast, only 5 of 10 *MLL* fusion transcripts detected in normal donors were in-frame, suggesting this to be a random event. Moreover, these fusion transcripts from normal samples could be amplified only in the total RNA fraction, and not in the polyA+ RNA, suggesting that they are not translated into a partially duplicated protein. Finally, no rearrangement of the *MLL* gene could be identified at the genomic level by Southern analysis or DNA PCR amplification in the normal individuals otherwise positive for the fusion transcripts. Collectively, these results suggested that the genesis and the composition of the *MLL* fusion transcripts found in normal cells are distinct from those found in leukemic cells, reflecting the different biological significance of each product. It appears that the fusion transcripts in normal samples are not derived from a mutated *MLL* gene, but, rather, may be generated during a mRNA splicing process termed "exon scrambling." Recently, these results were confirmed by two other groups *(60,61)*. In the study by Schnittger et al., however, the incidence of *MLL* fusion transcript in normal donors was higher and the PTD of *MLL* gene was detected by genomic PCR, whereas in the second study, Caldas et al. confirmed the presence of *MLL* "scrambled" transcripts in normal BM without detecting the PTD of *MLL* at the genomic level. Although the reasons for these differences remain to be resolved, these studies underscore that the presence of *MLL* fusion transcripts detected by RT-PCR may not be sufficiently specific for diagnosis of AML associated with the PTD of *MLL* associated and, in addition, may not correlate with a correct assessment of MRD during remission.

## UNIVERSAL MARKERS FOR MRD

Despite its limitation, the use of specific chimeric genes or their fusion transcripts by RT-PCR–based methodologies may represent an important step in understanding the significance of MRD and implement a risk-adapted strategy in those AML patients who achieve CR. Unfortunately, this approach can be used only in the context of fully characterized genomic abnormalities, whereas it cannot be used in AML patients who present with normal cytogenetics or other chromosome rearrangements that fail to generate chimeric transcripts. For these patients, the demand for "universal" molecular markers that could consistently be used to assess treatment response and predict clinical outcome independently of specific genomic rearrangements has remained, thus far, unanswered.

In the search for disease-specific markers, the prognostic value of *WT1* gene expression at diagnosis or during remission has been assessed in patients with acute leukemia. *WT1* is a tumor suppressor gene that encodes a zinc-finger DNA-binding protein. This gene plays a key role in the carcinogenesis of Wilms' tumor, but its expression has also been demonstrated in embryologic development of genitourinary organs and during normal hematopoiesis. *WT1* transcripts have been demonstrated in the majority of patients with acute leukemia and CML *(62)*. In about 80% of patients with acute leukemia, the *WT1* transcript was detectable by RT-PCR, and in some studies, an association between *WT1* expression and an increased risk of relapse was shown. Therefore, detection of *WT1* transcript by RT-PCR has been suggested to be a potential marker for MRD in acute leukemia regardless of the presence or absence of other tumor-specific DNA markers *(63)*. Inoue et al. monitored *WT1* expression in nine acute leukemia patients during remission. In four patients, *WT1* transcripts were detected at 2–8 mo before clinical relapse *(62)*. The same group has recently updated their initial results by reporting 31 patients (27 with AML, 2 with acute lymphocytic leukemia [ALL], and 2 with acute mixed lineage leukemia) treated with conventional chemotherapy, and 23 patients (13 AML, 5 ALL, and 5 with CML) treated with alloBMT *(64)*. In these patients, expression of *WT1* transcript was assessed in serial samples by RT-PCR. Sixteen patients in the chemotherapy group and three patients in the alloBMT group relapsed following achievement of CR. In 10 of these patients, *WT1* expression that had returned to low levels during remission, significantly increased at 1–18 mo before clinical relapse. In another nine patients, the level of *WT1* transcript never significantly decreased after achievement of CR, and the subsequent relapse was accompanied by a further rapid increase in *WT1* expression. Levels of *WT1* mRNA in the remaining 35 patients who continued in CR instead remained significantly low during remission.

In contrast, Geigeret et al. found no correlation between *WT1* expression and probability of relapse *(65)*. These authors analyzed *WT1* gene expression by RT-PCR in serial blood or BM samples from patients with *de novo* AML up to 95 mo after diagnosis. Of those patients with *WT1*-positive AML, 44 were treated with chemotherapy, whereas 24 patients underwent unrelated donor (*n* = 4), sibling donor (*n* = 13), or autologous (*n* = 7) BMT. After achieving CR, 62% of these patients became *WT1* negative, whereas 38% remained *WT1* positive. There was no difference in DFS or OS between *WT1*-positive and *WT1*-negative patients. Following BMT, 32% of the patients analyzed in CR within the first 100 d after transplantation were *WT1* positive by RT-PCR. Detection of *WT1* transcripts within 100 d following BMT, however, did not affect DFS and OS after transplantation. Ten of 11 patients who were in CCR for more than 3 yr had been transiently *WT1* positive during the observation period. Thirteen relapsed patients were *WT1* negative at 4 mo before disease recurrence, and eight of them were *WT1* negative at the time of relapse. These data indicate that (1) achievement of *WT1* negativity is not associated with longer DFS and OS, (2) not all patients who relapse become *WT1* positive again, and (3) patients in long-term CR frequently display the *WT1* transcript. Similar results were reported by Elmaagacli et al. in 46 patients with acute leukemia after alloBMT or PSCT *(65a)*. Prior to alloBMT, *WT1* transcripts were detected by RT-PCR in 38 of 46 patients (83%). In 14 of 38 patients (37%), *WT1* transcripts were detected at least once posttransplant (range: 1–89 mo). Twelve of the 38 patients relapsed after transplant, but only 7 of the 12 were *WT1* positive. In five relapsed patients, the *WT1* RT-PCR status remained negative 0–3 mo prior to relapse. On the other hand, only 7 of 14 patients with a positive test for *WT1* after transplant relapsed. In 17 of the 46 study patients, chromosomal abnormalities had been found prior to transplant. In these 17 patients, the *WT1* transcript was simultaneously expressed with other fusion transcripts specific for the corresponding chromosomal abnormality. In 32 of 45 samples (71%), the results for the fusion transcripts and *WT1* transcript were concordant, but differed in 13 patients. On the basis of these data, therefore, it is possible to conclude that the value of *WT1* transcript detection to predict leukemic relapse remains, at the very least, controversial. Other more recent fusion products such as the PTD of *FLT3* detected in AML patients will be important to assess for predictability in a prospective fashion *(66–69)*.

Finally, another area of potential interest for disease "universal" markers is represented by detection of genes that become methylated in AML. Recent data have suggested that hypermethylation of the promoter area of a few selected genes is an important mechanism of inactivating growth control and/or tumor suppressor genes during different phases of leukemogenesis *(70–72)*. Because these epigenetic mutations are independent of specific chromosome rearrangement, the use of PCR-based methodologies could be used to detect methylated genes as "universal" markers to predict disease relapse. These methodologies are based on the introduction of methylation-dependent sequence differences into the genomic DNA by sodium bisulfite treatment and PCR amplification *(73)*. The combination of bisulfite treatment and PCR amplification results in the conversion of unmethylated cytosine (C) residues to thymine (T) and in the conversion of methylated cytosine (m-C) to cytosine (C). The net result are two possible distinct sequences of the same DNA site, depending on the methylated or unmethylated status of the original sequence, that can be exploited as a marker for MRD by using specific primers and restriction enzyme analysis of the amplified product. Furthermore, the methylation-dependent sequence modifications of target genes can be quantified by applying the quantitative real-time PCR technology *(74,75)*. Thus, as new methylated genes are identified and characterized, these bisulfite–PCR-based assays will be tested for their usefulness in determining the incidence and the prognostic significance of genes methylated in AML at diagnosis and during remission.

## CONCLUSION

In summary, analysis of MRD is an appealing strategy to stratify AML patients for risk of relapse during remission. The applicability of this strategy, however, suffers from technical limitations, which could be overcome by the systematic utilization of standardized methodologies and their prospective evaluation in larger patient populations. In addition, it will be important to develop markers that can be utilized independently from specific chromosome rearrangements. Unfortunately, despite numerous studies, these goals have not been met and, thus, the usefulness of MRD analysis by RT-PCR for the management of AML in remission remains undetermined. Moreover, because it is unlikely that the presence of a chimeric gene by itself is causative of leukemogenesis, but rather is important in addition to other genomic changes, detection of chimeric clone in remission may not be predictive of a clonal cell potential to express a leukemia phenotype *(2)*. This hypothesis is supported by studies showing the presence of hemetopoietic precursors carrying chimeric fuson genes in patients in long-term remission and by the inability of fusion genes by themselves to induce leukemia in transgenic mouse models *(24–26,76)*. Monitoring just the fusion transcript and not also monitoring other genomic rearrangements such as deletions or epigenetic mutations such as methylation may lead to incorrect identification of the true residual leukemic blasts. In this regard, innovative gene microarray technologies are being developed and applied to the study of the molecular biology of hematopoietic clonal disease *(77)*. It is conceivable, therefore, that the use of these methodologies may identify additional structural and functional genomic changes occurring with the fusion genes, providing additional important characterizations of the malignant potential of residual blasts detected at initial presentation of that may be used singly or in combination to follow the progression of the disease as a marker of MRD during remission.

## ACKNOWLEDGMENTS

This work was supported in part by the National Cancer Institute (grant no. P30CA16058) and The American Cancer Society (grant no. IRG-98-278-01).

# REFERENCES

1. Mrózek K and Bloomfield C. Chromosome aberrations in de novo acute myeloid leukemia in adults: clinical implications, *Rev. Clin. Exp. Hematol.*, **5** (1998) 44.
2. Caligiuri M and Bloomfield C. The molecular biology of leukemia, in *Principles and Practice of Oncology Cancer.* DeVita VJ, Hellman S, and Rosenberg S. (eds). Philadelphia: JB Lippincott, 2000, p. 2389.
3. Yin JA and Tobal K. Detection of minimal residual disease in acute myeloid leukaemia: methodologies, clinical and biological significance, *Br. J. Haematol.*, **106** (1999) 578.
4. Willman CL. Molecular evaluation of acute myeloid leukemias, *Semin. Hematol.*, **36** (1999) 390.
5. Radich JP. Clinical applicability of the evaluation of minimal residual disease in acute leukemia, *Curr. Opin. Oncol.*, **12** (2000) 36.
6. Lion T. Monitoring of residual disease in chronic myelogenous leukemia by quantitative polymerase chain reaction and clinical decision making, [letter; comment], *Blood*, **94** (1999) 1486.
7. Diverio D, Rossi V, Avvisati G, De Santis S, Pistilli A, Pane F, et al. Early detection of relapse by prospective reverse transcriptase–polymerase chain reaction analysis of the PML/ RARalpha fusion gene in patients with acute promyelocytic leukemia enrolled in the GIMEMA-AIEOP multicenter "AIDA" trial. GIMEMA–AIEOP Multicenter "AIDA" Trial, *Blood*, **92** (1998) 784.
8. Jurlander J, Caligiuri MA, Ruutu T, Baer MR, Strout MP, Oberkircher AR, et al. Persistence of the AML1/ETO fusion transcript in patients treated with allogeneic bone marrow transplantation for t(8;21) leukemia, *Blood*, **88** (1996) 2183.
9. Marcucci G, Strout MP, Bloomfield CD, and Caligiuri MA. Detection of unique ALL1 (MLL) fusion transcripts in normal human bone marrow and blood: distinct origin of normal versus leukemic ALL1 fusion transcripts, *Cancer Res.*, **58** (1998) 790.
10. Marcucci G, Caligiuri MA, and Bloomfield CD. Molecular and clinical advances in core binding factor primary acute myeloid leukemia: a paradigm for translational research in malignant hematology, *Cancer Invest.*, **18** (2000) 768.
11. Bloomfield CD, Lawrence D, Byrd JC, Carroll A, Pettenati MJ, Tantravahi R, et al. Frequency of prolonged remission duration after high-dose cytarabine intensification in acute myeloid leukemia varies by cytogenetic subtype, *Cancer Res.*, **58** (1998) 4173.
11a. Ferrant A, Labopin M, Frassoni F, et al. Karyotype in acute myeloblastic leukemia: prognostic significance for bone marrow transplantation in first remission: a European Group for Blood and Marrow Transplantation study. Acute Leukemia Working Party of the European Group for Blood and Marrow Transplantation (EBMT), *Blood*, **90(8)** (1997) 2931–2938.
12. Downing JR. The AML1-ETO chimaeric transcription factor in acute myeloid leukaemia: biology and clinical significance, *Br. J. Haematol.*, **106** (1999) 296.
13. Nucifora G, Birn DJ, Erickson P, Gao J, LeBeau MM, Drabkin HA, et al. Detection of DNA rearrangements in the AML1 and ETO loci and of an AML1/ETO fusion mRNA in patients with t(8;21) acute myeloid leukemia, *Blood*, **81** (1993) 883.
14. Nucifora G, Larson RA, and Rowley JD. Persistence of the 8;21 translocation in patients with acute myeloid leukemia type M2 in long-term remission, *Blood*, **82** (1993) 712.
15. Chang KS, Fan YH, Stass SA, Estey EH, Wang G, Trujillo JM, et al. Expression of AML1-ETO fusion transcripts and detection of minimal residual disease in t(8;21)-positive acute myeloid leukemia, *Oncogene*, **8** (1993) 983.
16. Kusec R, Laczika K, Knobl P, Friedl J, Greinix H, Kahls P, et al. AML1/ETO fusion mRNA can be detected in remission blood samples of all patients with t(8;21) acute myeloid leukemia after chemotherapy or autologous bone marrow transplantation, *Leukemia*, **8** (1994) 735.

17. Saunders MJ, Tobal K, and Yin JA. Detection of t(8;21) by reverse transcriptase polymerase chain reaction in patients in remission of acute myeloid leukaemia type M2 after chemotherapy or bone marrow transplantation, *Leukemia Res.*, **18** (1994) 891.

18. Sakata N, Okamura T, Inoue M, Yumura-Yagi K, Hara J, Tawa A, et al. Rapid disappearance of AML1/ETO fusion transcripts in patients with t(8;21) acute myeloid leukemia following bone marrow transplantation and chemotherapy, *Leuk. Lymphoma*, **26** (1997) 141.

19. Miyamoto T, Nagafuji K, Akashi K, Harada M, Kyo T, Akashi T, et al. Persistence of multipotent progenitors expressing AML1/ETO transcripts in long-term remission patients with t(8;21) acute myelogenous leukemia, *Blood*, **87** (1996) 4789.

20. Elmaagacli AH, Beelen DW, Stockova J, Trzensky S, Kroll M, Schaefer UW, et al. Detection of AML1/ETO fusion transcripts in patients with t(8;21) acute myeloid leukemia after allogeneic bone marrow transplantation or peripheral blood progenitor cell transplantation, [letter]; comment, *Blood*, **90** (1997) 3230.

21. Morschhauser F, Cayuela JM, Martini S, Baruchel A, Rousselot P, Socie G, et al. Evaluation of minimal residual disease using reverse-transcription polymerase chain reaction in t(8;21) acute myeloid leukemia: a multicenter study of 51 patients, *J. Clin. Oncol.*, **18** (2000) 788.

22. Lo Coco F, Diverio D, Falini B, Biondi A, Nervi C, and Pelicci PG. Genetic diagnosis and molecular monitoring in the management of acute promyelocytic leukemia, *Blood*, **94** (1999) 12.

23. Tobal K, Saunders MJ, Grey MR, and Yin JA. Persistence of RAR alpha-PML fusion mRNA detected by reverse transcriptase polymerase chain reaction in patients in long-term remission of acute promyelocytic leukaemia, *Br. J. Haematol.*, **90** (1995) 615.

24. Saunders MJ, Tobal K, Keeney S, and Liu Yin JA. Expression of diverse AML1/MTG8 transcripts is a consistent feature in acute myeloid leukemia with t(8;21) irrespective of disease phase, *Leukemia*, **10** (1996) 1139.

25. Miyamoto T, Weissman IL, and Akashi K. AML1/ETO-expressing nonleukemic stem cells in acute myelogenous leukemia with 8;21 chromosomal translocation, *Proc. Natl. Acad. Sci. USA*, **97** (2000) 7521.

26. Higuchi M, O'Brien D, Lenny N, Yang S, Cai Z, and Downing J. Expression of AML1-ETO immortalizes myeloid progenitors and cooperates with secondary mutations to induce granulocytic sarcoma/acute myeloid leukemia, *Blood*, **96** (2000) 222a.

27. Marcucci G, Livak KJ, Bi WL, Strout MP, Bloomfield CD, and Caligiuri MA. Detection of the *AML1/ETO* fusion transcript in patients with t(8;21)-associated AML using a novel "real time" quantitative RT-PCR assay, *Leukemia*, **12** (1998) 1482.

28. Muto A, Mori S, Matsushita H, Awaya N, Ueno H, Takayama N, et al. Serial quantification of minimal residual disease of t(8;21) acute myeloid leukaemia with RT-competitive PCR assay, *Br. J. Haematol.*, **95** (1996) 85.

29. Tobal K and Yin JA. Monitoring of minimal residual disease by quantitative reverse transcriptase-polymerase chain reaction for AML1-MTG8 transcripts in AML-M2 with t(8; 21), *Blood*, **88** (1996) 3704.

30. Tobal K, Newton J, Macheta M, Chang J, Morgenstern G, Evans PA, et al. Molecular quantitation of minimal residual disease in acute myeloid leukemia with t(8;21) can identify patients in durable remission and predict clinical relapse, *Blood*, **95** (2000) 815.

31. Heid CA, Stevens J, Livak KJ, and Williams PM. Real time quantitative PCR, *Genome Res.*, **6** (1996) 986.

32. Gibson UE, Heid CA, and Williams PM. A novel method for real time quantitative RT-PCR, *Genome Res.*, **6** (1996) 995.

33. Marcucci G, Livak KJ, Bi W, Strout MP, Bloomfield CD, and Caligiuri MA. Detection of minimal residual disease in patients with AML1/ETO-associated acute myeloid leukemia using a novel quantitative reverse transcription polymerase chain reaction assay, *Leukemia*, **12** (1998) 1482.

34. Krauter J, Wattjes MP, Nagel S, Heidenreich O, Krug U, Kafert S, et al. Real-time RT-PCR for the detection and quantification of AML1/MTG8 fusion transcripts in t(8;21)-positive AML patients, *Br. J. Haematol.*, **107** (1999) 80.
35. Sugimoto T, Das H, Imoto S, Murayama T, Gomyo H, Chakraborty S, et al. Quantitation of minimal residual disease in t(8;21)-positive acute myelogenous leukemia patients using real-time quantitative RT-PCR, *Am. J. Hematol.*, **64** (2000) 101.
36. Wattjes MP, Krauter J, Nagel S, Heidenreich O, Ganser A, and Heil G. Comparison of nested competitive RT-PCR and real-time RT-PCR for the detection and quantification of AML1/MTG8 fusion transcripts in t(8;21) positive acute myelogenous leukemia, *Leukemia*, **14** (2000) 329.
37. Liu P, Tarle SA, Hajra A, Claxton DF, Marlton P, Freedman M, et al. Fusion between transcription factor CBFb/PEBP2b and a myosin heavy chain in acute myeloid leukemia, *Science*, **261** (1993) 1041.
38. Liu PP, Hajra A, Wijmenga C, and Collins FS. Molecular pathogenesis of the chromosome 16 inversion in the M4Eo subtype of acute myeloid leukemia, *Blood*, **85** (1995) 2289.
39. Dissing M, Le Beau MM, and Pedersen-Bjergaard J. Inversion of chromosome 16 and uncommon rearrangements of the CBFB and MYH11 genes in therapy-related acute myeloid leukemia: rare events related to DNA-topoisomerase II inhibitors?, *J. Clin. Oncol.*, **16** (1998) 1890.
40. Marcucci G, Caligiuri M, and Bloomfield C. Defining the "absence" of the *CBFb/MYH11* fusion transcript in patients with acute myeloid leukemia and inversion of chromosome 16 to predict long-term complete remission: a call for definitions, *Blood*, **90** (1997) 5022.
41. Claxton DF, Liu P, Hsu HB, Marlton P, Hester J, Collins F, et al. Detection of fusion transcripts generated by the inversion 16 chromosome in acute myelogenous leukemia, *Blood*, **83** (1994) 1750.
42. Martinelli G, Ottaviani E, Testoni N, Visani G, Terragna C, Amabile M, et al. Molecular remission in PCR-positive acute myeloid leukemia patients with inv(16): role of bone marrow transplantation procedures, *Bone Marrow Transplant.*, **24** (1999) 694.
43. Poirel H, Radford-Weiss I, Rack K, Troussard X, Veil A, Valensi F, et al. Detection of the chromosome 16 CBF beta-MYH11 fusion transcript in myelomonocytic leukemias, *Blood*, **85** (1995) 1313.
44. Hebert J, Cayuela JM, Daniel MT, Berger R, and Sigaux F. Detection of minimal residual disease in acute myelomonocytic leukemia with abnormal marrow eosinophils by nested polymerase chain reaction with allele specific amplification, *Blood*, **84** (1994) 2291.
45. Costello R, Sainty D, Blaise D, Gastaut JA, Gabert J, Poirel H, et al. Prognosis value of residual disease monitoring by polymerase chain reaction in patients with CBF beta/MYH11-positive acute myeloblastic leukemia, *Blood*, **89** (1997) 2222.
46. Martin G, Barragan E, Bolufer P, Chillon C, Garcia-Sanz R, Gomez T, et al. Relevance of presenting white blood cell count and kinetics of molecular remission in the prognosis of acute myeloid leukemia with CBFbeta/MYH11 rearrangement, *Haematologica*, **85** (2000) 699.
47. Tobal K, Johnson PR, Saunders MJ, Harrison CJ, and Liu Yin JA. Detection of CBFB/MYH11 transcripts in patients with inversion and other abnormalities of chromosome 16 at presentation and remission, *Br. J. Haematol.*, **91** (1995) 104.
48. Elmaagacli AH, Beelen DW, Kroll M, Trzensky S, Stein C, and Schaefer UW. Detection of CBFbeta/MYH11 fusion transcripts in patients with inv(16) acute myeloid leukemia after allogeneic bone marrow or peripheral blood progenitor cell transplantation, *Bone Marrow Transplant.*, **21** (1998) 159.
49. Evans PA, Short MA, Jack AS, Norfolk DR, Child JA, Shiach CR, et al. Detection and quantitation of the CBFbeta/MYH11 transcripts associated with the inv(16) in presentation and follow-up samples from patients with AML, *Leukemia*, **11** (1997) 364.
50. Laczika K, Novak M, Hilgarth B, Mitterbauer M, Mitterbauer G, Scheidel-Petrovic A, et al. Competitive CBFbeta/MYH11 reverse-transcriptase polymerase chain reaction for quantita-

tive assessment of minimal residual disease during postremission therapy in acute myeloid leukemia with inversion(16): a pilot study, *J. Clin. Oncol.*, **16** (1998) 1519.

51. Marcucci G, Caligiuri M, Maghraby E, Archer K, Dohner K, Schlenk R, et al. Quantification of the CBFb/MYH11 fusion transcript in inv(16) acute myeloid leukemia by real time RT-PCR, *Blood*, **94** (1999) 625a.

52. Strout MP, Marcucci G, Caligiuri MA, and Bloomfield CD. Core-binding factor (CBF) and MLL-associated primary acute myeloid leukemia: biology and clinical implications, *Ann. Hematol.*, **78** (1999) 251.

53. Caligiuri MA, Schichman SA, Strout MP, Mrozek K, Baer MR, Frankel SR, et al. Molecular rearrangement of the *ALL-1* gene in acute myeloid leukemia without cytogenetic evidence of 11q23 chromosomal translocations, *Cancer Res.*, **54** (1994) 370.

54. Schichman SA, Canaani E, and Croce CM. Self-fusion of the ALL1 gene. A new genetic mechanism for acute leukemia, [review], *JAMA*, **273** (1995) 571.

55. Mrozek K, Heinonen K, Lawrence D, Carroll AJ, Koduru PRK, Rao KW, et al. Adult patients with de novo acute myeloid leukemia and t(9;11)(p22;q23) have a superior outcome to patients with other translocations involving 11q23: a Cancer and Leukemia Group B study, *Blood*, **90** (1997) 4532.

56. Mitterbauer G, Zimmer C, Pirc-Danoewinata H, Haas OA, Hojas S, Schwarzinger I, et al. Monitoring of minimal residual disease in patients with MLL-AF6-positive acute myeloid leukaemia by reverse transcriptase polymerase chain reaction, *Br. J. Haematol.*, **109** (2000) 622.

57. Mitterbauer G, Zimmer C, Fonatsch C, Haas O, Thalhammer-Scherrer R, Schwarzinger I, et al. Monitoring of minimal residual leukemia in patients with MLL-AF9 positive acute myeloid leukemia by RT-PCR, *Leukemia*, **13** (1999) 1519.

58. Caligiuri MA, Strout MP, Schichman SA, Mrozek K, Arthur DC, Herzig GP, et al. Partial tandem duplication of *ALL1* as a recurrent molecular defect in acute myeloid leukemia with trisomy 11, *Cancer Res.*, **56** (1996) 1416.

59. Caligiuri MA, Strout MP, Lawrence D, Arthur DC, Baer MR, Yu F, et al. Rearrangement of *ALL1* in acute myeloid leukemia with normal cytogenetics, *Cancer Res.*, **58** (1998) 55.

60. Caldas C, So CW, MacGregor A, Ford A, McDonald B, and Wiedermann LM. Exon scrambling of MLL transcripts occur commonly and mimic partial genomic duplication of the gene, *Gene*, **208** (1998) 167.

61. Schnittger S, Wormann B, Hiddemann W, and Griesinger F. Partial tandem duplications of the MLL gene are detectable in peripheral blood and bone marrow of nearly all healthy donors, *Blood*, **92** (1998) 1728.

62. Inoue K, Sugiyama H, Ogawa H, Nakagawa M, Yamagami T, Miwa H, et al. WT1 as a new prognostic factor and a new marker for the detection of minimal residual disease in acute leukemia, *Blood*, **84** (1994) 3071.

63. Sugiyama H. Wilms tumor gene (WT1) as a new marker for the detection of minimal residual disease in leukemia, *Leuk. Lymphoma*, **30** (1998) 55.

64. Inoue K, Ogawa H, Yamagami T, Soma T, Tani Y, Tatekawa T, et al. Long-term follow-up of minimal residual disease in leukemia patients by monitoring WT1 (Wilms tumor gene) expression levels, *Blood*, **88** (1996) 2267.

65. Gaiger A, Schmid D, Heinze G, Linnerth B, Greinix H, Kalhs P, et al. Detection of the WT1 transcript by RT-PCR in complete remission has no prognostic relevance in de novo acute myeloid leukemia, *Leukemia*, **12** (1998) 1886.

65a. Elmaagacli AH, Beelen DW, Trenschel R, and Schaefer UW. The detection of wt-1 transcripts is not associated with an increased leukemic relapse rate in patients with acute leukemia after allogeneic bone marrow or peripheral blood stem cell transplantation, *Bone Marrow Transplant*, **25** (2000) 91–96.

66. Nakao M, Janssen JW, Erz D, Seriu T, and Bartram CR. Tandem duplication of the FLT3 gene in acute lymphoblastic leukemia: a marker for the monitoring of minimal residual disease, [letter], *Leukemia*, **14** (2000) 522.
67. Nakao M, Yokota S, Iwai T, Kaneko H, Horiike S, Kashima K, et al. Internal tandem duplication of the flt3 gene found in acute myeloid leukemia, *Leukemia*, **10** (1996) 1911.
68. Yokota S, Kiyoi H, Nakao M, Iwai T, Misawa S, Okuda T, et al. Internal tandem duplication of the FLT3 gene is preferentially seen in acute myeloid leukemia and myelodysplastic syndrome among various hematological malignancies. A study on a large series of patients and cell lines, *Leukemia*, **11** (1997) 1605.
69. Xu F, Taki T, Yang HW, Hanada R, Hongo T, Ohnishi H, et al. Tandem duplication of the FLT3 gene is found in acute lymphoblastic leukaemia as well as acute myeloid leukaemia but not in myelodysplastic syndrome or juvenile chronic myelogenous leukaemia in children, *Br. J. Haematol.*, **105** (1999) 155.
70. Baylin SB, Herman JG, Graff JR, Vertino PM, and Issa JP. Alterations in DNA methylation: a fundamental aspect of neoplasia, *Adv. Cancer Res.*, **72** (1998) 141.
71. Issa JP, Baylin SB, and Herman JG. DNA methylation changes in hematologic malignancies: biologic and clinical implications, *Leukemia*, **11** (1997) S7.
72. Plass C, Yu F, Yu L, Strout MP, El-Rifai W, Elonen E, et al. Restriction landmark genome scanning for aberrant methylation in primary refractory and relapsed acute myeloid leukemia; involvement of the WIT-1 gene, *Oncogene*, **18** (1999) 3159.
73. Xiong Z and Laird PW. COBRA: a sensitive and quantitative DNA methylation assay, *Nucleic Acids Res.*, **25** (1997) 2532.
74. Eads CA, Danenberg KD, Kawakami K, Saltz LB, Blake C, Shibata D, et al. MethyLight: a high-throughput assay to measure DNA methylation, *Nucleic Acids Res.*, **28** (2000) E32.
75. Lo YM, Wong IH, Zhang J, Tein MS, Ng MH, and Hjelm NM. Quantitative analysis of aberrant p16 methylation using real-time quantitative methylation-specific polymerase chain reaction, *Cancer Res.*, **59** (1999) 3899.
76. Castilla LH, Garrett L, Adya N, Orlic D, Dutra A, Anderson S, et al. The fusion gene Cbfb-MYH11 blocks myeloid differentiation and predisposes mice to acute myelomonocytic leukaemia, [letter], *Nat. Genet.*, **23** (1999) 144.
77. Golub TR, Slonim DK, Tamayo P, Huard C, Gaasenbeek M, Mesirov JP, et al. Molecular classification of cancer: class discovery and class prediction by gene expression monitoring, *Science*, **286** (1999) 531.

# 10 Minimal Residual Disease in Acute Promyelocytic Leukemia

## Francesco Lo Coco and Daniela Diverio

### INTRODUCTION

Acute promyelocytic leukemia (APL) is a unique subtype of acute myeloid leukemia (AML) with specific genetic and clinical features, which include the frequent association at diagnosis of a life-threatening hemorrhagic diathesis, the presence in leukemic blasts of a specific chromosome translocation that has never been detected outside the APL context, and a striking response in vitro and in vivo to retinoids such as all-*trans* retinoic acid (ATRA) *(1–5)*. In light of the associated risk of massive bleeding (approx 10% of early hemorrhagic death are still reported even in patients receiving state-of-the-art modern treatments) *(6–14)*, APL should be considered a medical emergency. Together, the above characteristics contribute to classifying this disease as a unique leukemic subset requiring immediate recognition by means of genetic diagnosis and early onset of tailored treatment.

Detection of the APL-specific chromosome aberration (or of its molecular counterpart) permits identification of virtually 100% of patients responsive to ATRA, which, in turn, is known to exert its action through targeting the same product of the t(15;17) (i.e., the PML/RARα protein) *(1–5)* (see below). In addition, by inducing cell differentiation, ATRA therapy may effectively counteract the hemorrhagic syndrome and improve the coagulation parameters *(15)*. According to recently reported multicenter trials, combined ATRA and anthracycline-based chemotherapy results in long-term remission and potential cure in up to 70% of cases *(6–14)*, whereas prior to 1990, no more than 30% of patients were reported as long-term survivors after receiving conventional chemotherapy *(16)*. Two major advances have contributed to this impressive improvement: the identification of the APL-specific genetic lesion and the introduction of retinoids in frontline therapy.

From: *Leukemia and Lymphoma: Detection of Minimal Residual Disease*
Edited by: T. F. Zipf and D. A. Johnston © Humana Press Inc., Totowa, NJ

In 1990, only a few months after the report of first clinical experiences with ATRA *(17)*, several groups cloned the t(15;17) and demonstrated that two genes, the retinoic acid receptor-α (RARα) and the newly described *PML* gene (for promyelocytic), were joined together to form a hybrid protein as a result of the chromosomal recombination *(18–20)*. As it occurred with the BCR-ABL hybrid underlying the Philadelphia chromosome detected in chronic myeloid leukemia, the identification of such novel abnormality led to an impressive series of basic and applied studies. The latter included development of polymerase chain reaction (PCR)-based strategies for improving diagnosis and for analysis of minimal residual disease *(21–29)*. In addition to the important progress in diagnostic recognition, it was soon demonstrated that use of the PCR technology to assess response to therapy and clinical outcome could be helpful in the management of APL. In fact, a number of studies published in the early 1990s indicated that patients who converted from PCR negative to PCR positive for PML/RARα while in clinical remission were at higher relapse risk and, conversely, that negativization of PML/RARα below PCR sensitivity levels was associated with improved outcome *(28–34)*. More recently, large cooperative studies in which patients were prospectively monitored have confirmed these results and several groups worldwide are currently using PCR results to guide therapy *(7,35,36)*. In light of this possibility and considering the availability of a disease-specific agent targeting the genetic lesion, APL is now regarded as a paradigm for molecularly targeted and PCR-driven therapy in hematooncology. However, a number of issues related to the technique itself and to its reproducibility and standardization have been raised and actually deserve special attention *(37)*. The objective of solving these controversies is, obviously, that of allowing clinicians a better comparison of PCR results among studies, in order to feel more confident with respect to PCR-based therapeutic decision.

We will describe here methodologic and clinical aspects of PCR studies applied to APL diagnosis and monitoring. Furthermore, we will review critically the results reported so far in clinical trials and relevant investigational areas for future research.

## MOLECULAR ARCHITECTURE OF THE t(15;17) AND ROLE IN APL PATHOGENESIS

APL is cytogenetically characterized by reciprocal translocations that constantly involve chromosome 17, with breaks within the locus encoding for the retinoic acid receptor-α (RARα) *(18–20)*. Usually, the chromosome partner is the 15, with the break located within the PML locus. The t(15;17) originates several aberrant proteins, including PML/RARα on the 15q+, RARα/PML on the 17q–, and a truncated PML gene *(26)*. The RARα/PML fusion gene is expressed in approx 70% of APLs, whereas the reciprocal PML/RARα is detected in almost 100% of cases, being, therefore, more suitable for routine molecular diagnosis and monitoring *(38)*. On the 17q, the breakpoints are consistently located in RARα intron 2 *(39,40)*, whereas on 15q, the breakpoints may be located at three different sites of the PML locus *(26)*. Based on this variability, three different PML/RARα isoforms are formed *(26–28)*. Of these, the so-called "long transcript," derived from PML bcr1, is detected in 55–60% of cases; the "short transcript" created as a consequence of bcr3 PML breakpoints is described in 35–40% of patients, and, finally, a bcr2 PML breakpoint (or "variable" transcript, derived from breaks in PML exon 6) is found in approx 8% of cases *(7,11,12)*.

The hybrid PML/RARα transcript retains both the PML RING finger and dimerization domains and the RARα DNA-binding and retinoic-acid-binding domains. In the presence of physiological concentrations of ATRA, PML/RARα acts as a transcription repressor on target genes, interfering with normal RAR, RXR, and PML functions *(1–5)*. When analyzed with specific antibodies, the PML protein shows, in normal cells and in non-t(15;17) leukemias, a characteristic nuclear staining in nuclear bodies (also named PODs). Interestingly, this pattern is abrogated in t(15;17)-positive cells and replaced by a microspeckled nuclear distribution. The identification of microspeckled structures correlates with the presence of the PML/RARα protein as determined by RT-PCR analysis, and is therefore suitable for the purpose of correct diagnosis *(41,42)*.

In rare cases, the APL phenotype might be associated with translocations involving RARα at 17q and other chromosome regions (i.e., 11q23, 5q32, 11q13 and 17q21 with breaks in the PLZF, NPM, NuMA, and STAT5b loci, respectively). The resulting hybrid genes encode PML/RARα, PLZF/RARα, NPM/RARα, or STAT5b/RARα fusion proteins, all of which retain the same portion of RARα *(43–46)*. Among the APL variants associated with distinct fusion genes, only the PML/RARα and the PLZF/RARα forms have been characterized in detail at the biological and clinical level *(1–5,47)*. Despite the fact that PML/RARα and PLZF/RARα APLs show clinical similarity, ATRA treatment induces differentiation only in PML/RARα APLs *(1–5,47)*. Moreover, both PML/RARα and PLZ/RARα transgenic mice develop leukemias; however, only leukemias from PML/RARα mice are ATRA sensitive *(48–52)*.

The potential of PML/RARα to interfere with hematopoietic differentiation is thought to involve transcriptional deregulation of retinoic acid (RA)-target genes. RARs are RA-dependent transcription factors that, in adult hematopoietic cells, are involved in the control of terminal differentiation *(53)*. In the absence of RA, RARs repress transcription by recruiting the nuclear corepressor (N-CoR)–histone deacetylase (HD) complex. Low levels of histone acetylation are thought to lead to a repressive chromatin conformation. RA releases the HD complex from RARs and recruits multiple coactivators, thus resulting in activation of gene expression *(54–57)*. PML/RARα retains the ability of RARα to regulate transcription of RA-target genes. Indeed, the integrity of the PML/RARα DNA-binding domain is essential for both the transcriptional regulation properties on RA-target genes and the effects on differentiation of the fusion protein. PML/RARα and PLZF/RARα fusion proteins recruit the N-CoR/HD complex through their RARα moiety. PLZF/RARα contains a second, RA-resistant binding site in the PLZF N-terminal region. This might explain why high doses of RA release HD activity from PML/RARα, but not from PLZF/RARα *(54–57)*.

## GENETIC CHARACTERIZATION OF APL AND UTILITY OF REVERSE TRANSCRIPTION–PCR AT DIAGNOSIS

Based on the equation specific lesion = specific therapy, modern diagnosis of APL must aim at rapidly identifying the genetic abnormality. This can be demonstrated at the chromosome, DNA, RNA, or protein level. Karyotyping on banded metaphases allows identification of the pathognomonic t(15;17) in the majority of cases; however, false-negative results are not uncommon, as a result of the analysis of cells not belonging to the neoplastic clone or, alternatively, to poor quality metaphases or occurrence of cryptic rearrangements *(1–5)*. This clearly indicates that lack of a t(15;17) by conventional cytogenetics does not necessarily preclude a diagnosis of APL. The use of fluorescence *in situ* hybridization (FISH) with specific probes frequently allows one to overcome the drawbacks of karyotyping by identifying the PML/RARα rearrangement in cases with cryptic translocations or apparently normal karyotype *(58)*.

Southern blot might be employed to identify rearrangements in the PML and RARα loci, although it is a laborious approach. In fact, several probes must be used to confirm the involvement of both PML and RARα *(39,59,60)*. Anti-PML polyclonal or monoclonal antibodies to analyze the PML distribution pattern in leukemic cells provide a rapid and simple diagnostic tool. This latter method exploits the characteristic aberrant distribution of the PML protein deriving form the translocation t(15;17), often referred to as "microspeckled," which differs considerably from that observed in normal cells and in non-t(15;17) leukemias (so-called "nuclear body" PML distribution) *(41,42,60)*. In light of their poor sensitivity, conventional karyotyping, Southern blot, and PML immunostaining are not suitable for MRD assessment.

Diagnostic detection of PML/RARα in leukemic cells by reverse transcription (RT)–PCR is the most specific and sensitive method for establishing patient eligibility into state-of-the-art ATRA-containing regimens *(21–29)*. In light of this and because it is the only technique that defines precisely the PML breakpoint type allowing one to establish a correct strategy for successive MRD monitoring, RT-PCR of PML/RARα should be mandatory at diagnosis in every APL patient. Recent results of large multicenter studies have indicated complete remission rates close to 100% for patients who had diagnosis confirmed by RT-PCR *(6,7,11,12)*. Updated results of the Italian GIMEMA study show that, of 480 patients PML/RARα positive by RT-PCR who completed the induction phase, only 1 (0.2%) was resistant to a treatment combining ATRA and idarubicin (unpublished data).

The main technical approaches for genetic diagnosis of APL, together with advantages and pitfalls of each method, are shown in Table 1.

## RT-PCR AMPLIFICATION OF PML/RARα: TECHNICAL ASPECTS

The quality of RNA and efficiency of the reverse transcription (RT) step are the most important determinants for successful RT-PCR analysis of PML/RARα *(58,61)*. Analysis of the extracted RNA by running into a minigel is recommended for detecting degradation and/or gross DNA contamination. At diagnosis, blood or marrow samples taken from an APL patient are particularly prone to rapid clotting, cell damage release of enzymes that could affect RNA yield and integrity. Rapid isolation of mononuclear cells and storage in a guanidium–isothiacyanate (GTC) solution is important in order to prevent RNA degradation. As for the reverse-transcription (RT) step, improved specificity of the reaction and amplification of cleaner products have been reported using the hot-start method, which contributes to minimize primer misannealing and enhances sensitivity of the reaction *(29)*. Controls of the diagnostic assay should include both the NB4 cell line (long transcript) and RNA derived from a patient with the short PML/RARα isoform. Negative controls should include a water lane and a no-RT lane to distinguish between possible RNA or cDNA contamination, respectively. To further verify RNA integrity and efficiency of the RT step using patient RNA ("internal control"), some authors amplify one of the two normal genes involved in the translocation, whereas others analyze a gene with a ubiquitous but low expressions gene *(62)*. Choice of the internal control is particularly relevant in the context of MRD studies. Figure 1 shows the location of PML and RARα primers and the distinct types of PML/RARα isoforms that may be detected in t(15;17) APL. Given two alternative splicings of PML exons downstream of exon 3 and two distinct locations of breakpoints, external PML primers would amplify a single band in bcr3 (short or S transcript) cases and a multiple band pattern in bcr1-2 (long or L transcript) cases *(26)*. In these latter, the successive use of an internal PML primer allows the resolution of a single band. Thus, the appropriate primer set capable of amplifying a single fragment will be preferably used after induction treatment for MRD monitoring.

As concerns MRD tests, the most critical issues are the timing of sampling, the sensitivity of the assay, and the controls of the reaction *(58)*. The timing of sampling is strictly dependent on the type of clinical context (e.g., ATRA, ATRA

Table 1
Techniques Used for Genetic Diagnosis of APL

| Method | Target lesion | Advantages | Pitfalls |
|---|---|---|---|
| Karyotype | t(15;17) | Highly specific; widely available | Frequent "normal" K (cryptic PML/RARα) |
| Southern blot | PML and RARα rearrangements | Highly specific | Time-consuming and laborious (several hybridizations required) |
| RT-PCR | PML/RARα hybrid | Rapid; specific; highly sensitive | Prone to false positive (contaminations, artifacts); poor RNA yield |
| PML immunostaining | PML nuclear pattern | Rapid; specific | Artifacts resulting from cell degradation; poorly sensitive |

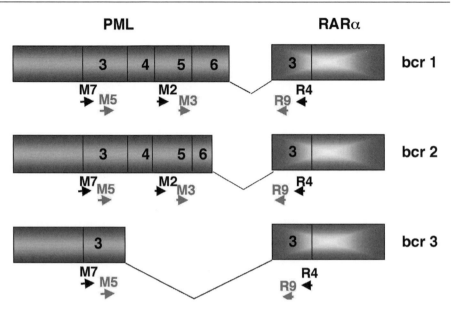

**Fig. 1.** Schematic representation of the three major PML/RARα isoforms and location of oligoprimers (arrows) used for the RT-PCR amplification of the hybrid transcript.

plus chemotherapy, allogeneic transplantation). Moreover, the frequency of PCR testing might be adapted to the relapse risk, which, in turn, may be considerably different from patient to patient. For example, a higher risk has been calculated for hyperleukocytic APL *(63)*. Finally, the first 6–8 mo after the end of frontline induction and consolidation represents a higher relapse risk *(6–14)*, and during which a more stringent monitoring might be justified. Thus, establishing appropriate time intervals for MRD evaluations is relevant to obtaining useful clinical information.

False-negative PCR has been attributed to the limited sensitivity of the assays used. This, in turn, depends largely on reasons intrinsic to the disease biology. In fact, it has been shown that the PML/RARα hybrid is expressed at extremely low levels in APL cells and is more unstable than the two wild-type genes. To increase the efficiency of reverse transcription, Seale et al. *(61)* suggested the use of greater amounts of RNA (up to 20 µg), initial denaturation of RNA (65°C for 5 min), and elongation of the incubation time to 2 h. Such modifications and the application of the hot-start principle allow one to increase the cDNA yield, as reproduced by others and by our group. Internal controls to be chosen in the context of MRD should be low-expressed genes devoid of pseudogenes and should be diluted in order to quantitatively reproduce the minimal amounts of MRD *(62)*.

# CLINICAL SIGNIFICANCE
# OF THE DISTINCT PML/RARα ISOFORMS

Initial studies published in the early 1990s suggested that patients with the short (bcr3) isoform had an inferior outcome, as compared to those carrying the long PML/RARα transcript *(64,65)*. In addition, a study by Gallagher et al. *(66)* indicated a poorer response to ATRA in vitro for patients with the bcr2 (or variable) isoform. More recently, the same analysis in a larger series published in Europe *(7,11,12)* and in the United States *(67)* did not report a significant difference in the outcome of APL patients according to PML/RARα junction type, although a trend toward a poorer clinical outcome was found for patients with the short isoform. One important difference explaining such apparent discrepancies is related to the different therapeutic context. In fact, although patients with bcr2 and bcr3 isotypes might be less responsive to ATRA alone, such difference seems to be abrogated with modern combinatorial regimens, including chemotherapy and ATRA, as shown by the US Intergroup *(67)*, the Italian GIMEMA *(7)*, the British MRC *(11)*, and the Spanish PETHEMA studies *(12)*. However, it has to be emphasized that in the reported series the techniques used fail to distinguish the bcr1 from bcr2 PML/RARα isoforms. Hence, the prognostic significance of including bcr2 patients in the long-transcript group is unknown. However, the bcr2 patient cohort accounts for only 8% of APL cases *(58)*. A recently reported in vivo study in patients enrolled in the US Intergroup trial did not clarify this issue, given the low patient number and the fact that half of them received chemotherapy alone *(67)*. A longer follow-up of large clinical trials will probably clarify better the prognostic significance of PML/RARα isoforms.

## LONGITUDINAL PCR STUDIES OF MRD IN APL

The first technical reports on RT-PCR strategies to amplify the PML/RARα hybrid were reported in 1992 by Miller et al. *(21)*, Biondi et al. *(22)*, Castaigne et al. *(24)*, and Borrow et al. *(23)*. These were immediately followed by a number of studies on MRD assessment after therapy, which included mostly retrospective evaluations performed in patients receiving ATRA alone or with chemotherapy *(25–34)*. Together, these showed that treatment with ATRA given as a single agent was almost uniformly associated with persistence of PCR positivity. Confirming previous clinical observation, this indicated that ATRA given orally was unable to eradicate the leukemic clone. By contrast, chemotherapy and/or bone marrow transplantation was associated in approximately half of the cases with negativization of the PCR test. Moreover, using techniques with sensitivity $10^{-4}$–$10^{-3}$, patients in long-term remission invariably tested PCR negative, whereas conversion from negative to positive during hematologic remission was strongly predictive of subsequent relapse *(25–34)*. This suggested, in turn, that

Table 2
Results of Prospective RT-PCR Monitoring of PML/RARα
in APL Patients Treated in the GIMEMA, MRC, and PETHEMA Trials

| Study group (ref.) | % Patients PCR positive/ PCR negative after induction | Difference in relapse risk in patients positive vs negative postinduction | % Positive postconsolidation | Relapse risk at 2 yr (all patients) |
|---|---|---|---|---|
| GIMEMA (7) | 40 | NS | 5 | 20 |
| MRC (11) | 60 | NS | 6 | 25 |
| PETHEMA (12) | 51 | NS | 7 | 10 |

Note: NS = not significant.

molecular remission represents a more appropriate and advanced therapeutic objective in APL. Following publication of these preliminary reports, several groups initiated prospective PCR monitoring in patients enrolled in large multicenter trials of ATRA and chemotherapy, including the GIMEMA, PETHEMA, and MRC groups (7,11,12,35,36). Based on the notion that ATRA alone was insufficient for cure, these trials included several combinatorial regimens in which conventional chemotherapy was added to differentiating treatment (7,11,12,35,36).

Approximately 50% of patients receiving ATRA plus chemotherapy had detectable PML/RARα transcript in their marrow after completing induction in the GIMEMA (7), MRC (11), and PETHEMA (12) studies, although no correlations were found between PCR status at the time of remission achievement after induction and relapse risk (Table 2). After completion of consolidation, 93–95% of cases tested PCR negative in the marrow in the above series (7,11,12). As to tests performed in between consolidation cycles, the MRC data indicated that patients remaining positive after three chemotherapy courses (of four total cycles) had increased risk of hematologic relapse as compared to patients who achieved earlier negativization of PML/RARα. Interestingly, this finding had independent prognostic significance together with white blood cell count in the multivariate analysis of relapse risk. Unfortunately, this evaluation was available for only a minor proportion of patients enrolled in the MRC study (11). A rather distinct kinetics of PML/RARα negativization was observed in the German AMLCG study, where patients were given a double induction strategy including high-dose cytarabine (TAD/HAM protocol) in combination with ATRA. In fact, up to 91% of patients studied after this induction tested negative by RT-PCR performed in the bone marrow. Given the low patient number and limited follow-up, it cannot be established at this time whether such a high percentage of early PCR negativization translates into better relapse-free and overall survival as compared with results published by others *(68)*.

Postconsolidation monitoring studies have been prospectively performed at pre-established time intervals in patients enrolled in the GIMEMA study *(35)*. The results on 163 homogeneously treated and longitudinally evaluated cases showed that 20 of 21 who converted from PCR negative to PCR positive after consolidation therapy underwent hematologic relapse at a median time of 3 mo from PCR conversion, whereas only 8 (or 5.6%) in the group of patients who tested PCR negative in two or more tests after consolidation relapsed after a median time of 18 mo. These results led the Italian group to anticipate salvage therapy in such patients *(35)*.

A comparison of marrow versus peripheral blood (PB) PCR testing for PML/RARα has been performed in some of the patients enrolled in the GIMEMA study. This showed that although the hybrid transcript is always detectable at diagnosis in both PB and marrow (even in cases with very low leukocyte count and absence of PB blasts), MRD is better identified during remission in marrow samples (unpublished observations). Therefore, for the purpose of MRD evaluation, marrow testing rather than PB is recommended.

Although there is general consensus on the value of PCR positivity during remission as a predictor of relapse, several cautionary issues have to be considered before a therapeutic decision is based on molecular tests. The above results are, in fact, based on studies performed in the context of uniform clinical trials and employing PCR tests with $10^{-4}$ sensitivity. Persistence of residual disease in long-term remission using more sensitive assays have been occasionally reported *(69)*. In addition, in order to rule out the occurrence of contamination, confirmation of molecular relapse in an additional marrow sample is required in the GIMEMA study prior to initiate salvage therapy *(35)*. Finally, one major limitation of the employed assays is their failure to precisely quantitate the amount of residual disease, which, in turn, makes difficult a comparison among the reported studies. The use in the near future of the newly developed real-time PCR technology may hold promise to provide adequate standardization at the quantitative level and more objective comparison of results.

## PCR-DRIVEN THERAPY IN APL

Based on results of prospective PCR studies, several groups have designed therapeutic strategies for APL that include longitudinal PCR monitoring of PML/RARα and adaptation of treatment intensity to the results of molecular evaluations *(36,70)*. Treatment intensification for patients who convert to PCR positive is currently adopted by the GIMEMA, PETHEMA, Japan Acute Leukemia Study Group (JALSG), and MD Anderson Cancer Center (MDACC) groups *(36,70)*. Following frontline induction and consolidation with ATRA and anthracycline-based chemotherapy, the GIMEMA and PETHEMA groups have adapted the stringency of PCR controls according to relapse risk. Thus, patients at higher risk of relapse (e.g., those with initial leukocyte counts above $10 \times 10^6$) are monitored more frequently as compared to patients in the low-risk category. Then, patients who show conversion from PCR negative to positive are given salvage therapy (following confirmation of molecular relapse in another marrow sample), and the same treatment is administered to those rare cases of molecularly resistant disease (i.e., patients who after frontline induction and consolidation do not achieve PCR negativity).

In a recently published study of the MDACC *(36)*, patients with newly diagnosed APL were given intravenous liposomal ATRA as a single agent for a total time of 9 mo and were monitored prospectively from the time of diagnosis. Patients who had a PCR-positive test in two successive controls during Atragen therapy were administered additional treatment with idarubicin, whereas those remaining PCR negative were maintained on Atragen alone *(36)*. Hence, PCR monitoring not only is intended as a tool for identifying patients in need of additional treatments but also may function as a means of avoiding unnecessary toxicity in a highly curable leukemia.

## FUTURE PERSPECTIVES

During the past decade, basic and clinical research have contributed important advances in our understanding of APL pathogenesis and this has been paralleled by a significant improvement in clinical results. The use in APL of treatment targeted at an abnormal leukemia-associated protein represent the first example of genetic-tailored therapy in human cancer and have fostered basic and clinical research aimed at extending the potential of differentiation and molecularly driven therapy to other leukemia subsets. In addition to these important advances, several issues still remain to be addressed and will be the subject of future investigation. Among these, the precise biochemical mechanisms of APL leukemogenesis, the role of other APL-associated abnormal products, and the significance of additional genetic alterations need to be clarified. Moreover, mechanisms associated with the development of ATRA resistance are poorly understood, and in spite of receiving modern state-of-the-art therapies, a sizable proportion of APL patients still succumb to their disease and/or suffer from severe chemotherapy-related toxicity. In this context, the use of a well-designed and standardized molecular monitoring is not only relevant to better identify patients at risk of relapse and therefore intensifying or anticipating treatment, but also appears important in order to spare unnecessary toxicity in patients presumably cured. It is hoped that cooperation at the multinational level, including efforts aimed at improving PCR technology and interlaboratory standardization, will further contribute to better risk-adapted protocols to increase the cure rate of this once inevitably fatal disease.

## REFERENCES

1. Grignani F, Fagioli M, Alcalay M, Longo L, Pandolfi PP, Donti E, et al. Acute promyelocytic leukemia: from genetics to treatment, *Blood*, **83** (1994) 10–25.
2. Chen S-J, Wang Z-Y, and Chen Z. Acute promyelocytic leukemia: from clinic to molecular biology, *Stem Cells*, **13** (1995) 22–31.
3. Warrell RP Jr. Pathogenesis and management of acute promyelocytic leukemia, *Annu. Rev. Med.*, **47** (1996) 555–565.
4. Fenaux P, Chomienne C, and Degos L. Acute promyelocytic leukemia: biology and treatment, *Semin. Oncol.*, **24** (1997) 92–102.
5. Lo Coco F, Nervi C, Avvisati A, and Mandelli F. Acute promyelocytic leukemia: a curable disease, *Leukemia*, **12** (1998) 1866–1880.
6. Soignet S, Fleischauer A, Polyak T, Heller G, and Warrell RP Jr. All-trans retinoic acid significantly increases 5-year survival in patients with acute promyelocytic leukemia: long-term follow-up of the New York study, *Cancer Chemother. Pharmacol.*, **40** (1997) S25–S29.
7. Mandelli F, Diverio D, Avvisati G, Luciano A, Barbui T, Bernasconi C, et al. Molecular remission in PML/RARa positive acute promyelocytic leukemia by combined all-trans retinoic acid and idarubicin (AIDA) therapy, *Blood*, **90** (1997) 1014–1021.
8. Estey E, Thal PG, Pierce S, Kantarjian H, and Keating M. Treatment of newly diagnosed acute promyelocytic leukemia without cytarabine, *J. Clin. Oncol.*, **15** (1997) 483–490.
9. Tallman MS, Andersen JW, Schiffer CA, Appelbaum FR, Feusener JH, Ogden A, et al. All-trans retinoic acid in acute promyelocytic leukemia, *N. Engl. J. Med.*, **337** (1997) 1201–1208.
10. Asou N, Adachi J, Tamura J, Kanamuru S, Kageyama S, Hirakoa A, et al., for the Japan Adult Leukemia Study Group. Analysis of prognostic factors in newly diagnosed acute promyelocytic leukemia treated with all-trans retinoic acid and chemotherapy, *J. Clin. Oncol.*, **16** (1998) 78–85.
11. Burnett AK, Grimwade D, Solomon E, Wheatley K, and Goldstone AH, on behalf of the MRC Adult Leukemia Working Party. Presenting white blood cell count and kinetics of molecular remission predict prognosis in acute promyelocytic leukemia treated with all-trans retinoic acid: result of the randomized MRC trial, *Blood*, **93** (1999) 4131–4143.
12. Sanz MA, Martin G, Rayon C, Esteve J, Gonzalez M, Diaz-Mediavilla J, et al. A modified AIDA protocol with anthracycline-based consolidation results in high antileukemic efficacy and reduced toxicity in newly diagnosed PML/RARa-positive acute promyelocytic leukemia, *Blood*, **94** (1999) 3015–3021.
13. Wang Z, Sun G, Shen Z, Chen S, and Chen Z. Differentiation therapy for acute promyelocytic leukemia with all-trans retinoid acid: 10-year experience of its application, *Chin. Med. J.*, **112** (1999) 963–967.
14. Fenaux P, Chastang C, Chevret S, Sanz MA, Dombret H, Archimbaud E, et al. A randomized comparison of ATRA followed by chemotherapy and ATRA plus chemotherapy, and the role of maintenance therapy in newly diagnosed acute promyelocytic leukemia, *Blood*, **94** (1999) 1192–1200.
15. Barbui T, Finazzi G, and Falanga A. The impact of all-trans retinoic acid on the coagulopathy of acute promyelocytic leukemia, *Blood*, **91** (1998) 3093–3102.
16. Stone R and Mayer RJ. The unique aspects of acute promyelocytic leukemia, *J. Clin. Oncol.*, **8** (1990) 1913–1921.
17. Huang ME, Yu-Chen Y, Shou-Rong C, Lu MX, Zhoa L, Gu LJ, et al. Use of all-trans retinoic acid in treatment of acute promyelocytic leukemia, *Blood*, **72** (1988) 567–572.

18. Borrow J, Goddard AD, Sherr D, and Solomon E. Molecular analysis of acute promyelocytic leukemia breakpoint cluster region on chromosome 17, *Science*, **249** (1990) 1577–1580.
19. de Thé H, Chomienne C, Lanotte M, Degos L, and Dejean A. The t(15;17) translocation of acute promyelocytic leukemia fuses the retinoic acid receptor α gene to a novel transcribed locus, *Nature*, **347** (1990) 558–561.
20. Alcalay M, Zangrilli D, Pandolfi PP, Longo L, Mencarelli A, Giacomucci A, et al. Translocation breakpoint of acute promyelocytic leukemia lies within retinoic acid receptor α locus, *Proc. Natl. Acad. Sci. USA*, **88** (1991) 1977–1981.
21. Miller WH, Kakizuka A, Frankel SR, Warrell RP, DeBlasio A, Levine K, et al. Reverse transcription polymerase chain reaction for the rearranged retinoic acid receptor alpha clarifies diagnosis and detects minimal residual disease in acute promyelocytic leukemia, *Proc. Natl. Acad. Sci. USA*, **89** (1992) 2694–2698.
22. Biondi A, Rambaldi A, Alcalay M, Pandolfi PP, Lo Coco F, Diverio D, et al. RARa rearrangements as a genetic marker for diagnosis and monitoring in acute promyelocytic leukemia, *Blood*, **77** (1991) 1418–1422.
23. Borrow J, Goddard AD, Gibbons B, Katz F, Swirsky D, Fioretos T, et al. Diagnosis of acute promyelocytic leukemia by RT-PCR detection of PML/RARa and RARa /PML fusion transcript, *Br. J. Haematol.*, **82** (1992) 529–540.
24. Castaigne S, Balitrand N, de Thé H, Dejean A, Degos L, and Chomienne C. A PML/retinoic acid receptor a fusion transcript is constantly detected by RNA-based polymerase chain reaction in acute promyelocytic leukemia, *Blood*, **79** (1992) 3110–3115.
25. Chang KS, Lu J, Wang G, Trujillo JM, Estey E, Cork A, et al. The t(15;17) breakpoint in acute promyelocytic leukemia cluster within two different sites of the myl gene. Targets for the detection of minimal residual disease by polymerase chain reaction, *Blood*, **79** (1992) 554–558.
26. Pandolfi PP, Alcalay M, Fagioli M, Zangrilli D, Mencarelli A, Diverio D, et al. Genomic variability and alternative splicing generate multiple PML-RARα transcripts that encode aberrant PML proteins and PML-RARα isoforms in acute promyelocytic leukemia, *EMBO J.*, **11** (1992) 1397–1407.
27. Chen SJ, Chen Z, Chen A, Tong JH, Dong S, Wang ZY, et al. Occurrence of distinct PML-RARα fusion gene isoforms in patients with acute promyelocytic leukemia detected by reverse transcriptase/polymerase chain reaction, *Oncogene*, **7** (1992) 1223–1232.
28. Huang W, Sun GL, Li XS, Cao Q, Lu Y, Jang GS, et al. Acute promyelocytic leukemia: clinical relevance of two major PML-RARα isoforms and detection of minimal residual disease by retrotranscriptase polymerase chain reaction to predict relapse, *Blood*, **82** (1993) 1264–1269.
29. Diverio D, Riccioni R, Pistilli A, Buffolino S, Avvisati G, Mandelli F, et al. Improved rapid detection of the PML/RARa fusion gene in acute promyelocytic leukemia, *Leukemia*, **10** (1996) 1214–1216.
30. Lo Coco F, Diverio D, Pandolfi PP, Biondi A, Rossi V, Avvisati G, et al. Molecular evaluation of residual disease as a predictor of relapse in acute promyelocytic leukemia, *Lancet*, **340** (1992) 1437–1438.
31. Miller WH, Levine K, DeBlasio A, Frankel SR, Dmitrovsky E, and Warrell RP. Detection of minimal residual disease in acute promyelocytic leukemia by reverse transcription polymerase chain reaction for the PML/RARa fusion mRNA, *Blood*, **82** (1993) 1689–1694.
32. Diverio D, Pandolfi PP, Biondi A, Avvisati G, Petti MC, Mandelli F, et al. Absence of RT-PCR detectable residual disease in acute promyelocytic leukemia in long term remission, *Blood*, **85** (1993) 3556–3559.
33. Fukutani H, Naoe T, Ohno R, Yoshida H, Kiyoi H, Miyawaki S, et al. Prognostic significance of the RT-PCR assay of PML/RARa transcripts in acute promyelocytic leukemia, *Leukemia*, **9** (1995) 588–593.

34. Martinelli G, Remiddi C, Visani G, Farabegoli P, Testoni N, Zaccaria A, et al. Molecular analysis of PML/RARa fusion mRNA detected by reverse transcription-polymerase chain reaction assay in long-term disease-free acute promyelocytic leukemia patients, *Br. J. Haematol.*, **90** (1995) 966–968.

35. Diverio D, Rossi V, Avvisati G, De Santis S, Pistilli A, Pane F, et al. Early detection of relapse by prospective reverse transcriptase–polymerase chain reaction analysis of the PML/RARa fusion gene in patients with acute promyelocytic leukemia enrolled in the GIMEMA-AIEOP multicenter AIDA trial, *Blood*, **92** (1998) 784–789.

36. Estey EH, Giles FJ, Kantarjian H, O'Brien S, Cortes J, Freireich EJ, et al. Molecular remissions induced by liposomal-encapsulated all-trans retinoic acid in newly diagnosed acute promyelocytic leukemia, *Blood*, **94** (1999) 2230–2235.

37. Lo Coco F, Diverio D, Falini B, Biondi A, Nervi C, and Pelicci PG. Genetic diagnosis and molecular monitoring in the management of acute promyelocytic leukemia, *Blood*, **94** (1999) 12–22.

38. Alcalay M, Zangrilli D, Fagioli M, Pandolfi PP, Mencarelli A, Lo Coco F, et al. Expression pattern of the RARα/PML fusion gene in acute promyelocytic leukemia, *Proc. Natl. Acad. Sci. USA*, **89** (1992) 4840–4845.

39. Diverio D, Lo Coco F, D'Adamo F, Biondi A, Fagioli M, Grignani F, et al. Identification of DNA rearrangements at the RARa locus in all patients with acute promyelocytic leukemia and mapping of APL breakpoints within the RARa second intron, *Blood*, **79** (1992) 3331–3336.

40. Chen SJ, Zhu YJ, Tong JH, Dong S, Huang W, Chen Y, et al. Rearrangements in the second intron of the RARα gene are present in a large majority of patients with acute promyelocytic leukemia and are used as molecular marker for retinoic acid-induced leukemic cell differentiation, *Blood*, **78** (1991) 2696–2701.

41. Dyck J, Warrell RP, Evans RM, and Miller WH. Rapid diagnosis of acute promyelocytic leukemia by immunohistochemical localization of PML/RARa protein, *Blood*, **86** (1995) 862–867.

42. Falini B, Flenghi L, Fagioli M, Lo Coco F, Cordone I, Diverio D, et al. Immunocytochemical diagnosis of acute promyelocytic leukemia (M3) with the monoclonal antibody PG-M3 (anti-PML), *Blood*, **90** (1997) 4046–4053.

43. Chen SJ, Zelent A, Tong JH, Yu HQ, Wang ZY, Derre J, et al. Rearrangements of the retinoic acid receptor alpha and promyelocytic zing finger genes resulting from t(11;17)(q23;q21) in a patient with acute promyelocytic leukaemia, *J. Clin. Invest.*, **91** (1993) 2260–2267.

44. Redner RL, Rush EA, Faas S, Rudert WA, and Corey SJ. The t(5;17) variant of acute promyelocytic leukemia expresses a nucleophosmin-retinoic acid receptor fusion, *Blood*, **87** (1996) 882–886.

45. Wells RA, Catzavelos C, and Kamel-Reid S. Fusion of retinoic acid receptor a to NUMA, the nuclear mitotic apparatus protein, by a variant translocation in acute promyelocytic leukemia, *Nat. Genet.*, **17** (1997) 109–113.

46. Arnould C, Philippe C, Bourdon V, Gregoire MJ, Berger R, and Jonveaux P. The signal transducer and activator of transcription STAT5b gene is a new partner of retinoic acid receptor [alpha] in acute promyelocytic leukemia, *Hum. Mol. Genet.*, **8** (1999) 1741–1749.

47. Licht JD, Chomienne C, Goy A, Chen A, Scott AA, Head DR, et al. Clinical and molecular characterization of a rare syndrome of acute promyelocytic leukemia associated with translocation (11;17), *Blood*, **85** (1995) 1083–1094.

48. Early E, Moore MAS, Kakizuka A, Nason-Burchenal K, Martin P, Evans RM, et al. Transgenic expression of PML/RARa impairs myelopoiesis, *Proc. Natl. Acad. Sci. USA*, **93** (1996) 7900–7905.

49. He LZ, Tribioli C, Rivi R, Peruzzi D, Pelicci PG, Soares V, et al. Acute leukemia with promyelocytic features in PML/RARa transgenic mice, *Proc. Natl. Acad. Sci. USA*, **94** (1997) 5302–5307.

50. Brown D, Kogan S, Lagasse E, Weissman I, Alcalay M, Pelicci PG, et al. A PML/RARa transgene initiates murine acute promyelocytic leukemia, *Proc. Natl. Acad. Sci. USA*, **94** (1997) 2551–2556.
51. Grisolano JL, Wesselschmidt RL, Pelicci PG, and Ley TJ. Altered myeloid development and acute leukemia in transgenic mice expressing PML/RARa under control of cathepsin G regulatory sequences, *Blood*, **89** (1997) 2322–2333.
52. Cheng G-X, Meng X-Q, Jin X-L, Wang L, Zhu J, Xiong SM, et al. Establishment of transgenic mice models with acute promyelocytic leukemia-specific fusion genes PLZF-RARa and NPM-RARa, *Blood*, **92** (1998) 213a
53. Chambon P. A decade of molecular biology of retinoic acid receptors, *FASEB J.*, **10** (1996) 940–954.
54. Grignani F, Matteis SD, Nervi C, Tommasoni L, Gelmetti V, Cioce M, et al. Fusion proteins of the retinoic acid receptor-a recruit histone deacetylase in promyelocytic leukemia, *Nature*, **391** (1998) 815–818.
55. Lin R, Nagy L, Inoue S, Shao W, Miller WH, and Evans RM. Role of the histone deacetylase complex in acute promyelocytic leucemia, *Nature*, **391** (1998) 811–814.
56. Hong SH, David G, Wong CW, Dejean A, and Privalsky ML. SMRT corepressor interacts with PLZF and with the PML-retinoic acid receptor a (RARa) and PLZF/RARa oncoproteins associated with acute promyelocytic leukemia, *Proc. Natl. Acad. Sci. USA*, **94** (1997) 9028–9033.
57. He LZ, Guidez F, Tribioli C, Peruzzi D, Ruthardt M, Zelent A, et al. Distinct interactions of PML/RARalpha and PLZF/ RARalpha with co-repressors determine differential responses to RA in APL, *Nat. Genet.*, **18** (1998) 126–134.
58. Lo Coco F, Diverio D, Falini B, Biondi A, Nervi C, and Pelicci PG. Genetic diagnosis and molecular monitoring in the management of acute promyelocytic leukemia, *Blood*, **94** (1999) 12–22.
59. Chen SJ, Zhu Y-J, Dong S, Huang W, Chen Y, Xiang W-M, et al. Rearrangements in the second intron of the RARA gene are present in a large majority of patients with acute promyelocytic leukemia and are used as molecular marker for retinoic acid-induced leukemic cell differentiation, *Blood*, **78** (1991) 2696–2701.
60. Grimwade D, Howe K, Langabeer S, Davies L, Oliver F, Walker H, et al. Establishing the presence of the t(15;17) in suspected acute promyelocytic leukemia: cytogenetic, molecular and PML immunofluorescence assessment of patients entered into the M.R.C. ATRA trial, *Br. J. Haematol.*, **94** (1996) 557–573.
61. Seale JRC, Varma S, Swirsky DM, Pandolfi PP, Goldman JM, and Cross NCP. Quantification of PML/RARa transcript in acute promyelocytic leukemia: explanation for lack of sensitivity of RT-PCR for the detection of minimal residual disease and induction of the leukemia specific mRNA by alpha interferon, *Br. J. Haematol.*, **95** (1996) 95–101.
62. Kidd V and Lion T. Debate round-table: appropriate controls for RT-PCR, *Leukemia*, **11** (1997) 871–881.
63. Sanz MA, Lo Coco F, Martin G, Avvisati G, Rayon C, Barbui T, et al, for the Spanish PETHEMA and the Italian GIMEMA Cooperative Groups. Definition of relapse risk and role of non anthracycline drugs for consolidation in patients with acute promyelocytic leukemia: a joint study of the PETHEMA and GIMEMA cooperative groups, *Blood*, **96** (2000) 1247–1253.
64. Vahdat L, Maslak P, Miller WH, Eardley A, Heller G, Scheinberg DA, et al. Early mortality and retinoic acid syndrome in acute promyelocytic leukemia: impact of leucocytosis, low-dose chemotherapy, PML/RARα isoform, and CD13 expression in patients treated with all-trans retinoic acid, *Blood*, **84** (1994) 3843–3849.
65. Slack JL, Arthur DC, Lawrence D, Mrozek K, Mayer RJ, Davey FR, et al. Secondary cytogenetic changes in acute promyelocytic leukemia: prognostic importance in patients treated

with chemotherapy alone and association with the intron 3 breakpoint of the PML gene. A Cancer and Leukemia Group B study, *J. Clin. Oncol.*, **15** (1997) 1786–1795.

66. Gallagher RE, Li Y-P, Rao S, Paietta E, Andersen J, Etkind P, et al. Characterization of acute promyelocytic leukemia cases with PML/RARα break/fusion sites in PML exon 6: Identification of a subgroup with decreased in vitro responsiveness to all-trans retinoic acid, *Blood*, **86** (1995) 1540–1547.

67. Gallagher RE, Willman CL, Slack JL, Andersen JW, Li YP, Viswanatha D, et al. Association of PML-RAR alpha fusion mRNA type with pretreatment hematologic characteristics but not treatment outcome in acute promyelocytic leukemia: an intergroup molecular study, *Blood*, **90** (1997) 1656–1663.

68. Lengfelder E, Reichert A, Schoch C, Haase D, Haferlach T, Loffler H, et al. Double induction strategy including high dose cytarabine in combination with all-trans retinoic acid: effects in patients with newly diagnosed acute promyelocytic leukemia. German AML Cooperative Group, *Leukemia*, **14** (2000) 1362–1370.

69. Tobal K, Saunders MJ, Grey MR, and Liu Yin JA. Persistence of RARa/PML fusion mRNA detected by reverse polymerase chain reaction in patients in long-term remission of acute promyelocytic leukemia, *Br. J. Haematol.*, **90** (1995) 615–618.

70. Lo Coco F, Diverio D, Avvisati G, Petti MC, Meloni G, Pogliani EM, et al. Therapy of molecular relapse in acute promyelocytic leukemia, *Blood*, **94** (1999) 2225–2229.

# 11 Minimal Residual Disease in Chronic Myelogenous Leukemia

## Results of RT-PCR Detection of BCR-ABL Transcripts

### *Nicholas C. P. Cross and Andreas Hochhaus*

## INTRODUCTION

### *Aims of MRD Analysis in CML*

The degree of treatment-induced tumor load reduction is an important prognostic factor for patients with CML. Response to treatment may be determined at three levels: (1) hematologic response, defined as the normalization of peripheral blood counts and spleen size; (2) cytogenetic response, defined as the reduction in the proportion of Ph-positive metaphases detected by conventional karyotypic analysis or fluorescence *in situ* hybridization; and (3) molecular response, defined as the reduction in BCR-ABL DNA, mRNA, or protein.

Minimal residual disease (MRD) refers to the presence of cells derived from the malignant clone in patients who are in conventional remission; in CML this is usually defined by cytogenetic criteria. The aim of MRD analysis is to enable a better assessment of the response of individual patients to treatment or to evaluate the efficacy of a particular treatment protocol on a group of patients. Measurements of residual disease may potentially be used to stratify patients according to risk of relapse prior to conventional relapse diagnosis and to adopt risk-oriented or individualized treatment protocols. In the context of CML, this stratification could mean a reduced or increased dosage of interferon-$\alpha$ (IFN) and whether or not to undergo bone marrow transplantation (BMT) or the use of immunotherapy (e.g., donor lymphocyte infusion) post-BMT for impending relapse. The same techniques can also be used to assess the extent to which enriched "stem" cell harvests or selected cells for autografting are contaminated

From: *Leukemia and Lymphoma: Detection of Minimal Residual Disease*
Edited by: T. F. Zipf and D. A. Johnston © Humana Press Inc., Totowa, NJ

with malignant cells. MRD analysis is likely to play an important role in the initial assessment of the efficacy of new treatments, such as the tyrosine kinase inhibitor ST1571.

## Molecular Genetics of CML

The standard Ph chromosome is seen in approx 90% of cases of CML, and cytogenetic visible variants account for a further 5%. The remaining 5% of cases have a visibly normal karyotype, and on molecular analysis, roughly half turn out to be BCR-ABL positive; the rest are considered to have a BCR-ABL-negative chronic myeloproliferative disorder (1).

The t(9;22) genomic translocation breakpoints cluster within the 5.8-kb major breakpoint cluster region of the BCR gene but are widely dispersed within ABL, principally because the first intron of this gene is extremely large (2,3). However, after splicing of the primary transcript, at least 98% of CML patients have a chimeric mRNA in which either BCR exon b2 (exon 13) or b3 (exon 14) is fused to ABL exon 2 (b2a2 or b3a2 transcripts) (4,8). Both transcripts give rise to a 210-kDa BCR-ABL protein and roughly 5–10% of patients express both b2a2 and b3a2 mRNA (see Fig. 1). About 0.5–1% of patients express p190 BCR-ABL, which results from the fusion of BCR exon 1 to ABL exon 2 and which is more typically found in Ph-positive acute lymphoblastic leukemia (5). p190 BCR-ABL mRNA is also detectable in most or all p210 patients at a low level and probably arises through missplicing (6,7). The remaining cases, perhaps 1–2% of the total, are accounted for by a number of rare BCR-ABL fusions, the majority of which lack ABL exon 2 (3,4). BCR-ABL transcript types are stable over time in individual patients and there is no convincing evidence that clonal evolution may occur.

There is believed to be no clinical difference between those cases that are positive for p210 BCR-ABL without a discernible Ph-chromosome and those cases with typical Ph-positive disease (9). Patients who express high levels of p190 BCR-ABL usually have distinct hematological features, principally monocytosis (5). However, because of the small number of cases reported, the impact on prognosis for these individuals, or patients who express other variant fusions, is unclear.

## METHODS TO DETECT CML CELLS

### Cytogenetic Techniques

#### CONVENTIONAL CYTOGENETICS

Several studies have shown that cytogenetic response to IFN is significantly correlated with clinical outcome (10–12), and this technique therefore remains the standard method to ascertain the quality of remission in CML patients. Bone marrow metaphase chromosomes, derived from dividing cells, are scored for the

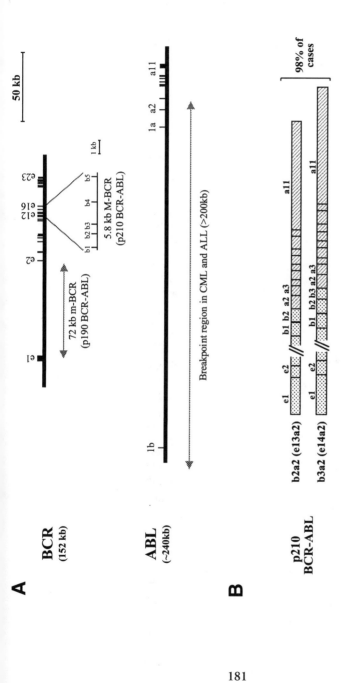

**Fig. 1.** (A) Structure of the BCR and ABL loci. The minor breakpoint cluster region (m-BCR) and major breakpoint cluster regions (M-BCR) are indicated. (B) Structure of b2a2, b3a2, and e1a2 BCR-ABL transcripts in CML.

presence or absence of the Ph-chromosome and/or any other abnormalities. Complete cytogenetic remission or response is usually defined as the finding of a normal karyotype in at least 20 or 30 consecutive metaphases for those patients who were Ph-chromosome (or variant Ph-chromosome) positive at diagnosis. In CML, this technique therefore has an abnormal metaphase detection probability of about 3–5%, although it is possible that the selection in culture for dividing cells means that the real sensitivity is greater.

Cytogenetic analysis does, however, have a number of disadvantages. First, it is usually necessary to obtain a bone marrow sample. Not only is this invasive, but in some patients, the marrow may be inseparable. Second, patients at presentation who are negative for the Ph chromosome or an easily recognizable variant are not amenable to analysis. Third, although the results of cytogenetic analysis are quantitative, the large statistical errors resulting from analysis of small numbers of metaphases are considerable *(13)*. Fourth, it cannot be used in cases that have a normal karyotype. Fifth, it is relatively insensitive. In its favor, cytogenetics is very well established and it is the only technique that detects prognostically significant secondary chromosomal abnormalities.

## FLUORESCENCE *IN SITU* HYBRIDIZATION

Fluorescence *in situ* hybridization (FISH) analysis detects the juxtaposition of BCR and ABL sequences in metaphase or interphase cells *(14,15)*. Probes are usually large genomic clones, such as cosmids or YACs, and are labeled with different fluorochromes so that they can be readily distinguished. Because it is the colocalization of BCR and ABL that is scored, FISH analysis does not depend on the presence of the Ph chromosome and will detect rare BCR-ABL variant fusions. Interphase FISH has further advantages over conventional cytogenetics in that it can be performed on peripheral blood samples and a larger number of nuclei, at least 100, are scored, resulting in smaller sampling errors *(16–19)*. The use of hypermetaphase FISH routinely enables 500 bone-marrow-derived metaphases to be analyzed *(20,21)*.

The sensitivity of interphase FISH is limited by the false-positive rate (i.e., the frequency with which BCR and ABL signals randomly colocalize in normal cells). For standard two-color FISH, the limit of detection of CML cells is typically 1–10% and depends, in part, on which probes are used, the size of the nucleus, the precise position of the breakpoint within the ABL gene, and the criteria used to define colocalization *(22)*. The false-positive rate can be reduced by addition of a third or fourth probe that enables the reciprocal 9q+ to be detected in addition to the Ph chromosome *(23–25)*. In many cases, however, the presence of large deletions surrounding the ABL-BCR breakpoint on the 9q+ chromosome preclude the use of this more sensitive assay *(26,27)*.

It has been claimed that FISH is capable of detecting BCR-ABL-positive cells in substantial proportion of patients who have very low or undetectable levels of residual disease as determined by reverse transcription–polymerase chain reaction (RT-PCR) *(28)*. Potentially, these cells could be dormant components (not producing mRNA transcripts) that might have the capacity to contribute to late relapse. However, detection of low level of disease by FISH is problematical as a result the intrinsic false-positive rate, and other groups have failed to confirm these findings *(29,30)*.

## *Molecular Techniques*

### SOUTHERN BLOTTING

Southern blotting is used to detect a rearrangement within the BCR gene. Once a rearrangement has been identified in a diagnostic specimen, subsequent samples from patients on treatment are analyzed with the same restriction enzyme/probe combination. The intensity of the rearranged allele is measured relative to the nonrearranged allele to estimate the proportion of malignant cells *(31,32)*. Apart from some very rare exceptions *(33)*, the level of disease detected in contemporaneous peripheral blood and bone marrow samples is essentially identical, and, therefore, peripheral blood is normally used for analysis *(32,34)*. The typical sensitivity of Southern blot analysis is 5–10%, but this technique is routinely used in only a small number of centers.

### WESTERN BLOTTING

Western blotting is used to detect BCR-ABL protein. BCR-ABL isoforms can be distinguished with a maximum sensitivity of about 1–10% and quantified relative to the amount of normal p145 ABL protein *(35,36)*. As above, this technique is not widely used for routine monitoring of patient response to treatment.

### QUALITATIVE RT-PCR

*RT-PCR Assays and Controls.* Reverse transcription–PCR is used to detect BCR-ABL mRNA. With all PCR amplification assays, stringent precautions have to be employed to prevent false-positive results that can arise by contamination of patient samples and reaction substrates by previously amplified products. In outline, the procedure involves extraction of peripheral blood or bone marrow leukocyte RNA, reverse transcription to form cDNA, and PCR amplification using a BCR and an ABL primer. This single-step PCR amplification is relatively insensitive but is useful to determine the BCR-ABL transcript type at diagnosis and to test for the presence or absence of BCR-ABL in patients who have a normal or ambiguous karyotype *(37)*. To achieve the maximum sensitivity for remission specimens, a small portion of this reaction is reamplified in a second PCR using primers that are internal to the first set. This procedure is referred to as "nested PCR." To control for adequate cDNA quality for each specimen, a housekeeping gene such as ABL, b2M, G6PD, or PBGD is amplified by single-step PCR. Because genomic DNA frequently contaminates RNA preparations, it is essential to ensure that the primers employed are specific to cDNA. Although some groups have used β-actin as a control, this is generally considered to be unsatisfactory in the context of MRD because of its high level of expression and the presence of multiple processed pseudogenes *(38)*. It is also customary to include dilute positive controls, such as dilutions of BCR-ABL-positive cell lines, to control for adequate sensitivity. Given adequate controls, patient samples are scored as positive or negative for BCR-ABL transcripts.

*Sensitivity of RT-PCR.*    Nested RT-PCR can routinely enable a single BCR-ABL-positive cell to be detected in a background of $10^5$–$10^6$ normal cells *(39)*. However, although RT-PCR is up to four orders of magnitude more sensitive than conventional methods, patients who have no residual disease detectable by this technique may still harbor up to a million malignant cells that could contribute to subsequent relapse *(39)*. Attainment of RT-PCR negativity is therefore not tantamount to cure.

*Variability in Clinical Specimens.*    The quality of cDNA samples from clinical specimens may vary considerably. Obviously, an effectively smaller sample will appear to contain less of a particular target sequence compared to a similar sample that is in good condition. The problem is particularly serious for RT-PCR because of the susceptibility of RNA to degradation and the variable efficiency of the reverse-transcription step. This has led to considerable confusion in the literature and makes it difficult to compare studies between centers. In particular, the term "PCR negative" has limited meaning because the sensitivity of the assay for each negative sample is not generally known. However, this problem can be solved by the use of quantitative assays.

There has been some debate on whether bone marrow is more sensitive that peripheral blood for analysis. This question can only be answered satisfactorily by quantitative techniques and results indicate a similar level of BCR-ABL relative to control genes in both tissues after treatment with BMT or IFN *(40,41)*. Many groups, therefore, prefer to use peripheral blood for analysis because this is readily obtainable.

## QUANTITATIVE RT-PCR

*Kinetics of PCR Amplification.*    Analysis of patient samples after treatment by qualitative RT-PCR gives only very limited information (see above). Quantitative PCR aims to estimate the number of BCR-ABL molecules in a sample and thus, by implication, the amount of detectable MRD. Because of the nature of the amplification process, accurate quantification has proved to be technically challenging, for three reasons: (1) the amplification efficiency may vary between samples, (2) the kinetics of PCR amplification, and (3) the amount and "amplifiability" of cDNA derived from patient samples may be highly variable *(42)*.

Because the products of each cycle become substrates for the subsequent cycles, template amplification initially proceeds exponentially. However, replication at each step is not perfect and, therefore, the number of molecules that accumulate ($N$) is described by the equation $N = N_0(1 + E)^n$, where $N_0$ is the initial number of target molecules, $E$ is the efficiency (the fraction of templates that are replicated per cycle), and $n$ is the number of cycles. Small variations in the amplification efficiency can make large differences in the amount of product that accumulates. The efficiency may vary substantially from tube to tube even when reactions are performed at the same time using identical reagents. As increasing numbers of cycles are performed, amplification no longer proceeds exponentially. The efficiency eventually drops to zero, leading to a plateau in the amount of product that accumulates. Once the amount of product begins to plateau off, which may often occur before the product is visible on an agarose gel, information about the number of starting molecules is lost *(42)*.

*Units of MRD Detected by Quantitative RT-PCR.* The only effective way to control for the variables described above is to quantify the number of transcripts of a housekeeping gene as an internal control for each sample. For positive specimens, the number of BCR-ABL transcripts are then normalized to the number of transcripts of the control gene and expressed as a ratio (e.g., BCR-ABL/ABL, BCR-ABL/β2M, etc.) or the number of control transcripts is used to estimate the effective amount of RNA analyzed and results expressed as BCR-ABL transcripts per microgram of RNA. Because the number of BCR-ABL and control gene transcripts per cell is unknown and, furthermore, this number is likely to vary depending on cell type and cycling status, it is not possible to accurately translate these figures into the number of CML cells that are being detected. For negative specimens, results are expressed as negative per number of control transcripts or effective amount of RNA actually analyzed, which then gives an indication of the level at which MRD can be excluded for each sample. Unfortunately, it is not obvious what is the best control gene to be used and different groups have tended to set up different systems. Again, this means that it is difficult to accurately compare results between centers.

*Quantitative RT-PCR Methods.* The most commonly used method in the literature for quantification of BCR-ABL transcripts is competitive PCR *(42–44)*. Known numbers of molecules of a synthetic template are added to fixed aliquots of BCR-ABL-positive cDNA and subjected to nested PCR (*see* Fig. 2). Provided that conditions are established whereby the competitor and BCR-ABL are amplified with equal efficiency, the number of BCR-ABL transcripts in the sample is indicated by the amount of competitor added that produces equal molar amounts of target and competitor PCR products. Although this methodology has provided much useful information, it is highly laborious and, consequently, has not been widely adopted.

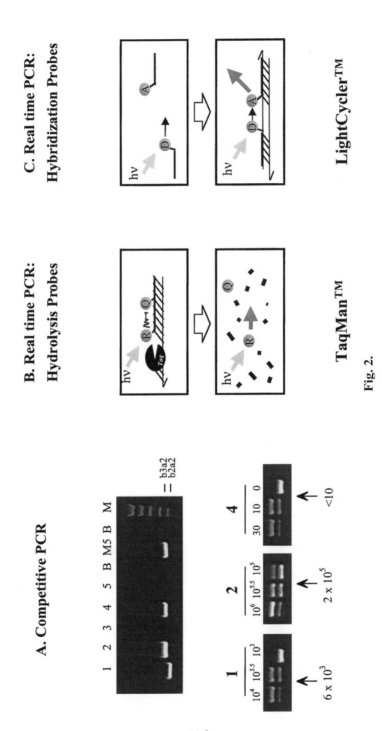

**A. Competitive PCR**

**B. Real time PCR: Hydrolysis Probes**

**C. Real time PCR: Hybridization Probes**

TaqMan™

LightCycler™

Fig. 2.

186

Recently, real-time PCR procedures have been developed that simplify existing protocols (*see* Fig. 2). These techniques employ a single-step amplification of the target sequence in conjunction with specific fluorescent detection probes that enable the amount of product to be determined accurately during the exponential phase of the amplification reaction. Several independent assays for quantification of BCR-ABL mRNA using the TaqMan™ system have been developed *(45–48)*. The assay is based on the use of the 5' nuclease activity of *Taq* polymerase to cleave a nonextendible dual-labeled hybridization probe during the extension phase of PCR. One fluorescent dye serves as a reporter and its emission spectra is quenched by the second fluorescent dye. Degradation of the probe during the extension phase releases the quenching, resulting in an increase of fluorescent emission. The point at which the fluorescence for each sample exceeds a threshold limit is compared to a standard curve in order to determine the number of BCR-ABL or control gene transcripts.

An alternative real-time RT-PCR approach for detection of BCR-ABL mRNA has been established using the LightCycler™ technology *(49)*. Fluorescence monitoring of PCR amplification is based on fluorescence resonance energy transfer between two adjacent hybridization probes carrying donor and acceptor fluorophores. Excitation of the donor fluorophore results in energy transfer to the acceptor, which then emits a fluorescence at a different wavelength, the intensity of which is proportional to the amount of PCR product.

## RESULTS OF RT-PCR ANALYSIS

### Detection of BCR-ABL in Normal Individuals

If the RT-PCR method is pushed to extreme, principally by analyzing a larger number of leukocytes, BCR-ABL mRNA can be detected at a level of 1–10 transcripts per $10^8$ cells in many normal adults *(50,51)*. It has been suggested

---

**Fig. 2.** *(previous page)* Quantitative PCR techniques. **(A)** Competitive PCR. Remission samples are initially subject to nested PCR (top panel). In this example, samples 1, 2, and 4 are positive for BCR-ABL transcripts; samples 3 and 5 are negative. B = blank; M5 = dilute positive control. Fixed amounts of BCR-ABL-positive cDNA are coamplified with different numbers of competitor molecules (bottom panel, samples 1, 2, and 4). The number of BCR-ABL transcripts in each specimen is estimated by the number of competitor molecules added to give equimolar competitor and BCR-ABL products **(B)**. Real-time quantitative PCR using hydrolysis probes. The probe hybridizes to BCR-ABL PCR products during the annealing phase (top panel) and is degraded during extension phase (bottom panel). Hydrolysis of the probe dissociates the reporter (R) from the quencher (Q) resulting in a fluorescent signal on excitation. **(C)** Real-time quantitative PCR using hybridization probes. The two probes are initially free in solution (top panel) but hybridize to BCR-ABL products during the annealing phase (bottom panel). Hybridization brings the two probes together, enabling the donor (D) to excite the acceptor (A).

that BCR-ABL and, probably, several other fusion genes are being continuously formed at a low frequency during cell division, but only the combination of an in-frame BCR-ABL fusion in the correct primitive hematopoietic progenitor would have the potential to confer a selective advantage. Alternatively, it is possible that BCR-ABL alone is not sufficient to result in the expansion of myeloid cell numbers and that other cooperating genetic events may be required. Whatever the explanation of BCR-ABL in normal individuals, there is general agreement that it is only detectable at a very low level. Using routine RT-PCR methodologies, the chance of detecting background "normal" BCR-ABL is approx 1 in 40 and, therefore, this phenomenon is unlikely to impinge significantly on MRD analysis which is principally concerned with kinetic changes on sequential assays *(51)*.

## *Allogeneic BMT*

### QUALITATIVE RT-PCR

The primary aim of MRD analysis post-BMT is to distinguish those patients who will relapse from those destined to remain in sustained remission. Indeed, the first evidence that RT-PCR could detect early relapse was made as long ago as 1990 *(52)*. Several investigators have since reported on the detection of residual disease in patients in cytogenetic remission after allogeneic BMT *(53–67)*. To summarize some of the principal studies, Miyamura et al. studied 64 patients but found no association between BCR-ABL positivity and subsequent relapse *(53)*. Cross et al. studied 61 patients and found that RT-PCR positivity was frequent in the first 9 mo but was not associated with relapse, whereas positivity at 1 yr or later was weakly predictive of subsequent relapse *(54)*. Lee et al. studied 26 patients and found no significant association between RT-PCR positivity and relapse *(55)*. Delage et al. studied 26 patients who underwent CD6 T-cell-depleted transplants and found that early detection of BCR-ABL or persistent PCR positivity was significantly associated with subsequent relapse *(56)*. Roth et al. studied 64 patients and found that the sequential pattern of RT-PCR results defined subgroups with a low, intermediate, or high risk of relapse *(57)*. Guerassio et al. found a very low incidence of BCR-ABL positivity in 48 patients who were in long-term remission (approx 4 yr) after transplant *(58)*. Van Rhee et al. found 2 of 18 patients more than 10 yr after BMT remained BCR-ABL positive *(59)*. For 36 patients who had undergone T-cell-depleted transplants, Mackinnon et al. found that two consecutive positive RT-PCR assays was highly predictive of relapse *(60)*. Radich et al. studied 346 patients and found that BCR-ABL positivity at 6–9 mo was a highly significant independent predictor of relapse, but positivity later than this time was of no prognostic significance *(61)*. Despite the impressive association between RT-PCR positivity and subsequent relapse found here, it is worth noting that disease recurrence was seen in less than 50% of patients who were BCR-ABL positive at 6–9 mo.

The reasons for the discrepancies between studies are probably twofold. First, differences could be caused by heterogeneity of treatment regimens and of the patients analyzed. In particular, some of the studies showing a strong predictive value of a positive assay had a high proportion of patients at relatively high risk of relapse (i.e., patients who had undergone T-cell-depleting transplantation or who were transplanted in advanced phases of the disease). Second, it is possible that the assays in those laboratories finding a strong association between PCR positivity and relapse were less sensitive than those laboratories that found a poor association. Nevertheless, some clear points of consensus have emerged:

- BCR-ABL transcripts can be detected in most patients for some months after transplant, indicating that some CML cells commonly survive the conditioning regimen.
- RT-PCR detectable disease correlates with either absent or less severe graft-versus-host disease.
- Patients who are persistently RT-PCR negative, particularly more than 6 mo after transplant, have a low risk of relapse, but this finding is no guarantee that remission will be sustained.
- Patients who relapse by hematologic or cytogenetic criteria are RT-PCR positive several months prior to relapse.
- Qualitative RT-PCR cannot generally be used to predict relapse for individual patients.

More recently, Serrano et al. found that reappearance of alternatively spliced p190 BCR-ABL mRNA in p210 patients and increases of lineage-specific chimerism preceded cytogenetic relapse *(68)*. This finding needs to be confirmed by other studies but might prove to be useful as an alternative to quantitative assays.

## Quantitative RT-PCR

The first suggestion that a quantitative rise in BCR-ABL transcripts might be a useful predictor of relapse was made by Delage et al. and Thompson et al. *(56,69)*. Subsequently, it has been clearly demonstrated that rising or persistently high levels of BCR-ABL mRNA can be detected several months prior to cytogenetic relapse provided that assays are performed relatively frequently (*see* Fig. 3). In contrast, patients who remain in remission have low, stable, or falling BCR-ABL levels on sequential analysis *(44,70,71)*.

## Response of Patients Treated for Relapse by Donor Lymphocyte Infusion

An important aim of MRD analysis is to diagnose early relapse. It is hoped that treatment of relapse while the burden of disease is relatively low might be more effective and/or allow relatively mild treatment that might lead to fewer side effects. Quantitative RT-PCR data have been used to initiate early treatment for relapse by donor lymphocyte infusion (DLI) and preliminary evidence suggests

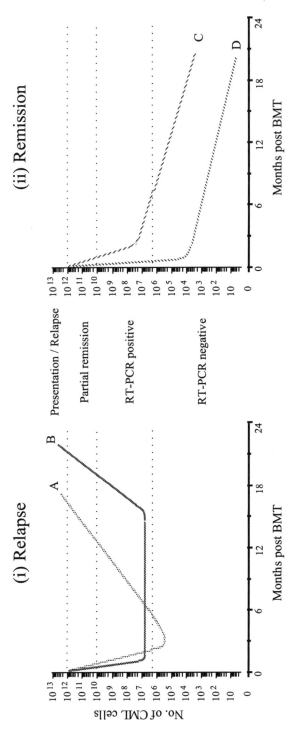

**Fig. 3.** Representative courses in the levels of disease in patients who relapse (A and B) or remain in sustained remission (C and D) after allogeneic BMT. Patient A was RT-PCR negative shortly after transplant but then became RT-PCR positive. Patient B remained persistently RT-PCR positive at a low level for several months, but rising BCR-ABL transcript levels preceded frank relapse in both cases. Patient C was initially RT-PCR positive but, subsequently, became RT-PCR negative. Patient D was persistently RT-PCR negative. Because nothing is known about the level of disease when patients are RT-PCR negative, the lines below a total of approx $10^6$ CML cells are hypothetical. Other patterns of the disease course, such as intermittent low-level positivity, are seen occasionally.

that early intervention is of therapeutic benefit *(72,73)*. Dazzi et al. found that the great majority of patients who respond to DLI achieve durable molecular remission (RT-PCR negativity) with a median followup of 29 mo *(74)*.

## DEFINITIONS OF MOLECULAR RELAPSE

A definition of molecular relapse would ideally be a level of disease at which patients had a very high probability of progressing to cytogenetic relapse. Defining such a level of disease needs to take kinetic changes and the sensitivity of detection into account, which depends on the frequency of analysis and the quantification of control genes, respectively. In the absence of a standardized assay, defining molecular relapse has proved to be difficult. We have suggested a level of 0.02% BCR-ABL/ABL (equivalent to 100 BCR-ABL transcripts per microgram of RNA) as a threshold for relapse. This corresponds to a level of disease approx 50-fold less than that present at early cytogenetic relapse. In practice, the criteria we currently use for molecular relapse are somewhat cumbersome, a minimum of 4 wk in which the BCR-ABL/ABL ratio exceeded 0.02% in three samples, or exceeded 0.05% in two samples, or showed rising levels, with the last two higher than 0.02%. These criteria were adopted to avoid classifying as relapse the occasional patient who had fluctuating low levels of BCR-ABL transcripts *(74)*.

A more general definition of molecular relapse has been suggested as a 10-fold rise in the level of BCR-ABL transcripts, which does not depend on the use of a specific control gene *(70,75)*. However, this definition also clearly depends on the frequency of analysis, and it is unclear how to consider a patient who converts from negative to positive, particularly if the RT-PCR positivity is at a relatively high level. A complete definition of molecular relapse would ideally be framed in the context of a defined assay at specified intervals and take into account both increases in BCR-ABL expression and a threshold above which subsequent cytogenetic relapse is almost certain.

## TOWARD A STANDARDIZED RT-PCR ASSAY AFTER ALLOGRAFTING

The issue of how frequently to monitor patients post-BMT is relatively straightforward. There is a general consensus that patients should be monitored as a baseline at 3-monthly intervals for the first year and then at 6-monthly intervals for at least 5 yr, or perhaps indefinitely. Patients who are BCR-ABL positive at any time-point should have additional assays, ideally monthly, to determine if levels of disease are rising, falling, or static.

Defining the precise parameters of quantitative RT-PCR assays is much more problematical. Although it is probably not necessary for all centers to use identical primers and amplification conditions, it is becoming increasingly important to define a unit of residual disease in CML that is readily comparable between laboratories. Such a unit must necessarily involve the quantification of one or more control genes in order to normalize levels of detectable BCR-ABL or to indicate the sensitivity with which MRD can be excluded if BCR-ABL is undetectable. As mentioned above, there is currently little consensus on what reference gene to use. This situation is unlikely to progress much further until, for example, participation in international trials or cooperative studies compels participating laboratories to define common protocols. Alternatively, it is possible in the future that commercially available kits will become the preferred method of analysis.

## *Interferon-α*

A substantial minority of patients (6–38%) with CML achieve a complete response to treatment with IFN defined as the disappearance of Ph-positive metaphases or, for patients who are Ph negative but BCR-ABL positive, the disappearance of the leukemia clone as assayed by FISH or Southern or Western analysis. For the great majority of patients treated with IFN, qualitative RT-PCR is of very limited value in determining patient response. For those patients who have achieved a complete cytogenetic response, several groups have reported that a substantial proportion are also PCR negative (reviewed in ref. 76). Other studies, however, have shown that the great majority of complete responders do, in fact, have PCR-detectable residual disease. Hochhaus et al. studied 54 patients and found that all were RT-PCR positive, although 3 were intermittently negative *(77)*. Similarly Martinelli et al. detected MRD in all 34 patients analyzed while in complete cytogenetic remission *(78)*. Again, different findings between studies are almost certainly attributable to the sensitivity with which BCR-ABL transcripts have been detected, but in the absence of internal quantitative controls, it is not possible to estimate the magnitude of different sensitivities between laboratories.

Patients who achieve a complete response to IFN have levels of residual disease that differ by as much as 10,000-fold; Hochhaus et al. have shown that the level of MRD on IFN therapy is related to the probability of relapse *(77)*. Consistent with this, analysis of granulocyte–macrophage colony-forming units from patients with a complete response has indicated that detectable BCR-ABL transcripts are at least partly derived from clonogenic myeloid cells *(79,80)*. Sequential analysis of patients in complete remission has indicated a slow decline in levels of BCR-ABL transcripts over time, suggesting an ongoing process of quantitative disease depletion by IFN treatment *(77,81)*. However, these levels appear to plateau at about 5 yr, which brings into question whether or not IFN is really capable of entirely eradicating the disease in any patient. On the other hand, several patients have been described who maintain remission long term despite cessation of treatment, suggesting that they may be "operationally" cured *(81)*.

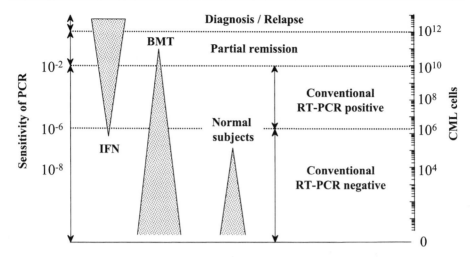

**Fig. 4.** Summary of BCR-ABL RT-PCR results. Almost all IFN-treated patients remain RT-PCR positive, whereas the majority of patients after allogeneic BMT become RT-PCR negative. Normal healthy individuals may be RT-PCR positive for BCR-ABL transcripts using an optimized, very sensitive PCR strategy.

## *Autografting*

There has been considerable interest in recent years in autografting for CML using purged marrow or mobilized peripheral blood stem cells (PBSC). Corsetti et al. have shown that quantitative RT-PCR reveals considerable heterogeneity in the extent to which Ph-negative PBSC are contaminated with CML cells and that the first one or two collections generally contain significantly lower levels of BCR-ABL transcripts. Furthermore, there was a significant correlation between the degree of PBSC contamination and the probability that an autografted patient will achieve cytogenetic remission *(82)*. Waller et al. have suggested that a DNA-based PCR assay for BCR-ABL may be more sensitive than RT-PCR for detecting contamination of PBSC with CML cells *(83)*; however, in the absence of internal quantitative controls, this remains speculative.

## CONCLUSIONS

Qualitative RT-PCR is useful for clarification of diagnosis but has very limited value for monitoring CML patients after treatment. For patients in cytogenetic remission after treatment by allografting, the results of serial quantitative RT-PCR analysis can alert the clinician to the need for further antileukemia therapy. For patients treated with IFN, BCR-ABL transcript numbers very seldom fall below the level of detection, but their actual level correlates with the probability that remission will be maintained *(see* Fig. 4).

New real-time quantitative RT-PCR procedures promise to greatly simplify the cumbersome protocols that are currently in use. They also offer a unique opportunity to standardize the assay and to develop rigorous standards and controls. We believe that quantitative RT-PCR will shortly become a routine and widely used basis for clinical decision making in CML.

## REFERENCES

1. Shepherd P, Suffolk R, Halsey J, and Allan N. Analysis of molecular breakpoint and m-RNA transcripts in a prospective randomized trial of interferon in chronic myeloid leukaemia, no correlation with clinical features, cytogenetic response, duration of chronic phase, or survival, *Br. J. Haematol.*, **89** (1995) 546–554.
2. Groffen J, Stephenson JR, Heisterkamp N, de Klein A, Bartram CR, and Grosveld G. Philadelphia chromosomal breakpoints are clustered within a limited region, bcr, on chromosome 22, *Cell*, **36** (1984) 93–99.
3. Bernards A, Rubin CM, Westbrook CA, Paskind M, and Baltimore D. The first intron in the human c-abl gene is at least 200 kilobases long and is a target for translocations in chronic myelogenous leukemia, *Mol. Cell Biol.*, **7** (1987) 3231–3236.
4. Melo JV. The diversity of BCR-ABL fusion proteins and their relationship to leukemia phenotype. *Blood* **88** (1996) 2375–2384.
5. Melo JV, Myint H, Galton DA, and Goldman JM. p190BCR-ABL chronic myeloid leukaemia, the missing link with chronic myelomonocytic leukaemia?, *Leukemia*, **8** (1994) 208–211.
6. van Rhee F, Hochhaus A, Lin F, Melo JV, Goldman JM, and Cross NCP. A9 p190 BCR-ABL mRNA is expressed at low levels in p210-positive chronic myeloid and acute lymphoblastic leukemias, *Blood*, **87** (1996) 5213–5217.
7. Saglio G, Pane F, Gottardi E, Frigeri F, Buonaiuto MR, Guerrasio A, et al. Consistent amounts of acute leukemia-associated p190BCR/ABL transcripts are expressed by chronic myelogenous leukemia patients at diagnosis, *Blood*, **87** (1996) 1075–1080.
8. Hochhaus A, Reiter A, Skladny H, Melo JV, Sick C, Berger U, et al. A novel BCR-ABL fusion gene (e6a2) in a patient with Philadelphia chromosome negative chronic myelogenous leukemia, *Blood*, **88** (1996) 2236–2240.
9. Shtalrid M, Talpaz M, Blick M, Romero P, Kantarjian H, Taylor K, et al. Philadelphia-negative chronic myelogenous leukemia with breakpoint cluster region rearrangement, molecular analysis, clinical characteristics, and response to therapy, *J. Clin. Oncol.*, **6** (1988) 1569–1575.
10. Allan NC, Richards SM, and Shepherd PC. UK Medical Research Council randomised, multicenter trial of interferon-alpha n1 for chronic myeloid leukaemia, improved survival irrespective of cytogenetic response. The UK Medical Research Council's Working Parties for Therapeutic Trials in Adult Leukaemia, *Lancet*, **345** (1995) 1392–1397.
11. The Italian Cooperative Study Group on Chronic Myeloid Leukemia. Interferon alfa-2a as compared with conventional chemotherapy for the treatment of chronic myeloid leukemia, *N. Engl. J. Med.*, **330** (1994) 820–825.
12. Hehlmann R, Heimpel H, Hasford J, Kolb HJ, Pralle H, Hossfeld DK, et al., and the German CML Study Group. Randomized comparison of interferon-alpha with busulfan and hydroxyurea in chronic myelogenous leukemia. The German CML Study Group, *Blood*, **84** (1994) 4064–4077.
13. Hook EB. Exclusion of chromosomal mosaicism, tables of 90%, 95%, and 99% confidence limits and comments on use, *Am. J. Hum. Genet.*, **29** (1977) 94–97.
14. Tkachuk DC, Westbrook CA, Andreeff M, Donlon TA, Cleary ML, Suryanarayan K, et al. Detection of bcr-abl fusion in chronic myelogenous leukemia by in situ hybridization, *Science*, **250** (1990) 559–562.

15. Arnoldus EPJ, Wiegant J, Noordermeer JA, Wessels JW, Beverstock GC, Grosveld GC, et al. Detection of the Philadelphia chromosome in interphase nuclei, *Cytogenet. Cell Genet.*, **54** (1990) 108–111.

16. Zhao L, Kantarjian HM, Van Oort J, Cork A, Trujillo JM, and Liang JC. Detection of residual proliferating leukemic cells by fluorescence in situ hybridization in CML patients in complete remission after interferon treatment, *Leukemia*, **7** (1993) 168–171.

17. Nacheva E, Holloway T, Brown K, Bloxham D, and Green AR. Philadelphia-negative chronic myeloid leukaemia, detection by FISH of BCR-ABL fusion gene localized either to chromosome 9 or chromosome 22, *Br. J. Haematol.*, **87** (1994) 409–412.

18. Cox Froncillo MC, Maffei L, Cantonetti M, Del Poeta G, Lentini R, Bruno A, et al. FISH analysis for CML monitoring?, *Ann. Hematol.*, **73** (1996) 113–119.

19. Tchirkov A, Giollant M, Tavernier F, Briancon G, Tournilhac O, Kwiatkowski F, Philippe P, et al. Interphase cytogenetics and competitive RT-PCR for residual disease monitoring in patients with chronic myeloid leukaemia during interferon-a therapy, *Br. J. Haematol.*, **101** (1998) 552–557.

20. Seong DC, Kantarjian HM, Ro JY, Talpaz M, Xu J, Robinson JR, et al. Hypermetaphase fluorescence in situ hybridization for quantitative monitoring of Philadelphia chromosome-positive cells in patients with chronic myelogenous leukemia during treatment, *Blood*, **86** (1995) 2343–2349.

21. Seong D, Giralt S, Fischer H, Hayes K, Glassman A, Arlinghaus R, et al. Usefulness of detection of minimal residual disease by "hypermetaphase" fluorescent *in situ* hybridization after allogeneic BMT for chronic myelogenous leukemia, *Bone Marrow Transplant.*, **19** (1997) 565–570.

22. Chase A, Grand F, Zhang JG, Blackett N, Goldman JM, and Gordon M. Factors influencing the false positive and negative rates in fluorescence in situ hybridization, *Genes Chromosom. Cancer*, **18** (1997) 246–253.

23. Sinclair PB, Green AR, Grace C, and Nacheva EP. Improved sensitivity of BCR-ABL detection, A triple-probe three-color fluorescence in situ hybridization system, *Blood*, **90** (1997) 1395–1402.

24. Dewald GW, Wyatt WA, Juneau AL, Carlson RO, Zinsmeister AR, Jalal SM, et al. Highly sensitive fluorescence in situ hybridization method to detect double BCR/ABL fusion and monitor response to therapy in chronic myeloid leukemia, *Blood*, **91** (1998) 3357–3365.

25. Grand FH, Chase A, Iqbal S, Nguyen DX, Lewis JL, Marley SB, et al. A two-color BCR-ABL probe that greatly reduces the false positive and false negative rates for fluorescence in situ hybridization in chronic myeloid leukemia, *Genes Chromosom Cancer*, **23** (1998) 109–115.

26. Grand F, Kulkarni S, Chase A, Goldman JM, Gordon M, and Cross NCP. Frequent deletion of hSNF5/INI1, a component of the SWI/SNF complex, in chronic myeloid leukemia, *Cancer Res.*, **59** (1999) 3870–3874.

27. Sinclair PB, Nacheva EP, Leversha M, Telford N, Chang J, Reid A, et al. Large deletions at the t(9;22) breakpoint are common and may identify a poor-prognosis subgroup of patients with chronic myeloid leukemia, *Blood*, **95** (2000) 738–743.

28. Chomel JC, Brizard F, Veinstein A, Rivet J, Sadoun A, Kitzis A, et al. Persistence of BCR-ABL genomic rearrangement in chronic myeloid leukemia patients in complete and sustained cytogenetic remission after interferon-alpha therapy or allogeneic bone marrow transplantation, *Blood*, **95** (2000) 404–408.

29. Chase A, Parker S, Kaeda J, Sivalingam R, Cross NCP, and Goldman JM. Absence of host-derived cells in the blood of patients in remission after allografting for chronic myeloid leukemia, *Blood*, **96** (2000) 777–778.

30. Deininger M, Lehmann T, Krahl R, Hennig E, Müller C, and Niederwieser D. No evidence for persistence of BCR-ABL-positive cells in patients in molecular remission after conventional allogeneic transplantation for chronic myeloid leukemia, *Blood*, **96** (2000) 778–779.

31. Reiter A, Skladny H, Hochhaus A, Seifarth W, Heimpel H, Bartram CR, et al. Molecular response of CML patients treated with interferon-a monitored by quantitative Southern blot analysis, *Br. J. Haematol.*, **97** (1997) 86–93.
32. Stock W, Westbrook CA, Peterson B, Arthur DC, Szatrowski TP, Silver RT, et al. Value of molecular monitoring during treatment of chronic myeloid leukemia. A Cancer and Leukemia Group B Study, *J. Clin. Oncol.*, **15** (1997) 26–36.
33. Birnie GD, MacKenzie ED, Goyns MH, and Pollock A. Sequestration of Philadelphia-chromosome positive cells in the bone marrow of a chronic myeloid leukemia patient in very prolonged remission, *Leukemia*, **4** (1990) 452–454.
34. Verschraegen CF, Talpaz M, Hirsch Ginsberg CF, Pherwani R, Rios MB, Stass SA, et al. Quantification of the breakpoint cluster region rearrangement for clinical monitoring in Philadelphia chromosome-positive chronic myeloid leukemia, *Blood*, **85** (1995) 2705–2710.
35. Guo JQ, Lian JY, Xian YM, Lee MS, Deisseroth AB, Stass SA, et al. BCR-ABL protein expression in peripheral blood cells of chronic myelogenous leukemia patients undergoing therapy, *Blood*, **83** (1994) 3629–3637.
36. Guo JQ, Lian J, Glassman A, Talpaz M, Kantarjian H, Deisseroth AB, et al. Comparison of *bcr-abl* protein expression and Philadelphia chromosome analyses in chronic myelogenous leukemia patients, *Am. J. Clin. Pathol.*, **106** (1996) 442–448.
37. Cross NCP, Melo JV, Feng L, and Goldman JM. An optimized multiplex polymerase chain reaction (PCR) for detection of BCR-ABL fusion mRNAs in haematological disorders, *Leukemia*, **8** (1994) 186–189.
38. Lion T. Debate Round Table. Monitoring of residual disease in chronic myelogenous leukemia, methodological approaches and clinical aspects, *Leukemia*, **10** (1996) 896–906.
39. Cross NCP. Assessing residual leukaemia, *Bailliere's Clin. Haematol.*, **10** (1997) 389–403.
40. Lin F, Goldman JM, and Cross NCP. A comparison of the sensitivity of blood and bone marrow for the detection of minimal residual disease in chronic myeloid leukaemia, *Br. J. Haematol.*, **86** (1994) 683–685.
41. Hochhaus A, Lin F, Reiter A, Skladny H, Hehlmann R, Goldman JM, et al. Quantification of residual disease in chronic myelogenous leukemia patients on interferon-a therapy by competitive polymerase chain reaction, *Blood*, **87** (1996) 1549–1555.
42. Cross NCP. Quantitative PCR techniques and applications, *Br J Haematol.*, **89** (1995) 693–697.
43. Lion T, Izraeli S, Henn T, Gaiger A, Mor W, and Gadner H. Monitoring of residual disease in chronic myelogenous leukemia by quantitative polymerase chain reaction, *Leukemia*, **6** (1992) 495–499.
44. Cross NCP, Lin F, Chase A, Bungey J, Hughes TP, and Goldman JM. Competitive polymerase chain reaction to estimate the number of BCR-ABL transcripts in chronic myeloid leukemia patients after bone marrow transplantation, *Blood*, **82** (1993) 1929–1936.
45. Mensink E, van de Locht A, Schattenberg A, Linders E, Schaap N, Guerts van Kessel A, et al. Quantitation of minimal residual disease in Philadelphia chromosome positive chronic myeloid leukaemia patients using real-time quantitative RT-PCR, *Br. J. Haematol.*, **102** (1998) 768–774.
46. Preudhomme C, Révillion F, Merlat A, Hornez L, Roumier C, Duflos-Grardel N, et al. Detection of BCR-ABL transcripts in chronic myeloid leukemia (CML) using a "real time" quantitative RT-PCR assay, *Leukemia*, **13** (1999) 957–964.
47. Eder M, Battner K, Kafert SO, Stucki A, Ganser A, and Hertenstein B. Monitoring of BCR-ABL expression using real-time RT-PCR in CML after bone marrow or peripheral blood stem cell transplantation, *Leukemia*, **13** (1999) 1383–1389.
48. Branford S, Hughes TP, and Rudski Z. Monitoring chronic myeloid leukaemia therapy by real-time quantitative PCR in blood is a reliable alternative to bone marrow cytogenetics, *Br. J. Haematol.*, **107** (1999) 587–599.

49. Emig M, Saussele S, Wittor H, Weisser A, Reiter A, Willer A, Berger U, et al. Accurate and rapid analysis of residual disease in patients with CML using specific fluorescent hybridization probes for real time quantitative RT-PCR, *Leukemia*, **13** (1999) 1825–1832.

50. Biernaux C, Loos M, Sels A, Huez G, and Stryckmans P. Detection of major bcr-abl gene expression at a very low level in blood cells of some healthy individuals, *Blood*, **88** (1995) 3118–3122.

51. Bose S, Deininger M, Gora-Tybor J, Goldman JM, and Melo JV. The presence of typical and atypical BCR-ABL fusion genes in leukocytes of normal individuals, biological significance and implications for the assessment of minimal residual disease, *Blood*, **92** (1998) 3362–3367.

52. Sawyers CL, Timson L, Kawasaki ES, Clark SS, Witte ON, and Champlin R. Molecular relapse in chronic myelogenous leukemia patients after bone marrow transplantation detected by polymerase chain reaction, *Proc. Natl. Acad. Sci. USA*, **87** (1990) 563–567.

53. Miyamura K, Tahara T, Tanimoto M, Morishita Y, Kawashima K, Morishima Y, et al. Long persistent bcr-abl positive transcript detected by polymerase chain reaction after marrow transplant for chronic myelogenous leukemia without clinical relapse, a study of 64 patients, *Blood*, **81** (1993) 1089–1093.

54. Cross NCP, Hughes TP, Feng L, O'Shea P, Bungey J, Marks DI, et al. Minimal residual disease after allogeneic bone marrow transplantation for chronic myeloid leukaemia in first chronic phase, correlations with acute graft-versus-host disease and relapse, *Br. J. Haematol.*, **84** (1993) 67–74.

55. Lee M, Khouri I, Champlin R, Kantarjian H, Talpaz M, Trujillo J, et al. Detection of minimal residual disease by polymerase chain reaction of bcr/abl transcripts in chronic myelogenous leukaemia following allogeneic bone marrow transplantation, *Br. J. Haematol.*, **82** (1992) 708–714.

56. Delage R, Soiffer RJ, Dear K, and Ritz J. Clinical significance of *bcr-abl* gene rearrangement detected by polymerase chain reaction after allogeneic bone marrow transplantation in chronic myelogenous leukemia, *Blood*, **78** (1991) 2759–2767.

57. Roth MS, Antin JH, Ash R, Terry VH, Gotlieb M, Silver SM, et al. Prognostic significance of Philadelphia chromosome-positive cells detected by the polymerase chain reaction after allogeneic bone marrow transplant for chronic myelogenous leukemia, *Blood*, **79** (1992) 276–282.

58. Guerrasio A, Martinelli G, Saglio G, Rosso C, Zaccaria A, Rosti G, et al. Minimal residual disease status in transplanted chronic myelogenous leukemia patients, low incidence of polymerase chain reaction positive cases among 48 long disease-free subjects who received unmanipulated allogeneic bone marrow transplants, *Leukemia*, **6** (1992) 507–512.

59. van Rhee F, Lin F, Cross NCP, Reid CDL, Lakhani AKV, Szydlo RM, et al. Detection of residual leukaemia more than 10 years after allogeneic bone marrow transplantation for chronic myelogenous leukaemia, *Bone Marrow Transplant*, **14** (1994) 609–612.

60. Mackinnon S, Barnett L, and Heller G. Polymerase chain reaction is highly predictive of relapse in patients following T cell-depleted allogeneic bone marrow transplantation for chronic myeloid leukemia, *Bone Marrow Transplant*, **17** (1996) 643–647.

61. Radich JP, Gehly G, Gooley T, Bryant E, Clift RA, Collins S, et al. Polymerase chain-reaction detection of the bcr-abl fusion transcript after allogeneic marrow transplantation for chronic myeloid leukemia—results and implications in 346 patients, *Blood*, **85** (1995) 2632–2638.

62. Snyder DS, Rossi JJ, Wang JL, Sniecinski IJ, Slovak ML, Wallace RB, et al. Persistence of bcr-abl gene expression following bone marrow transplantation for chronic myelogenous leukemia in chronic phase, *Transplantation*, **51** (1991) 1033–1040.

63. Ely P and Miller WJ. bcr/abl mRNA detection following bone marrow transplantation for chronic myelogenous leukemia, *Transplantation*, **52** (1991) 1023–1028.

64. Pichert G, Roy DC, Gonin R, Alyea EP, Belanger R, Gyger M, et al. Distinct patterns of minimal residual disease associated with graft-versus-host disease after allogeneic bone

marrow transplantation for chronic myelogenous leukemia, *J. Clin. Oncol.*, **13** (1995) 1704–1713.

65. Arnold R, Janssen JW, Heinze B, Bunjes D, Hertenstein B, Wiesneth M, et al. Influence of graft-versus-host disease on the eradication of minimal residual leukemia detected by polymerase chain reaction in chronic myeloid leukemia patients after bone marrow transplantation, *Leukemia*, **7** (1993) 747–751.

66. Morgan GJ, Hughes T, Janssen JW, Gow J, Guo AP, Goldman JM, et al. Polymerase chain reaction for detection of residual leukaemia, *Lancet*, **1** (1989) 928–929.

67. Hughes TP, Morgan GJ, Martiat P, and Goldman JM. Detection of residual leukemia after bone marrow transplant for chronic myeloid leukemia, role of polymerase chain reaction in predicting relapse, *Blood*, **77** (1991) 874–878.

68. Serrano J, Roman J, Sanchez J, Jimenez A, Castillejo JA, Herrera C, et al. Molecular analysis of lineage-specific chimerism and minimal residual disease by RT-PCR of p210(BCR-ABL) and p190(BCR-ABL) after allogeneic bone marrow transplantation for chronic myeloid leukemia, increasing mixed myeloid chimerism and p190(BCR-ABL) detection precede cytogenetic relapse, *Blood*, **95** (2000) 2659–2665.

69. Thompson JD, Brodsky I, and Yunis JJ. Molecular quantification of residual disease in chronic myelogenous leukemia after bone marrow transplantation, *Blood*, **79** (1992) 1629–1635.

70. Lion T, Henn T, Gaiger A, Kalhs P, and Gadner H. Early detection of relapse after bone marrow transplantation in patients with chronic myelogenous leukaemia, *Lancet*, **341** (1993) 275–276.

71. Lin F, van Rhee F, Goldman JM, and Cross NCP. Kinetics of increasing BCR-ABL transcript numbers in chronic myeloid leukemia patients who relapse after bone marrow transplantation, *Blood*, **87** (1996) 4473–4478.

72. van Rhee F, Lin F, Cullis JO, Spencer A, Cross NCP, Chase A, et al. Relapse of chronic myeloid leukemia after allogeneic bone marrow transplant, the case for giving donor leukocyte transfusions before the onset of hematologic relapse, *Blood*, **83** (1994) 3377–3383.

73. Raanani P, Dazzi F, Sohal J, Szydlo R, van Rhee F, Reiter A, et al. The rate and kinetics of molecular response to donor leucocyte transfusions in chronic myeloid leukaemia patients treated for relapse after allogeneic bone marrow transplantation, *Br. J. Haematol.*, **99** (1997) 945–950.

74. Dazzi F, Szydlo RM, Cross NCP, Craddock C, Kaeda J, Kanfer E, et al. Durability of responses following donor lymphocyte infusions for patients who relapse after allogeneic stem cell transplantation for chronic myeloid leukemia, *Blood*, **96** (2000) 2712–2716.

75. Lion T. Clinical implications of qualitative and quantitative polymerase chain reaction analysis in the monitoring of patients with chronic myelogenous leukemia. The European Investigators on Chronic Myeloid Leukemia Group, *Bone Marrow Transplant.*, **14** (1994) 505–509.

76. Hochhaus A, Lin F, Reiter A, Skladny H, van Rhee F, Shepherd PC, et al. Variable numbers of BCR-ABL transcripts persist in CML patients who achieve complete cytogenetic remission with interferon alpha, *Br. J. Haematol.*, **91** (1995) 126–131.

77. Hochhaus A, Reiter A, Saussele S, Reichert A, Emig M, Kaeda J, et al. Molecular heterogeneity in complete cytogenetic responders after interferon-alpha therapy for chronic myelogenous leukemia, low levels of minimal residual disease are associated with continuing remission. German CML Study Group and the UK MRC CML Study Group, *Blood*, **95** (2000) 62–66.

78. Martinelli G, Testoni N, Amabile M, Bonifazi F, De Vivo A, Farabegoli P, et al. Quantification of BCR-ABL transcripts in CML patients in cytogenetic remission after interferon-alpha-based therapy, *Bone Marrow Transplant.*, **25** (2000) 729–736.

79. Talpaz M, Estrov Z, Kantarjian H, Ku S, Foteh A, and Kurzrock R. Persistence of dormant leukemic progenitors during interferon-induced remission in chronic myelogenous leukemia. Analysis by polymerase chain reaction of individual colonies, *J. Clin. Invest.*, **94** (1994) 1383–1389.

80. Reiter A, Marley SB, Hochhaus A, Sohal J, Raanani P, Hehlmann R, et al. BCR-ABL positive progenitors in chronic myeloid leukaemia patients in complete cytogenetic remission after treatment with interferon-a, *Br. J. Haematol.*, **102** (1998) 1271–1278.
81. Kurzrock R, Estrov Z, Kantarjian H, and Talpaz M. Conversion of interferon-induced, long-term cytogenetic remissions in chronic myelogenous leukemia to polymerase chain reaction negativity, *J. Clin. Oncol.*, **16** (1998) 1526–1531.
82. Corsetti MT, Lerma E, Dejana A, Basta P, Ferrara R, Benvenuto F, et al. Quantitative competitive reverse transcriptase-polymerase chain reaction for BCR-ABL on Philadelphia-negative leukaphereses allows the selection of low-contaminated peripheral blood progenitor cells for autografting in chronic myelogenous leukemia, *Leukemia*, **13** (1999) 999–1008.
83. Waller CF, Dennebaum G, Feldmann C, and Lange W. Long-template DNA polymerase chain reaction for the detection of the bcr/abl translocation in patients with chronic myelogenous leukemia, *Clin. Cancer Res.*, **5** (1999) 4146–4151.

# 12 Utility of PCR Assessment of Minimal Residual Disease After Stem Cell Transplantation in Non-Hodgkin's Lymphoma

*Angela M. Krackhardt
and John G. Gribben*

## CLINICAL UTILITY OF PCR IN LYMPHOMA

Although patients with advanced-stage non-Hodgkin's lymphoma (NHL) often achieve clinical complete remission (CR), the majority of these patients ultimately relapse. The source of such relapse in NHL is from residual lymphoma cells that are below the limit of detection using standard diagnostic techniques. Considerable efforts have been made over the past decade to develop new techniques that have greatly increased the sensitivity of detection of neoplastic cells. In particular, the identification of specific gene rearrangements and chromosomal translocations in neoplastic cells has permitted the development of sensitive molecular techniques that are capable of detecting minimal residual malignant cells. With the development of these more sensitive techniques, especially by the application of polymerase chain reaction (PCR) technology, the presence of residual neoplastic cells in patients in complete clinical remission, commonly called "minimal residual disease" (MRD), has been demonstrated clearly. High-dose therapy approaches with stem cell support are attractive mechanisms to attempt to eradicate residual lymphoma cells. In addition, it has been shown that quantitative detection of residual neoplastic cells on the molecular level may reflect the clinical course of the patients. Results obtained to date suggest that the goal following stem cell transplantation in lymphoma should be the achievement of a "molecular CR."

From: *Leukemia and Lymphoma: Detection of Minimal Residual Disease*
Edited by: T. F. Zipf and D. A. Johnston © Humana Press Inc., Totowa, NJ

## PCR After Stem Cell Transplantation
## in Lymphoma

The evaluation of minimal residual disease has found one of its most important applications in the field of stem cell transplantation (SCT). SCT is an important treatment approach in order to enhance tumor eradication by chemotherapy escalation followed by autologous or allogeneic stem cell rescue. SCT has become the treatment of choice for patients with relapsed aggressive NHL. The role of SCT in the management of patients with low-grade NHL as follicular lymphoma remains more controversial although increasing numbers of patients with advanced-stage follicular lymphoma, mantle cell lymphoma, and chronic lymphocytic leukemia are now undergoing SCT. The major obstacle to the use of autologous stem cells for transplantation is that residual tumor cells present in the graft may contribute to relapse. The assessment of residual lymphoma cells in the stem cell collection is, therefore, essential for this treatment approach. In addition, PCR assessment of MRD can be used to assess the efficacy of purging strategies used to attempt to eradicate such residual lymphoma cells. In addition to the risk of reinfusion of tumor cells, there is increasing concern regarding toxicity of autologous SCT, especially the higher than expected long-term risk of development of myelodysplastic syndrome. This has led to renewed interest in the role of allogeneic BMT for patients with NHL. In addition, a major advantage of allogeneic SCT is the potential to exploit a graft versus lymphoma effect to eradicate MRD, and many studies are underway exploring the possibility of manipulating donor cells and the host to maximize T-cell responsiveness against lymphoma. Assessment of MRD is proving useful for following the effects of infusion of donor lymphocytes to eradicate residual disease.

### Tissue Sources to Detect Minimal Residual Disease

Non-Hodgkin's lymphoma is primarily a disease of the lymph nodes, but lymph node biopsies are usually only performed at the time of initial diagnosis or at overt relapse and rarely when a patient is in clinical CR. Peripheral blood (PB) and bone marrow (BM) samples provide a readily available tissue source to detect MRD. BM involvement is common in NHLs and bilateral BM biopsies are a routine part of initial staging of disease (1). The likelihood of BM infiltration with lymphoma is determined by a number of clinical variables such as tumor type and stage of disease. In general, the higher the stage of the tumor, the more likely the BM is to be involved, and especially in follicular lymphomas, BM involvement is almost invariable and may even be the site of the clonogenic lymphoma cell (2). In some subtypes of NHL, and particularly in the low grade BM and PB will be as useful as lymph node samples for detecting residual disease in follicular lymphoma.

## MOLECULAR BIOLOGIC TECHNIQUES
## FOR THE DETECTION OF LYMPHOMA

Human malignancies are characterized by the proliferation of cells that have undergone transformation with subsequent clonal expansion, and the underlying principle for the application of molecular biologic techniques to the diagnosis and detection of these cancers is the detection of such clonal proliferation of malignant cells. Tumor-specific DNA sequences occur at the sites of nonrandom chromosomal translocations that are commonly found in NHL and are candidates for detection by PCR amplification if the sequences at the sites of the chromosomal breakpoints are known. Tumor-specific DNA sequences also occur at the site of gene rearrangements. Because of the specific nature of gene rearrangements occurring at the antigen receptors, the lymphoid malignancies have been studied most extensively. During lymphoid ontogeny, there is rearrangement of the genes that encode the antigen receptors. These rearrangements, although not causal in the malignancy, nonetheless provide useful markers of disease that can be used both to confirm the diagnosis and to detect MRD.

DNA restriction fragment analysis with Southern blot hybridization with immunoglobulin (Ig) and T-cell receptor (TCR) probes has demonstrated the presence of the clonal lymphoid populations in the majority of lymphoid neoplasms including NHL, acute and chronic leukemias, myeloma, and Hodgkin's disease *(3–6)*. DNA hybridization techniques confirmed that residual lymphoma cells could, indeed, be detected in the PB of patients who were judged to be in complete clinical remission by established diagnostic criteria *(7)*.

### *PCR Amplification of t(14;18)*

One of the most widely studied nonrandom chromosomal translocations in NHL is the t(14;18) occurring in 85% of patients with follicular lymphoma and in up to 30% of patients with diffuse lymphoma *(8–12)*. In the t(14;18), the bcl-2 proto-oncogene on chromosome 18 is juxtaposed with the IgH locus on chromosome 14. The breakpoints have been cloned and sequenced and have been shown to cluster at two main regions 3' to the bcl-2 coding region: the major breakpoint region (MBR) within the 3' untranslated region of the bcl-2 gene, and the minor cluster region (mcr) located 20 kb downstream *(13–16)*. The clustering of the breakpoints at these two main regions at the bcl-2 gene and the availability of consensus regions of the IgH joining (J) regions make this an ideal candidate for PCR amplification to detect lymphoma cells containing the t(14;18) translocation *(17–19)*. A major advantage in the detection of lymphoma cells bearing the bcl-2/IgH translocation is that DNA rather than RNA can be used to detect the translocation. In addition, because there is a variation at the site of the breakpoint at the bcl-2 gene, the PCR products for individual patients differ in size and have unique sequences. The size of the PCR product can be assessed by gel electrophoresis and used as confirmation that the expected size fragment is amplified from a specific patient.

## PCR Amplification of t(11;14)

The t(11;14)(q13;q32) is associated with a number of B-cell malignancies, particularly mantle cell lymphoma (MCL). In this translocation, the proto-oncogene bcl-1 (also known as PRAD-1) on chromosome 11 is juxtaposed to the IgH chain locus on chromosome 14 (20). Although the breakpoints on chromosome 11 have been shown to be widely scattered, the majority are clustered within a restricted fragment known as the major translocation cluster (MTC) (21–23), making this suitable for PCR amplification (22–25).

## PCR Amplification of t(8;14)

The reciprocal chromosomal translocation t(8;14) is characteristic of the high-grade NHL, Burkitt's lymphoma and a subset of cases of ALL. This rearrangement juxtaposes coding exons 2 and 3 of the oncogene c-myc on chromosome 8 to the joining regions if the IgH locus on chromosome 14. The breakpoints involved in this rearrangement have been cloned and sequenced (26). PCR has been used to detect the site of the translocation and was a highly sensitive technique capable of detecting MRD (27). However, the breakpoints are highly variable on chromosome 8 and may occur upstream, downstream, or at the site of c-myc, which limits the applicability of this technique in MRD detection (28).

## PCR Amplification of t(2;5)

Anaplastic large-cell NHL is characterized by the expression of CD30 (Ki-1). Approximately one-third of anaplastic lymphomas express the chromosomal translocation t(2;5)(p23;q35). This translocation appears to involve a novel protein tyrosine kinase and nucleophosmin, resulting in a p80 fusion protein. This translocation can be detected by reverse-transcriptase (RT) PCR in a subset of patients (29). It remains to be determined whether this technique will have clinical utility.

## PCR Amplification of t(11;18)

Extranodal MALT-type marginal zone lymphoma is characterized by the chromosomal translocation t(11;18)(q21;q21). This results in the expression of a chimeric API2-MLT transcript fusing 5' API2 on chromosome 11 to 3' MLT on chromosome 18. The finding that this translocation occurs in extranodal MALT-type lymphomas of the stomach and not in other marginal zone cell lymphomas suggests its recognition as a separate lymphoma entity. Moreover, the absence of the translocation in nodal and splenic marginal zone cell lymphoma challenges the idea of these lymphomas being secondary to MALT-type lymphomas of the gut (30).

## PCR Detection of Antigen Receptor Gene Rearrangements

For those cases of lymphoma in which there is no nonrandom chromosomal translocation or in which the translocation cannot be detected by PCR amplification, an alternative strategy must be developed to detect MRD. During normal lymphoid maturation, B-cells and T-cells undergo rearrangement of their antigen receptors, the Ig and T-cell receptor (TCR) genes respectively. Lymphomas rearrange either Ig genes or TCR, and their clonal progeny have this identical antigen-receptor rearrangement, providing a useful marker of clonality and stage of differentiation in these tumors *(3,31)*. Because most NHLs are of B-lineage, most work has focused on the use of Ig gene rearrangements to detect MRD in this disease.

Ig diversity in B-cells is generated by rearrangement of the germ-line sequences on chromosome 14. The third complementarity-determining region (CDR III) of the IgH gene is generated early in B-cell development and is the result of rearrangement of germ-line variable (V), diversity (D), and joining (J) region elements *(32–34)*. The first process is recombination of the D and J regions. The resulting D-J segment then joins one V-region sequence, producing a V-D-J complex. In a similar mechanism in both Ig and TCR genes, the enzyme terminal deoxynucleotidyl transferase (TdT) inserts random nucleotides (N regions) at two sites—the V-D and D-J junctions—and, at the same time, random deoxynucleotides are removed by exonucleases *(35)*. Rearrangement of the heavy-chain locus is followed by rearrangement of the κ light-chain genes, and if this occurs nonproductively, the λ light chain genes rearrange *(36)*. Antibody diversity is increased further by somatic mutation. The final V-N-D-N-J sequence is unique to that cell, and if the cell expands to form a clone, then this region may act as a unique marker for the lymphoma cell clone.

Polymerase chain reaction amplification of the CDR III sequence is possible as a result of the presence of conserved sequences within the V and J regions that are specific to the rearranged allele and serve as useful clonal markers for MRD detection. A variety of strategies can be employed to PCR amplify the rearranged IgH gene as shown in Fig. 1. In humans, there may be up to 250 VH segments, more than 30 DH segments, and 6 functional JH segments. The germ-line VH segments are grouped into six families (VH1 to VH6), with the family sizes varying from 1 (VH6) to more than 30 (VH3). It is not possible, therefore, to find consensus primers that are capable of amplifying all possible V-D-J recombinations. However, two strategies have been successfully applied to amplify the CDR III region. Consensus primers to the framework region (FR) 3 are capable of amplifying clonal products in to up 50% of cases and will result in PCR amplification of a product some 100–120 basepair (bp) in length. In cases that fail to amplify using consensus primers, the use of V-family-specific consensus primers to the FR1 region will result in a PCR product of 280–300 bp. Although

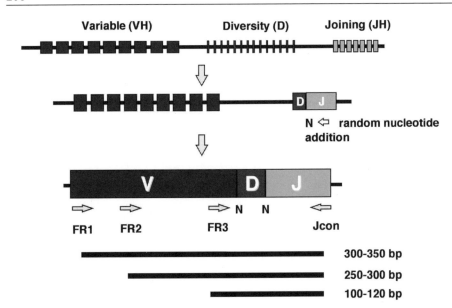

**Fig. 1.** IgH structure and PCR strategy. A variety of methods can be used to PCR amplify the CDR III region comprising the V-N-D-N-J region of the rearranged IgH gene. Consensus primers to the joining region (Jcon) are used with consensus primers to the framework region (FR) 1, FR2, or FR3. The resulting PCR product is directly sequenced.

these techniques have the advantage of being applicable to a larger number of patients, they are much less sensitive than the detection of chromosomal translocations. More highly sensitive tumor detection can be achieved by using primers directed against the unique junctional region sequences within the rearranged antigen-receptor genes *(37)*. These sequences can be cloned and sequenced from diagnostic tissue by first using primers for the conserved regions within the V and J regions for PCR amplification. Clone-specific oligonucleotides can then be constructed and used as primers for PCR amplification or as probes for hybridization in that patient. In designing patient-specific oligonucleotide probes, two regions within the CDR III complex may be used: V-N-D and D-N-J. The V-N-D sequence has a larger N region, but the D-N-J site may be preferable to use as a clone-specific probe, as there is less base deletion of the 3' end of the FR3 region than the 5' end of the J region. The N regions between D-J rather than V-D regions may be more suitable for patient-specific probe construction, as the D-J segments appear to be inherently more stable than V-D segments; and, in addition, where there is V-V switching, the D-J segment remains unchanged.

IgH genes show a high degree of somatic hypermutation in post-germinal-center lymphoid malignancies. Follicular lymphoma cells can also exhibit an oligoclonal pattern and characteristically have evidence of ongoing somatic mutation of the V genes *(38,39)*. Of note, the mutations tend to occur in the CDR regions while preserving the structural framework regions. This might suggest that the use of consensus primers will successfully amplify a clonal product even following somatic mutation. However, mutation at the site of the patient-specific oligonucleotide probe in the CDR III region might lead to a failure of hybridization with a subsequent false-negative result. Serial studies of follicular lymphomas that have progressed to diffuse lymphomas have shown shared mutations in both cell types, demonstrating a single origin *(40)*.

## QUANTITATION USING PCR

Although a number of quantitative methods have been developed, a major drawback of PCR is that it has been extremely difficult to quantitate the tumor cells in the original sample. Traditional methods for detection of MRD by PCR give a binary readout (i.e., the presence or absence of a PCR band). The semiquantitative nature of PCR is the result of minor differences in efficiency of amplification from tube to tube (e.g., a result of variation in temperature based on thermal cycling block position) that are accentuated during the logarithmic amplification of DNA samples. However, these variables can be controlled for amplification efficiency using an internal standard. Because variation in amplification efficiency can also be attributed to primer annealing efficiency, rate of template denaturation, and length of template among other variables, the best internal standard is primed by the same primers as the target DNA but can be distinguished from the starting template either by minor size differences or the presence of a single base-pair change adding or ablating a restriction endonuclease site. These quantitation strategies have been termed "competitive" PCR *(41,42)*.

### Real-Time PCR

Real-time quantitative PCR is a method that has been developed to address deficiencies of traditional quantitative PCR strategies *(43–45)*. This method exploits the 5'-3' nuclease activity associated with *Taq* polymerase and uses a fluorogenically labeled target-specific DNA probe (*see* Fig. 2). This probe is designed to anneal between the forward and reverse oligonucleotide primers used for PCR amplification. The nuclease activity of *Taq* polymerase cleaves the labeled probe during the extension phase of PCR amplification, producing a fluorescent signal that can be detected in solution. The amount of fluorescence produced in a reaction by this method is proportional to the starting DNA target number during the early phases of amplification. Thus, when this reaction is performed on a combined thermal cycler/sequence detector such as the PE Applied Biosystems 7700 (Foster City, CA), a quantitative assessment of input target DNA copy number can be made in the tube as the reaction proceeds. This method eliminates the need for post-PCR sample processing and thereby greatly

**Taq Polymerase**

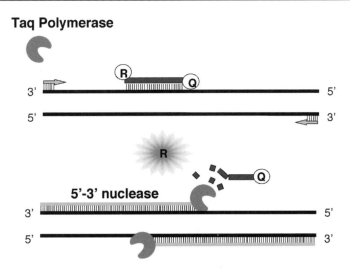

**Fig. 2.** Real-time quantitative PCR. The 5'-3' exonuclease activity of Taq polymerase is used to cleave the reporter (R) form the quencher activity (Q) of the probe. Upon laser activation, the reporter will fluoresce in proportion to the amount released, allowing quantitation of the PCR product.

increases throughput. Real-time PCR also reduces the potential for false-positive results by adding the additional level of specificity provided by the hybridization of a probe to sequences internal to amplification primers and offering a closed-tube assay system. Significant for purposes of MRD studies, real-time PCR has a relatively wide dynamic range. Thus, it is possible to accurately quantify MRD in samples with greatly differing levels of tumor contamination. Real-time PCR strategies have been developed to quantitate lymphomas expressing the t(14;18), t(11;14), and IgH rearrangements *(46–51)*.

## CLINICAL UTILITY OF MINIMAL DISEASE DETECTION AFTER STEM CELL TRANSPLANTATION

In patients with previously untreated advanced-stage low-grade lymphoma treated with combination chemotherapy to achieve a minimal disease state before proceeding to high-dose therapy and autologous BM transplantation (ABMT), PCR detection of minimal disease added little to morphologic assessment of the BM at the time of initial evaluation *(52)*. Of note, all patients with advanced-stage low-grade lymphoma who had a PCR-amplifiable bcl-2 translocation in their diagnostic tissue also had evidence of BM infiltration when assessed by PCR *(52)*. This study suggested that BM samples are a good tissue source for identifying PCR-detectable disease in patients treated with chemotherapy.

## PCR Detectable Disease Persists
## After Conventional Dose Chemotherapy

Long-term analysis after completion of conventional dose chemotherapy has suggested that conventional dose chemotherapy does not eradicate PCR-detectable disease, but that noneradicated disease might not be associated with poor outcome *(53,54)*. Because PCR analysis detects residual lymphoma cells after conventional dose chemotherapy in the majority of patients studied, it is hardly surprising that it has not been possible to determine any prognostic significance for the persistence of PCR-detectable lymphoma cells. Cells containing t(14;18) might not always represent residual lymphoma cells but, rather, cells with this translocation but without the additional necessary cellular changes required for malignant transformation. However, an alternative explanation is that conventional chemotherapy might not cure any patients with advanced-stage follicular lymphoma and that all patients with persistent lymphoma cells are destined to relapse. The long-term remission status of these small numbers of patients might therefore represent merely the very long tempo of their disease. These studies suggest that conventional dose chemotherapy does not result in a "molecular CR."

## Detection of Circulating Lymphoma Cells in PB

Peripheral blood is less frequently involved than BM at presentation, but is a more frequent finding as disease progresses *(55,56)*. Studies in patients at the time of presentation have suggested a high level of concordance between the detection of lymphoma cells in the PB and BM when assessed by PCR. However, other studies have found that the BM is more likely than PB to contain infiltrating lymphoma cells in previously untreated patients *(57)*. Multiple PB and BM samples were obtained from 45 patients at the time of BM harvest from patients undergoing ABMT to determine whether lymphoma cells could also be detected in PB at this time. Lymphoma cells were detected by PCR analysis in 44 of these patients (98%) in BM samples. In contrast, PCR analysis detected circulating lymphoma cells in 24 patients (53%) in PB samples. The presence of residual lymphoma in the BM but not in the PB argues strongly that the marrow is, indeed, infiltrated with lymphoma in these patients and does not simply represent contamination from the PB. The findings of PB contamination with NHL when assessed by PCR are likely to have profound implications because increasing interest is now being placed in the use of PB stem cells rather than BM as a source of hematopoietic progenitors. PB stem cell collections may also be contaminated with lymphoma cells when assessed by sensitive techniques in which it was found that almost 50% of patients had detectable lymphoma cells in PB stem cell collections *(58)*.

## PCR Detection of Tumor Cells in Stem Cells Collected
## at the Time of Transplantation

After combination chemotherapy, PCR-detectable lymphoma cells bearing the t(14;18) remain detectable in the BM *(52,59,60)*. In patients undergoing ABMT at the Dana-Farber Cancer Institute, the bcl-2/IgH translocation was identified in diagnostic tissue obtained from 212 patients, involving the MBR in 167 patients and the mcr in 45 patients. At the time of BM harvest, BM infiltration was detected by morphology in 96 of these patients (45%), whereas PCR analysis revealed BM infiltration in 211 of 212 patients (99.5%). Only one patient had no evidence of BM infiltration by PCR analysis in any of the four BM samples obtained at the time of BM harvest. Studies have compared the tumor burden in peripheral blood stem cells (PBSC) compared to BM *(61–63)*. These studies demonstrated that PBSC have a lower degree of tumor contamination than BM, but that a significant number of lymphoma patients have detectable lymphoma cells mobilized into PB at the time of stem cell collection. In addition, because approximately one log more PBSC than BM have to be collected, this decreases the difference in total tumor contamination *(62)*.

## Contribution of Reinfused Lymphoma Cells
## to Relapse After ABMT

The major obstacle to the use of autologous stem cells is that the reinfusion of occult tumor cells harbored within the marrow may result in a more rapid relapse of disease. To minimize the effects of the infusion of significant numbers of malignant cells, most centers obtain marrow for ABMT when the patient is either in CR or when there is no evidence by histologic examination of BM infiltration of disease. As described above, many patients with NHL have tumor cells detected within BM and PB at the time of transplantation, even in patients with no histologic evidence of disease in their BM. A variety of methods, including monoclonal antibodies (mAbs) to the proteins of the malignant cells, have therefore been developed to "purge" malignant cells from the marrow (Fig. 3). The aim of purging is to eliminate any contaminating malignant cells and leave intact the hematopoietic stem cells that are necessary for engraftment. The development of purging techniques has led, subsequently, to a number of studies of ABMT in patients with either a previous history of BM infiltration or even overt marrow infiltration at the time of BM harvest *(64,65)*. Because of their specificity, mAbs are ideal agents for selective elimination of malignant cells. Immunologic purging using mAbs was first performed at the Dana-Farber Cancer Institute *(66)* and has been most widely studied in patients with NHL *(59,64,65,67)*. These clinical studies have demonstrated that immunologic purging can deplete malignant cells in vitro without significantly impairing hematologic engraftment.

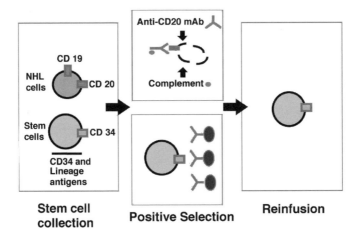

**Fig. 3.** Immunologic purging of tumor cells from autologous stem cell collections. Because of their specificity, monoclonal antibodies are ideal agents to attempt to eliminate contaminating tumor cells. This can be performed either by negative depletion of tumor cells by targeting antigens expressed on the tumor cell surface or by positive selection of hematopoietic stem cells using antibodies directed against CD34.

Whereas the rationale for removing any contaminating tumor cells from the autologous marrow appears to be compelling, there have been no clinical trials testing the efficacy of purging by comparison of infusion of purged versus unpurged autologous BM, primarily resulting from the large number of patients that would be required for such studies. Intense argument therefore persists as to whether attempts to remove residual tumor cells from the harvested BM have contributed to improving disease-free survival in these patients. In addition, the finding that the majority of patients who relapse after ABMT do so at sites of prior disease has led to the widespread view that purging of autologous marrow could contribute little to subsequent outcome after ABMT. Three independent lines of evidence have suggested that the reinfusion of tumor cells in autologous BM may, indeed, contribute to relapse. Gene marking studies performed at St. Jude Children's Hospital have demonstrated that, at the time of relapse, marked autologous marrow cells are detected, suggesting that the reinfused tumor cells contribute to relapse *(68–70)*. Studies at the University of Nebraska have demonstrated that those patients who are reinfused with morphologically normal BM containing clonogenic lymphoma cells have an increased incidence of relapse after ABMT *(71,72)*. Studies at the Dana-Farber Cancer Institute have demonstrated that those patients whose BM contain PCR detectable lymphoma cells after immunologic purging had an increased incidence of relapse after ABMT *(59,73)*.

## PCR Assessment of the Efficacy of Purging Lymphoma Cells from Autologous BM

Polymerase chain reaction has been used to assess the efficacy of immunologic purging in models using lymphoma cell lines *(74)*, demonstrating that PCR is a highly sensitive and efficient method to determine the efficacy of purging residual lymphoma cells. The efficacy of purging varies between the cell lines studied, making it likely that there would also be variability between patient samples.

Polymerase chain reaction amplification of the t(14;18) was used to detect residual lymphoma cells in the BM before and after purging in patients undergoing autologous BM transplantation to assess whether the efficiency of purging had any impact on disease-free survival *(59)*. In this study, 114 patients with B-cell NHL and the bcl-2 translocation were studied. Although these patients were highly selected on the basis of chemosensitivity and achieved either a CR or protocol eligible partial remission, residual lymphoma cells were detected in the harvested autologous BM of all patients. Following three cycles of immunologic purging using the anti-B-cell mAbs J5 (anti-CD10), B1 (anti-CD20), and B5 and complement-mediated lysis, PCR amplification detected residual lymphoma cells in 50% of these patients. The incidence of relapse was significantly increased in the patients who had residual detectable lymphoma cells compared to those in whom no lymphoma cells were detectable after purging. This finding was independent of the histology of the lymphoma, the degree of BM infiltration at the time of BM harvest, or remission status at the time of autologous BM transplantation. An updated follow-up of the outcome of patients who were reported in this chapter are shown in Fig. 4. In addition, we have published results from an expanded cohort of 202 patients and this continued to show a significantly improved disease-free survival of patients who are reinfused BM with no residual PCR detectable lymphoma cells. Of the 91 patients who were reinfused with marrow containing no detectable lymphoma cells, 11 patients have relapsed. In contrast, of the 111 patients who had detectable lymphoma cells after immunologic purging, 42 patients have relapsed ($p < 0.0005$) *(73)*. These studies have been confirmed from other centers *(75,76)*. However, other studies could not find a correlation between the PCR status of reinfused bone marrow and outcome in patients with follicular lymphoma *(77)*.

The majority of studies assessing purging have been performed in patients with follicular lymphoma. Studies have been performed at our own center in patients with follicular lymphoma who do not demonstrate a t(14;18) *(78)* and in patients with chronic lymphocytic leukemia *(79)* and have demonstrated similar results to those seen assessing the t(14;18). In contrast, our studies in mantle cell lymphoma demonstrated that the purging strategy used rarely eradicated residual lymphoma cells in patients with mantle cell lymphoma *(25)*.

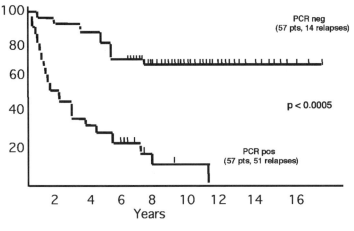

PCR neg
(57 pts, 14 relapses)

p < 0.0005

PCR pos
(57 pts, 51 relapses)

Years

12/00

**Fig. 4.** Successful purging is associated with improved outcome after autologous bone marrow transplant. Those patients who have successful eradication of PCR detectable tumor cells form their stem cell collections (PCR negative) have improved outcome compared to those patients who have residual PCR detectable tumor cells after immunologic purging (PCR positive).

The majority of patients who relapse do so at sites of previous disease, suggesting that the major contribution to subsequent relapse came from endogenous disease and not from the infused marrow. However, there was an association between the detection of residual lymphoma cells in the circulation and the detection of residual lymphoma cells within the reinfused BM *(80)*. Because follicular lymphoma cells use the same adhesion receptors as normal B cells to bind to the germinal center, circulating lymphoma *(81)* cells may, therefore, be capable of homing back to the sites of previous disease and it is these sites that provide the microenvironmental conditions conducive for cell growth.

We have used PCR analysis in preclinical studies to assess the efficacy of modifications to the purging procedure, including the use of additional monoclonal antibodies added to the cocktail of anti-B-cell monoclonal antibodies or the use of immunomagnetic bead depletion *(82)*. The finding that the use of immunomagnetic beads is significantly more efficient than complement-mediated lysis in depleting lymphoma cells suggests that the failure of complement-mediated lysis was not the result of failure to express the targeted antigen because the same mAbs were used for immunomagnetic bead depletion.

Studies have been performed using positive selection of CD34+ cells as a method to reduce tumor contamination *(83–85)*. The efficacy of purging can be increased by the use of combined positive selection and negative depletion steps

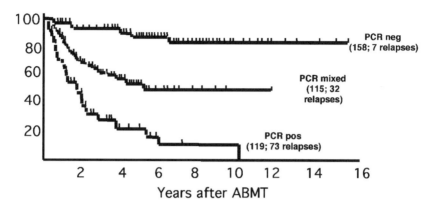

**Fig. 5.** Eradication of PCR-detectable disease is associated with improved outcome following autologous bone marrow transplant. Those patients in whom no PCR-detectable tumor cells are found after ABMT (PCR neg) have greatly improved outcome after ABMT than those patients in whom there is persistence of PCR detectable disease (PCR pos). Those patients who have PCR-detectable disease found intermittently (PCR mixed) have an intermediate prognosis.

*(86)*. More recently, a number of centers have used in vivo treatment with anti-B-cell monoclonal antibody to reduce tumor contamination *(84,87)*.

## Detection of Residual Lymphoma Cells in the BM After Transplantation Is Associated with Increased Incidence of Subsequent Relapse

At the Dana-Farber Cancer Institute, PCR analysis was performed on serial BM samples obtained after ABMT to assess whether high-dose therapy might be capable of depleting PCR-detectable lymphoma cells. The disease-free survival of patients in this study was adversely influenced by the persistence or reappearance of residual detectable lymphoma cells after high-dose therapy *(60)*. The failure to achieve or maintain a CR as assessed by PCR analysis of BM was predictive of which patients will relapse. In contrast to previous findings that all patients had BM infiltration following conventional dose therapy, no PCR-detectable lymphoma cells could be detected in the most recent BM sample obtained from 77 patients (57%) patients following high-dose chemoradiotherapy and ABMT and none of these patients relapsed. All 33 patients who relapsed had PCR-detectable lymphoma cells in the BM prior to relapse, irrespective of the site of relapse. The results of this study suggest that detection of MRD by PCR following ABMT in patients with lymphoma identifies those patients who require additional treatment for cure and also suggest that our therapeutic goal should be to eradicate all PCR-detectable lymphoma cells. Results to date on the patients treated at Dana-Farber Cancer Institute are shown in Fig. 5. These findings have been confirmed by the results from other centers. Absence of PCR-detectable Bcl-2/IgH rearrangements during follow-up was associated with a significantly lower risk of recurrence and death in studies at St. Bartholomew's in London *(88)* and from Germany *(89)*.

## Presence of Residual Lymphoma Cells in PB Is Predictive for Outcome After Autologous Stem Cell Transplantation

In a subsequent study at the Dana-Farber Cancer Institute, PB samples were obtained following ABMT and PCR analysis performed to determine whether the detection of residual lymphoma cells in the PB would also predict for subsequent relapse *(80)*. PB samples were analyzed from 168 patients of whom 36 had relapsed. No detectable lymphoma cells were found at any time after ABMT in PB samples analyzed from 95 patients (57%). Residual lymphoma cells were detected at some time after ABMT in samples obtained from 73 patients (43%). Of the 95 patients with no detectable lymphoma cells, 16 patients relapsed. Of the 73 patients (43%) in whom lymphoma cells were detected after ABMT, 20 patients relapsed with median disease-free survival of 43.5 mo. Although the presence of PCR-detectable lymphoma cells in the PB was associated with an increased likelihood of subsequent relapse. BM appeared to be a more sensitive tissue source to detect MRD because 16 patients relapsed with no detectable lymphoma cells in their PB. The persistence or reappearance of residual lymphoma in the BM may, therefore, provide more clinically relevant information.

## PCR Assessment After Allogeneic BMT

Allogeneic SCT offers the advantage of a tumor-free source of stem cells as well as exploitation of the graft versus lymphoma effect. However, few studies have assessed the impact of allogeneic stem cell transplantation on detection of MRD in patients with NHL. Results obtained in a small number of patients with mantle cell lymphoma demonstrated that allogeneic SCT resulted in eradication of PCR-detectable disease and improved outcome compared to autologous SCT *(25)*. These findings were confirmed in a larger series from MD Anderson Cancer Center *(90)*. T-Cell-depleted allogeneic SCT was also associated with low incidence of tumor relapse and eradication of PCR detectable disease *(91)*. As shown in Fig. 6, quantitative PCR analysis can be used to assess the impact of allogeneic BMT and the graft versus leukemia effect of infusion of donor lymphocytes. Of note, tumor reduction following DLI can continue for long periods following infusion of the donor cells.

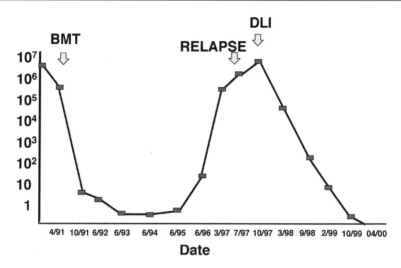

**Fig. 6.** Quantitative PCR analysis following allogeneic BMT. Quantitative PCR analysis can be used to follow patients following BMT. Shown here are the results of quantitative PCR analysis from a patient with chronic lymphocytic leukemia who has undergone allogeneic BMT. There is persistence of PCR-detectable disease following BMT, with a rising tumor burden documented before overt clinical relapse of disease. This patient was treated with DLI and had slow eradication of PCR-detectable disease over the next 2- to 3-yr period. By qualitative PCR analysis, only the last specimen was evaluated as PCR negative, demonstrating the increased power of quantification of minimal residual disease.

## CONCLUSIONS

Methodologies have been developed for the sensitive detection of MRD in lymphoma and are applicable to the majority of patients. The question that now remains to be answered is whether these techniques will have any clinical utility and will predict which patients will relapse. In NHL these studies are most advanced in patients with t(14;18). In these patients, conventional dose chemotherapy does not appear to be capable of depleting PCR-detectable lymphoma cells, although lymphoma cells were detectable in PB in only half of the patients studied. Following stem cell transplantation, the persistence or reappearance of PCR-detectable lymphoma cells in the BM was associated with an increased likelihood of relapse. Although detection of lymphoma cells by PCR in peripheral blood samples was also associated with an increased risk of relapse, the BM appears to be a more sensitive tissue source to detect minimal residual disease because a significant number of patients relapse who had no evidence of circulating lymphoma cells in their peripheral blood. The clinical significance of detection of lymphoma cells in the PB may well have different clinical implications than the detection of BM infiltration. In lymphomas that do not express the t(14;18), it is not yet clear whether failure to detect MRD in PB and BM will predict which patients will relapse because other subtypes of lymphoma may relapse in nodal sites without detectable lymphoma cells in the circulation.

It is, therefore, by no means clear whether our goal should really be to attempt to achieve a "molecular CR" in our patients to cure their underlying disease. Further studies in larger patient numbers are underway and will determine whether PCR detection of lymphoma cells has clinical significance. In addition, the recent introduction of real-time PCR analysis will allow serial quantitative assessment of MRD. It seems likely that a rising burden of MRD will be the most useful technique to predict relapse in these patients.

## REFERENCES

1. Juneja SK, Wolf MM, and Cooper IA. Value of bilateral bone marrow biopsy in non-Hodgkin's lymphoma, *J. Clin. Pathol.*, **43** (1990) 630–632.
2. Bertoli LF, Kubagawa H, Borzillo GV, Burrows PD, Schreeder MT, Carroll AJ, et al. Bone marrow origin of a B-cell lymphoma, *Blood*, **72** (1988) 94–101.
3. Cleary ML, Chao J, Warnke R, and Sklar J. Immunoglobulin gene rearrangement as a diagnostic criterion of B cell lymphoma, *Proc. Natl. Acad. Sci. USA*, **81** (1984) 593–597.
4. Aisenberg AC. Utility of gene rearrangements in lymphoid malignancies, *Annu. Rev. Med.*, **44** (1993) 75–84.
5. Bonati A. T Cell receptor genes: a glance at normal and malignant hematopoiesis, *Exp. Hematol.*, **21** (1993) 1408–1412.
6. Korsmeyer SJ and Waldmann TA. Immunoglobulin genes: rearrangement and translocation in human lymphoid malignancy, *J. Clin. Immunol.*, **4** (1984) 1–11.
7. Hu E, Trela M, Thompson J, Lowder J, Horning S, Levy R, et al. Detection of B cell lymphoma in peripheral blood by DNA hybridization, *Lancet*, **ii** (1985) 1092–1095.
8. Yunis JJ, Oken MM, Kaplan ME, Theologides RR, and Howe A. Distinctive chromosomal abnormalities in histological subtypes of non-Hodgkin's lymphoma, *N. Engl. J. Med.*, **307** (1982) 1231–1236.
9. Lee MS, Blick MB, Pathak S, Trujillo JM, Butler JJ, Katz RL, et al. The gene located at chromosome 18 band q21 is rearranged in uncultured diffuse lymphomas as well as follicular lymphomas, *Blood*, **70** (1987) 90–95.
10. Weiss LM, Warnke RA, Sklar J, and Cleary ML. Molecular analysis of the t(14;18) chromosomal translocation in malignant lymphomas, *N. Engl. J. Med.*, **317** (1987) 1185–1189.
11. Graninger WB, Seto M, Boutain B, Goldman P, and Korsmeyer SJ. Expression of Bcl-2 and Bcl-2-Ig fusion transcripts in normal and neoplastic cells, *J. Clin. Invest.*, **80** (1987) 1512–1515.
12. Aisenberg AC, Wilkes BM, and Jacobson JO. The bcl-2 gene is rearranged in many diffuse B-cell lymphomas, *Blood*, **71** (1988) 969–972.
13. Bakshi A, Jensen JP, Goldman P, Wright JJ, McBride OW, Epstein AL, et al. Cloning the chromosomal breakpoint of t(14;18) human lymphomas: clustering around $J_H$ on chromosome 14 and near a transcriptional unit on 18, *Cell*, **41** (1985) 899–906.
14. Tsujimoto Y, Gorman J, Jaffe E, and Croce CM. The t(14;18) chromosome translocations involved in B-cell neoplasms result from mistakes in VDJ joining, *Science*, **229** (1985) 1390–1393.
15. Cleary ML and Sklar J. Nucleotide sequence of a t(14;18) chromosomal breakpoint in follicular lymphoma and demonstration of a breakpoint cluster region near a transcriptionally active locus on chromosome 18, *Proc. Natl. Acad. Sci. USA*, **82** (1985) 7439–7443.

16. Cleary ML, Galili N, and Sklar J. Detection of a second t(14;18) breakpoint cluster region in human follicular lymphomas, *J. Exp. Med.*, **164** (1986) 315–320.
17. Lee MS, Chang KS, Cabanillas F, Freireich EJ, Trujillo JM, and Stass SA. Detection of minimal residual disease carrying the t(14;18) by DNA sequence amplification, *Science*, **237** (1987) 175–178.
18. Crescenzi M, Seto M, Herzig GP, Weiss PD, Griffith RC, and Korsmeyer SJ. Thermostable DNA polymerase chain amplification of t(14;18) chromosome breakpoints and detection of minimal residual disease, *Proc. Natl. Acad. Sci. USA*, **85** (1988) 4869–4873.
19. Ngan BY, Nourse J, and Cleary ML. Detection of chromosomal translocation t(14;18) within the minor cluster region of bcl-2 by polymerase chain reaction and direct genomic sequencing of the enzymatically amplified DNA in follicular lymphomas, *Blood*, **73** (1989) 1759–1762.
20. Tsujimoto Y, Yunis J, Onorato-Showe L, Erikson J, Nowell PC, and Croce CM. Molecular cloning of the chromosomal breakpoint of B-cell lymphomas and leukemias with the t(11;14) chromosome translocation, *Science*, **224** (1984) 1403–1406.
21. Tsujimoto Y, Jaffe E, Cossman J, Gorham J, Nowell PC, and Croce CM. Clustering of breakpoints on chromosome 11 in human B-cell neoplasms with the t(11;14) chromosome translocation, *Science*, **315** (1985) 340–343.
22. Rimokh R, Berger F, Delsol G, Digonnet I, Rouault JP, Tigaud JD, et al. Detection of the chromosomal translocation t(11;14) by polymerase chain reaction in mantle cell lymphomas, *Blood*, **83** (1994) 1871–1875.
23. Williams ME, Swerdlow SH, and Meeker TC. Chromosome t(11;14)(q13;q32) breakpoints in centrocytic lymphoma are highly localized at the bcl-1 major translocation cluster, *Leukemia*, **7** (1993) 1437–1440.
24. Molot RJ, Meeker TC, Wittwer CT, Perkins SL, Segal GH, Masih AS, et al. Antigen expression and polymerase chain reaction amplification of mantle cell lymphomas, *Blood*, **83** (1994) 1626–1631.
25. Andersen NS, Donovan JW, Borus JS, Poor CM, Neuberg D, Aster JC, et al. Failure of immunologic purging in mantle cell lymphoma assessed by PCR detection of minimal residual disease, *Blood*, **90** (1997) 4212–4221.
26. Haluska FG, Finver S, Tsujimoto Y, and Croce CM. The t(8;14) chromosomal translocation occurring in B-cell malignancies results from mistakes in V-D-J joining, *Nature*, **324** (1986) 158–161.
27. Shiramizu B and Magrath I. Localization of breakpoints by polymerase chain reaction in Burkitt's lymphoma with 8;14 translocations, *Blood*, **75** (1990) 1848–1852.
28. Joos S, Falk MH, Lichte RP, Haluska FG, Henglein B, Lenoir GM, et al. Variable breakpoints in Burkitt lymphoma cells with chromosomal t(8;14) translocation separate c-myc and the IgH locus up to several hundred kb, *Hum. Mol. Genet.*, **1** (1992) 625–632.
29. Shiota M, Mori S, Imajoh-Ohmi S, Nakamura M, Kanegasaki S, Serizawa H, et al. Expression of cytochrome b558 on B cell- and CD 30 positive-lymphomas, *Pathol. Res. Pract.*, **189** (1993) 985–991.
30. Maes B, Baens M, Marynen P, and De Wolf-Peeters C. The product of the t(11;18), an API2-MLT fusion, is an almost exclusive finding in marginal zone cell lymphoma of extranodal MALT-type, [in process citation], *Ann. Oncol.*, **11** (2000) 521–526.
31. Arnold A, Cossman J, Bakhshi A, Jaffe ES, Waldmann TA, and Korsmeyer SJ. Immunoglobulin gene rearrangements as unique clonal markers in human lymphoid neoplasms, *N. Engl. J. Med.*, **309** (1983) 1593–1599.
32. Seidman JG, Max EE, and Leder P. K-Immunoglobulin gene is formed by site specific recombination without further somatic mutation, *Nature*, **280** (1979) 280.
33. Early P, Huang H, Davis M, Calame K, and Hood L. An immunoglobulin heavy chain variable region gene is generated from three segments of DNA, *Cell*, **19** (1980) 281.

34. Sakano H, Kurosawa Y, Weigert M, and Tonegawa S. Identification and nucleotide sequence of a diversity DNA segment (D) of immunoglobulin heavy chain genes, *Nature*, **290** (1981) 562.

35. Tonegawa S. Somatic generation of antibody diversity, *Nature*, **302** (1983) 575–581.

36. Korsmeyer SJ, Hieter PA, Ravetch JV, Poplack DG, Waldman TA, and Leder P. Developmental hierarchy of immunoglobulin gene rearrangements in human leukemic pre-B cells, *Proc. Natl. Acad. Sci. USA*, **78** (1981) 7096.

37. Billadeau D, Blackstadt M, Greipp P, Kyle RA, Oken MM, Kay N, et al. Analysis of B-lymphoid malignancies using allele-specific polymerase chain reaction: a technique for sequential quantitation of residual disease, *Blood*, **78** (1991) 3021–3029.

38. Cleary ML, Nalesnik MA, Shearer WT, and Sklar J. Clonal analysis of transplant-associated lymphoproliferations based on the structure of the genomic termini of the Epstein-Barr virus, *Blood*, **72** (1988) 349–352.

39. Bahler DW and Levy R. Clonal evolution of follicular lymphoma: evidence for antigen selection, *Proc. Natl. Acad. Sci. USA*, **89** (1992) 6770–6774.

40. Zelenetz AD, Chen TT, and Levy R. Histologic transformation of follicular lymphoma to diffuse lymphoma represents tumor progression by a single malignant B cell, *J. Exp. Med.*, **173** (1991) 197–207.

41. Wang AM, Doyle MV, and Mark DF. Quantitation of mRNA by the polymerase chain reaction, *Proc. Natl. Acad. Sci. USA*, **86** (1989) 9717–9721.

42. Gilliland G, Perrin S, Balnchard K, and Bunn HF. Analysis of cytokine mRNA and DNA: detection and quantitation by competitive polymerase chain reaction, *Proc. Natl. Acad. Sci. USA*, **87** (1990) 2725–2729.

43. Holland PM, Abramson RD, Watson R, and Gelfand DH. Detection of specific polymerase chain reaction product by utilizing the 5'—>3' exonuclease activity of *Thermus aquaticus* DNA polymerase, *Proc. Natl. Acad. Sci. USA*, **88** (1991) 7276–7280.

44. Lee LG, Connell CR, and Bloch W. Allelic discrimination by nick-translation PCR with fluorogenic probes, *Nucleic Acids Res.*, **21** (1993) 3761–3766.

45. Gerard CJ, Arboleda MJ, Solar G, Mule JJ, and Kerr WG. A rapid and quantitative assay to estimate gene transfer into retrovirally transduced hematopoietic stem/progenitor cells using a 96-well format PCR and fluorescent detection system universal for MMLV-based proviruses, *Hum. Gene Ther.*, **10** (1996) 343–354.

46. Luthra R, McBride JA, Cabanillas F, and Sarris A. Novel 5' exonuclease-based real-time PCR assay for the detection of t(14;18)(q32;q21) in patients with follicular lymphoma, *Am. J. Pathol.*, **153** (1998) 63–68.

47. Dolken L, Schuler F, and Dolken G. Quantitative detection of t(14;18)-positive cells by real-time quantitative PCR using fluorogenic probes, *Biotechniques*, **25** (1998) 1058–1064.

48. Hirt C and Dolken G. Quantitative detection of t(14;18)-positive cells in patients with follicular lymphoma before and after autologous bone marrow transplantation, *Bone Marrow Transplant.*, **25** (2000) 419–426.

49. Luthra R, Sarris AH, Hai S, Paladugu AV, Romaguera JE, Cabanillas FF, et al. Real-time 5'—>3' exonuclease-based PCR assay for detection of the t(11;14)(q13;q32), *Am. J. Clin. Pathol.*, **112** (1999) 524–530.

50. Donovan JW, Ladetto M, Zou G, Neuberg D, Poor C, Bowers D, et al. Immunoglobulin heavy-chain consensus probes for real-time PCR quantification of residual disease in acute lymphoblastic leukemia, *Blood*, **95** (2000) 2651–2658.

51. Ladetto M, Donovan JW, Harig S, Trojan A, Poor C, Schlossnan R, et al. Real-time polymerase chain reaction of immunoglobulin rearrangements for quantitative evaluation of minimal residual disease in multiple myeloma, *Biol. Blood Marrow Transplant.*, **6** (2000) 241–253.

52. Gribben JG, Freedman A, Woo SD, Blake K, Shu RS, Freeman G, et al. All advanced stage non-Hodgkin's lymphomas with a polymerase chain reaction amplifiable breakpoint of bcl-2

have residual cells containing the bcl-2 rearrangement at evaluation and after treatment, *Blood*, **78** (1991) 3275–3280.

53. Price CGA, Meerabux J, Murtagh S, Cotter FE, Rohatiner AZS, Young BD, et al. The significance of circulating cells carrying t(14;18) in long remission from follicular lymphoma, *J. Clin. Oncol.*, **9** (1991) 1527–1532.

54. Lambrechts AC, de Ruiter PE, Dorssers LC, and van't Veer MB. Detection of residual disease in translocation (14;18) positive non-Hodgkin's lymphoma, using the polymerase chain reaction: a comparison with conventional staging methods, *Leukemia*, **6** (1992) 29–34.

55. Ault KA. Detection of small numbers of monoclonal B lymphocytes in the blood of patients with B cell lymphoma, *N. Engl. J. Med.*, **300** (1979) 1401–1405.

56. Horning SJ, Galila N, Cleary M, and Sklar J. Detection of non-Hodgkin's lymphoma in the peripheral blood by analysis of the antigen receptor gene rearrangements: results of a prospective trial, *Blood*, **75** (1990) 1139–1145.

57. Berinstein NL, Jamal HH, Kuzniar B, Klock RJ, and Reis MD. Sensitive and reproducible detection of occult disease in patients with follicular lymphoma by PCR amplification of t(14;18) both pre- and post-treatment, *Leukemia*, **7** (1993) 113–119.

58. Hardingham JE, Kotasek D, Sage RE, Dobrovic A, Gooley T, and Dale BM. Molecular detection of residual lymphoma cells in peripheral blood stem cell harvests and following autologous transplantation, *Bone Marrow Transplant.*, **11** (1993) 15–20.

59. Gribben JG, Freedman AS, Neuberg D, Roy DC, Blake KW, Woo SD, et al. Immunologic purging of marrow assessed by PCR before autologous bone marrow transplantation for B-cell lymphoma, *N. Engl. J. Med.*, **325** (1991) 1525–1533.

60. Gribben JG, Neuberg D, Freedman AS, Gimmi CD, Pesek KW, Barber M, et al. Detection by polymerase chain reaction of residual cells with the bcl-2 translocation is associated with increased risk of relapse after autologous bone marrow transplantation for B-cell lymphoma, *Blood*, **81** (1993) 3449–3457.

61. Lopez M, Lemoine FM, Firat H, Fouillard L, Laporte JP, Lesage S, et al. Bone marrow versus peripheral blood progenitor cells CD34 selection in patients with non-Hodgkin's lymphomas: different levels of tumor cell reduction. Implications for autografting, *Blood*, **90** (1997) 2830–2838.

62. Leonard BM, Hetu F, Busque L, Gyger M, Belanger R, Perreault C, et al. Lymphoma cell burden in progenitor cell grafts measured by competitive polymerase chain reaction: less than one log difference between bone marrow and peripheral blood sources, *Blood*, **91** (1998) 331–339.

63. Kanteti R, Miller K, McCann J, Roitman D, Morelli J, Hurley C, et al. Randomized trial of peripheral blood progenitor cell vs bone marrow as hematopoietic support for high-dose chemotherapy in patients with non-Hodgkin's lymphoma and Hodgkin's disease: a clinical and molecular analysis, *Bone Marrow Transplant.*, **24** (1999) 473–481.

64. Freedman AS, Takvorian T, Anderson KC, Mauch P, Rabinowe SN, Blake K, et al. Autologous bone marrow transplantation in B-cell non-Hodgkin's lymphoma: very low treatment-related mortality in 100 patients in sensitive relapse, *J. Clin. Oncol.*, **8** (1990) 784–791.

65. Freedman AS, Takvorian T, Neuberg D, Mauch P, Rabinowe SN, Anderson KC, et al. Autologous bone marrow transplantation in poor-prognosis intermediate-grade and high-grade B-cell non-Hodgkin's lymphoma in first remission: a pilot study, *J. Clin. Oncol.*, **11** (1993) 931–936.

66. Nadler LM, Takvorian T, Botnick L, Bast RC, Finberg R, Hellman S, et al. Anti-B1 monoclonal antibody and complement treatment in autologous bone-marrow transplantation for relapsed B-cell non-Hodgkin's lymphoma, *Lancet*, **2** (1984) 427–431.

67. Hurd DD, LeBien TW, Lasky LC, Haake RJ, Ramsay NKC, Kim TH, et al. Autologous bone marrow transplantation in non-Hodgkin's lymphoma: monoclonal antibodies plus complement for ex vivo marrow treatment, *Am. J. Med.*, **85** (1988) 829–834.

68. Brenner MK, Rill DR, Holladay MS, Heslop HE, Moen RC, Buschle M, et al. Gene marking to determine whether autologous marrow infusion restores long-term haemopoiesis in cancer patients, *Lancet*, **342** (1993) 1134–1137.
69. Rill DR, Moen RC, Buschle M, Bartholomew C, Foreman NK, Mirro J Jr, et al. An approach for the analysis of relapse and marrow reconstitution after autologous marrow transplantation using retrovirus-mediated gene transfer, *Blood*, **79** (1992) 2694–2700.
70. Rill DR, Santana VM, Roberts WM, Nilson T, Bowman LC, Krance RA, et al. Direct demonstration that autologous bone marrow transplantation for solid tumors can return a multiplicity of tumorigenic cells, *Blood*, **84** (1994) 380–383.
71. Sharp JG, Joshi SS, Armitage JO, Bierman P, Coccia PF, Harrington DS, et al. Significance of detection of occult non-Hodgkin's lymphoma in histologically uninvolved bone marrow by culture technique, *Blood*, **79** (1992) 1074–1080.
72. Sharp JG, Kessinger A, Mann S, Crouse DA, Armitage JO, Bierman P, et al. Outcome of high dose therapy and autologous transplantation in non-Hodgkin's lymphoma based on the presence of tumor in the marrow or infused hematopoietic harvest, *J. Clin. Oncol.*, **14** (1996) 214–219.
73. Freedman AS, Neuberg D, Mauch P, Soiffer RJ, Anderson KC, Fisher DC, et al. Long-term follow-up of autologous bone marrow transplantation in patients with relapsed follicular lymphoma, *Blood*, **94** (1999) 3325–3333.
74. Negrin RS, Kiem HP, Schmidt WI, Blume KG, and Cleary ML. Use of the polymerase chain reaction to monitor the effectiveness of ex vivo tumor cell purging, *Blood*, **77** (1991) 654–660.
75. Corradini P, Astolfi M, Cherasco C, Ladetto M, Voena C, Caracciolo D, et al. Molecular monitoring of minimal residual disease in follicular and mantle cell non-Hodgkin's lymphomas treated with high dose chemotherapy and peripheral blood progenitor cell autografting, *Blood*, **89** (1997) 724–731.
76. Blystad A, Kvalheim G, Torlakovic E, Holte H, Jacobsen E, Beiske K, et al. High-dose therapy supported with immunomagnetic purged autologous bone marrow in high-grade B cell non-Hodgkin's lymphoma, *Bone Marrow Transplant.*, **24** (1999) 865–872.
77. Pappa VI, Wilkes S, Salam A, Young BD, Lister TA, and Rohatiner AZ. Use of the polymerase chain reaction and direct sequencing analysis to detect cells with the t(14;18) in autologous bone marrow from patients with follicular lymphoma, before and after in vitro treatment, *Bone Marrow Transplant.*, **22** (1998) 553–558.
78. Zwicky CS, Maddocks AB, Andersen N, and Gribben JG. Eradication of polymerase chain reaction immunoglobulin gene rearrangement in non-Hodgkin's lymphoma as associated with decreased relapse after autologous bone marrow transplantation, *Blood*, **88** (1996) 3314–3322.
79. Provan D, Zwicky C, Bartlett-Pandite L, Maddocks A, Corradini P, Soiffer R, et al. Eradication of PCR detectable chronic lymphocytic leukemia cells is associated with improved outcome after bone marrow transplantation, *Blood*, **88** (1996) 2228–2235.
80. Gribben JG, Neuberg D, Barber M, Moore J, Pesek KW, Freedman AS, et al. Detection of residual lymphoma cells by polymerase chain reaction in peripheral blood is significantly less predictive for relapse than detection in bone marrow, *Blood*, **83** (1994) 3800–3807.
81. Freedman AS, Munro MJ, Rice GE, Bevilacqua MP, Morimoto C, McIntyre BW, et al. Adhesion of human B cells to germinal centers in vitro involves VLA-4 and INCAM-110, *Science*, **249** (1990) 1030–1033.
82. Gribben JG, Saporito L, Barber M, Blake KW, Edwards RM, Griffin JD, et al. Bone marrows of non-Hodgkin's lymphoma patients with a bcl-2 translocation can be purged of polymerase chain reaction-detectable lymphoma cells using monoclonal antibodies and immunomagnetic bead depletion, *Blood*, **80** (1992) 1083–1089.
83. Voso MT, Hohaus S, Moos M, and Haas R. Lack of t(14;18) polymerase chain reaction-positive cells in highly purified CD34+ cells and their CD19 subsets in patients with follicular lymphoma, *Blood*, **89** (1997) 3763–3768.

84. Voso MT, Pantel G, Weis M, Schmidt P, Martin S, Moos M, et al. In vivo depletion of B cells using a combination of high-dose cytosine arabinoside/mitoxantrone and rituximab for autografting in patients with non-Hodgkin's lymphoma, *Br. J. Haematol.*, **109** (2000) 729–735.

85. Voso MT, Hohaus S, Moos M, Pforsich M, Cremer FW, Schlenk RF, et al. Autografting with CD34+ peripheral blood stem cells: retained engraftment capability and reduced tumour cell content, *Br. J. Haematol.*, **104** (1999) 382–391.

86. Tarella C, Corradini P, Astolfi M, Bondesan P, Caracciolo D, Cherasco C, et al. Negative immunomagnetic ex vivo purging combined with high-dose chemotherapy with peripheral blood progenitor cell autograft in follicular lymphoma patients: evidence for long-term clinical and molecular remissions, *Leukemia*, **13** (1999) 1456–1462.

87. Magni M, Di Nicola M, Devizzi L, Matteucci P, Lombardi F, Gandola L, et al. Successful in vivo purging of CD34-containing peripheral blood harvests in mantle cell and indolent lymphoma: evidence for a role of both chemotherapy and rituximab infusion, *Blood*, **96** (2000) 864–869.

88. Apostolidis J, Gupta RK, Grenzelias D, Johnson PW, Pappa VI, Summers KE, et al. High-dose therapy with autologous bone marrow support as consolidation of remission in follicular lymphoma: long-term clinical and molecular follow-up, *J. Clin. Oncol.*, **18** (2000) 527–536.

89. Moos M, Schulz R, Martin S, Benner A, and Haas R. The remission status before and the PCR status after high-dose therapy with peripheral blood stem cell support are prognostic factors for relapse-free survival in patients with follicular non-Hodgkin's lymphoma, *Leukemia*, **12** (1998) 1971–1976.

90. Khouri IF, Lee MS, Romaguera J, Mirza N, Kantarjian H, Korbling M, et al. Allogeneic hematopoietic transplantation for mantle-cell lymphoma: molecular remissions and evidence of graft-versus-malignancy, *Ann. Oncol.*, **10** (1999) 1293–1299.

91. Juckett M, Rowlings P, Hessner M, Keever-Taylor C, Burns W, Camitta B, et al. T Cell-depleted allogeneic bone marrow transplantation for high-risk non-Hodgkin's lymphoma: clinical and molecular follow-up, *Bone Marrow Transplant.*, **21** (1998) 893–899.

# 13 Real-Time Polymerase Chain Reaction of Genomic DNA for Quantitation of t(14;18)

*Apostolia-Marie Tsimberidou, Yunfang Jiang, Richard J. Ford, Fernando Cabanillas, and Andreas H. Sarris*

## QUANTITATION OF MINIMAL RESIDUAL DISEASE BY CLASSICAL PCR

Polymerase chain reaction (PCR) has become a powerful tool in assessment of residual disease after treatment of leukemia and lymphoma, as well as in the detection of viral nucleic acid sequences. Quantitative PCR can be performed by measuring the product either after a given number of cycles (end-point quantitative PCR), which requires the generation and quantification of an internal standard for each tube. Alternatively, quantitation can be accomplished by sampling each reaction at regular intervals during the exponential phase and quantitating the amplification product for each aliquot (kinetic method). With this approach, an internal standard is not required, and quantitation is accomplished with an external standard curve. The kinetic method can quantitate samples over five orders of magnitude, but it is cumbersome and is rarely used *(1)*.

These methods, which depend on classical PCR, have several disadvantages. Sampling of the product requires opening the reaction tubes, and this introduces contamination into the work area. Detection of the product is accomplished by electrophoretic analysis of a fraction of the total reaction volume, thus limiting sensitivity. Ethidium bromide staining is not as sensitive as filter transfer followed by hybridization with radioactive probes. During transfer of DNA from

From: *Leukemia and Lymphoma: Detection of Minimal Residual Disease*
Edited by: T. F. Zipf and D. A. Johnston © Humana Press Inc., Totowa, NJ

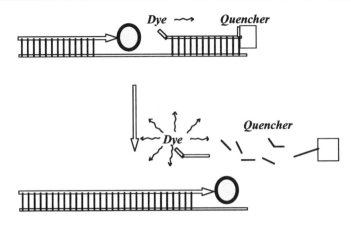

**Fig. 1.** Basic principles of real-time PCR.

agarose, only a fraction of DNA is bound to filters, additionally limiting sensitivity. Detection of radioactive product relies on autoradiography with X-ray films, where the response of a film to β- or γ-rays is linear only over one to two orders of magnitude, with prominent shoulders at both low and high concentrations (2,3).

## PRINCIPLES OF REAL-TIME QUANTITATIVE PCR

Real-time PCR uses Taqman DNA polymerase, which, in addition to its polymerase activity, has a 5'-exonuclease activity against double-stranded DNA and combines amplification and product detection. This is accomplished by the introduction of a third oligonucleotide, which is designed to hybridize to the amplified DNA internally to the two amplification primers. The third oligonucleotide cannot act as an amplification primer because it has a blocked 3'-OH end. As shown in Fig. 1, this nonextendable oligonucleotide has 6-carboxy-fluorescein (FAM) covalently linked to the 5' end (reporter dye), and 6-carboxy-tetramethylrhodamine (TAMRA) covalently linked close to the 3' end (quencher dye). As long as the probe is intact, the FAM fluorescence emission is quenched by its close proximity to TAMRA, and little or no signal is detectable. During DNA replication, the internal nonextendable probe hybridizes to the template internally to the amplification primers, and then it is digested via the 5' exonuclease activity of Taqman DNA polymerase. This digestion separates the reporter and the quencher dyes and results in an increase of fluorescence emission, without affecting the DNA replication reaction and the accumulation of the amplified product. Because the exonuclease activity of *Taq* polymerase degrades the fluorogenic probe only when it is annealed to the target, it is not degraded when the probe is free in solution. The increase of fluorescence is proportional to the amount of DNA template, which rises exponentially in the presence of DNA amplification but rises only linearly in its absence *(4)*. Fluorescence emission is monitored in real-time using the 7700 Sequence Detector (PE Applied Biosystems, Foster City, CA) *(5,6)*.

## Hardware Used in Real-Time PCR

The 7700 Sequence Detector combines a conventional 96-well thermal cycler, a laser for the excitation of fluorescent dyes, a fluorescent-emission-detection system, and a computer with software suitable for the automatic acquisition and calculation of specific fluorescence released during the 5'-exonuclease reaction. Reactions are placed in 96-well plates, with wells that are firmly closed with MicroAmp Optical caps (Perkin-Elmer), to avoid cross-contamination and allow monitoring the reaction in real time. Subsequently, the closed plates are loaded on the ABI Prism 7700 Sequence Detector. The amplification conditions vary, but usual starting points include 2 min at 50°C, 10 min at 95°C, followed by 40 cycles at 95°C for 15 sec and at 60°C for 1 min. Reaction conditions are programmed on a Macintosh desktop computer linked directly to the 7700 Sequence Detector.

The fluorescence emission is detected during real time through the closed tube caps with a CCD camera detector. For each sample, the CCD camera collects the emission data between wavelengths 520 and 660 nm once every few seconds. Using the fluorescence-emission coefficients of each dye, the computer calculates the concentration of reporter $(R)$ and the quenching dye $(Q)$. The $Rn$ values reflect the emission intensity of the reporter probe, as a function of cycle $(n)$. Emission intensity is usually expressed as $\Delta Rn$, which is defined as the difference of $Rn$ from baseline at cycle 14 and is displayed either in linear or in logarithmic scale against the number of amplification cycles. The threshold cycle at which the $\Delta Rn$ rises significantly above the base is designated as threshold cycle $(C_T)$ *(see* Fig. 2). The computer software automatically determines the $C_T$ on the basis of the mean baseline signal detected during the first 15 amplification cycles plus 10 standard deviations. The higher the starting number of the nucleic acid targets, the lower the $C_T$ value is *(see* Figs. 2 and 3). In order to quantitate unknown experimental samples, a standard curve is generated with serial dilutions of target DNA, which are amplified during the same PCR run. Linear regression between $C_T$ and the logarithm of the number of input DNA sequences yields an equation, which is used to quantitate unknowns on the basis of their $C_T$. Quantitation of DNA sequences *(7,8)* usually depends on cell line DNA as a standard, in which case results are usually expressed as number of copies per cell or microgram of DNA tested. With RNA quantitation, results are usually expressed as number of molecules per microgram of total RNA *(9)*.

Real-time PCR has several advantages over classical PCR methods. Workplace contamination is minimized because the fluorescent signal is monitored in

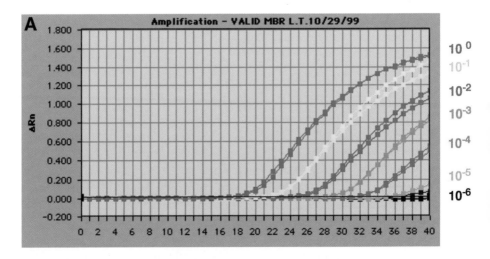

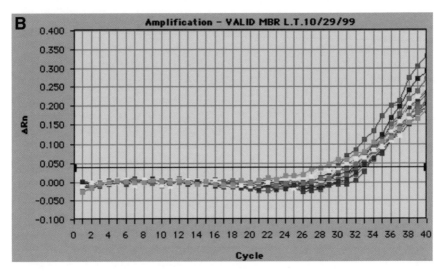

**Fig. 2.** Amplification of cell line DNA: **(a)** IgH-bcl-2 at MBR; **(b)** β-actin amplification. Cell-line DNA was serially diluted into normal genomic DNA and 1 μg from each dilution was tested in duplicate.

closed sample tubes, which do not need to be opened at the end of the assay. The $C_T$ is observed during the exponential phase and depends on the emission of the whole specimen, thus avoiding the reduced sensitivity, associated with quantitation of only part of the reaction volume with classical PCR, which relies on filter transfer, hybridization, and autoradiography *(9)*. In addition, the real-time probe has a long half-life and up to 80 specimens can be analyzed

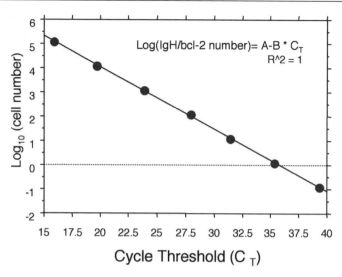

Fig. 3. Logarithm of target DNA sequences per reaction versus cycle threshold ($C_T$) from data in Fig. 2. Target DNA IgH/bcl-2 sequences are defined as number of cells multiplied by 4, which is the number of t(14;18) chromosomes (major breakpoint region), revealed by fluorescence *in situ* hybridization analysis in the JMcA cell line used for standardization. The equation is obtained by linear regression.

and quantitated in 1 d. Finally, the combination of amplification and product detection in real time yields results within a few hours.

## DESCRIPTION OF THE GENE t(14;18)(q32;q21)

The chromosomal translocation t(14;18)(q32;q21) is associated with follicular lymphoma *(10)* and juxtaposes the bcl-2 locus on the long arm of chromosome 18 to the immunoglobulin heavy-chain (IgH) locus on chromosome 14 *(11)*. The rearrangements involve the major breakpoint region (MBR) on chromosome 18q21, located within a 150-basepair (bp) region in the untranslated 3' end of the last bcl-2 exon *(12–14)* or the minor cluster region (mcr), located 30 kb downstream of the MBR. The rearrangements involve a region of 500 bases on chromosome 14q32 *(15)* at one of the six joining segments JH (1–6) of the heavy-chain locus *(16,17)*. The terminal transferase introduces a random number of deoxynucleotides at the JH breakpoints, which are unique for an individual tumor *(18,19)*. In follicular lymphoma (FL), 70% of bcl-2 rearrangements are detected at the MBR region and 15% at the mcr *(20)*. These rearrangements result in overexpression of bcl-2, which through its antiapoptotic properties causes accumulation of B-cells. This immortalization and accumulation of t(14;18) B-cells *(21)* is thought to allow additional transformation events to occur and to result in the emergence of frank B-cell lymphomas.

Table 1
Reports of Real-Time PCR in t(14;18)

| Author (ref.) | $N^a$ | Amplification control | Quantitation |
|---|---|---|---|
| Luthra et al. (22) | 53 | None | No |
| Dölken et al. (2) | 51 | β-Actin, external | Yes |
| Olsson et al. (23) | 134 | None | Yes |
| Voso et al. (24) | 28 | bcl-2, internal | Yes |
| Estalilla et al. (25) | 168 | β-Actin, external | No |
| Tsimberidou et al.[b] | 392 | β-Actin, internal | Yes |

$^a N$ = Number of specimens analyzed.
[b]Not published and cited in MedLine as of 1/07/2002.

## SUMMARY OF PUBLISHED REPORTS
## WITH REAL-TIME PCR OF t(14;18)

The first use of real-time PCR for the detection of IgH/bcl-2 was performed at our institution by Luthra and collaborators (*see* Table 1). They analyzed DNA from fresh or frozen lymph node biopsies, bone marrow, and peripheral blood from 53 patients, including 38 with B-cell non-Hodgkin's lymphoma, and from 15 subjects with non-neoplastic proliferations. They correlated results obtained with real-time and conventional PCR. No internal control was used to monitor for the presence of amplifiable DNA in a particular reaction tube. Twenty-four out of 25 samples positive with real-time PCR were also positive by conventional PCR. No fusion sequences could be detected in patients who were negative by conventional PCR. The overall concordance between classical and real-time PCR was 98% (52 of 53 cases either positive/positive or negative/negative) (22).

Dölken and collaborators have also used a real-time PCR technique to quantitate 51 samples of DNA. These samples were obtained from blood of patients with t(14;18)-positive follicular lymphoma, previously known to be PCR positive for IgH/bcl-2. A two-step, seminested PCR was used with an external control. The quantitation in 51 positive patients by classical and real-time PCR correlated quite well ($r^2 = 0.80$). Nineteen samples, which were negative by classical PCR, were also negative by real-time PCR. Only one sample deemed negative by classical PCR was positive by real-time PCR. The concordance between classical and real-time PCR was 98%. Circulating t(14;18)-positive cells were detectable in peripheral blood of six patients, who remained in continuous complete remission for more than 10 yr, but their number remained within one order of magnitude from baseline. Relapses in two patients were preceded or followed by a logarithmic increase in circulating t(14;18)-positive cells (2).

Olsson and collaborators performed a blinded comparison between real-time PCR and nested classical PCR to analyze cell line and DNA samples from patients treated on a phase I/II clinical trial for non-Hodgkin's lymphoma. They also assessed the efficacy of purging autologous stem cells for transplantation. Real-time PCR was able to detect a 4–6 log reduction on tumor cells. Concordance between real-time and classical PCR was observed in 122 of 134 samples analyzed (91%) (23).

Voso and collaborators used real-time and classical PCR to quantitate the number of t(14;18)-positive cells in blood and bone marrow. The sensitivity of real-time PCR was determined using a PCR-positive cell line and was one t(14;18)-positive cell in $10^5$–$10^6$ control cells for both PCR techniques. Amplification of bcl-2 sequences was used as an internal control in the same tube for real-time PCR. To quantitate the number of tumor cells, the ratio between the copy number of the internal bcl-2 gene and of the translocated IgH/bcl-2 was used. An increase in the $C_T$ reflected a decrease in the number of t(14;18)-positive cells. The $C_T$ obtained for the internal control was divided by the $C_T$ of the PCR for the t(14;18) translocation. A decrease in this ratio reflected a decrease in the number of t(14;18)-positive cells. A progressive decrease in the number of t(14;18)-positive cells in blood and bone marrow was observed with real-time PCR in four patients after treatment. Conversion to PCR negativity was achieved in the peripheral blood of seven patients. Concordant positive results were seen in 20 out of 28 samples with real-time and conventional PCR. Discordant results were observed in eight cases, of which four were positive only by real-time PCR and four only by classical PCR. The authors concluded that real-time PCR allowed quantitation of circulating cells. They felt that changes in minimal residual disease and the conversion to PCR negativity were better predicted by real-time than by conventional PCR (24).

Luthra and her collaborators have published updated results of real-time PCR analysis using samples from 135 patients with non-Hodgkin's lymphomas, 6 patients with Hodgkin's disease, 10 subjects with nonmalignant conditions, and peripheral blood specimens from 11 normal individuals. DNA from cell lines with t(14;18) involving MBR was amplified in duplicate to generate a standard curve of $C_T$ versus target DNA sequences. β-Actin was also included as an amplification control for each specimen, but was run in a separate tube. Overall concordance was noted in 160 out of 162 (99%) specimens between classical and real-time PCR. For non-Hodgkin's lymphoma (NHLs), concordance was found in 134 out of 135 specimens (99%). The tumor with discordant results had an IgH/bcl-2 in the mcr region sequences by real-time PCR, but was negative with classical PCR. The overall concordance for 10 benign biopsy specimens and 11 normal peripheral blood samples was 95% (20 out of 21). One lymph node with follicular hyperplasia was positive for the IgH/bcl-2 at the mcr region of bcl-2 by real-time PCR, but was negative by classical PCR methodology (25).

In our laboratory, we quantified genomic DNA extracted from peripheral blood of 102 volunteer blood donors, peripheral blood or bone marrow of

Table 2
Conditions of Real-Time PCR Reactions for IgH/bcl-2

| Reagents | Final concentration in 50 µL tube |
|---|---|
| Taqman buffer | 1x |
| MgCl$_2$ | 4 m$M$ |
| dATP | 200 µ$M$ |
| dGTP | 200 µ$M$ |
| dCTP | 200 µ$M$ |
| dUTP | 400 µ$M$ |
| Primers for β-actin (internal control) | 10 µ$M$ |
| Primers for IgH-bcl-2 | 120 n$M$ |
| Probe for β-actin (internal control) | 10 n$M$ |
| Probe for bcl-2 | 60 µ$M$ |
| *Taq* gold polymerase | 0.05 U/µL |
| Uracil *N*-Glycosylate | 0.01 U/µL |
| DNA (total) | 1 µg |

203 patients with follicular lymphoma, and 87 patients with nonfollicular lymphoma. We developed a real-time PCR method for IgH/bcl-2 using β-actin as the internal control to be amplified in the same tube with the IgH/bcl-2. This was needed in order to verify the presence of amplifiable DNA and the performance of amplification in a given reaction tube.

We optimized the reactions, using genomic DNA from a lymphoma cell line known to carry four copies of the IgH/bcl-2 rearrangement at MBR per genome. The primers and probes for both the IgH/bcl-2 and β-actin reaction were adjusted to maintain high sensitivity for the IgH/bcl-2 reaction. In order to accomplish this, the concentrations of the β-actin primers and probe were reduced to allow the detection of amplifiable DNA, but without interference with IgH/bcl-2 reaction (*see* Table 2). The cell-line DNA was serially diluted with germ-line DNA from normal blood donors, who were PCR negative. A constant amount of DNA (1 µg) was used for amplification *(26)*. Reaction conditions involved storage for 2 min at 50°C, denaturing for 10 min at 95°C, cycling 40 times at 95°C for 15 s only, and cooling at 60°C for 1 min. These cycling conditions were programmed on a Macintosh G3 linked directly to the 7700 Sequence Detector. Data analysis was performed on a Macintosh Power G3 using the Sequence Detector V1.6 program. All reactions were run in duplicate. The cell number was obtained from the $C_T$ of each reaction and linear regression between Δ$Rn$ and $C_T$ of the serial dilutions of the cell lines (*see* Fig. 3). Cell numbers were averaged from the cells obtained in each reaction and expressed as cells/µg DNA.

Amplification of serial dilutions of cell line DNA into normal genomic DNA (total, 1 µg) demonstrated that 100% of specimens diluted $10^{-5}$ (4 targets/tube) gave positive reactions. However, only 55% of specimens diluted $10^{-6}$ (0.4 targets/tube) gave positive reactions. These results are consistent with the Poisson distribution *(27)* and the four t(14;18) translocations present per genome in the standard cell line *(see* Figs. 2a,b and 3).

For analysis of patient samples, every experiment included duplicate tubes with a total of 1 μL of DNA from standard cell line, serially diluted from $10^0$ to $10^{-6}$ into normal genomic DNA. We analyzed duplicate 1 μL DNA reactions from patients with lymphoma. DNA from normal donors was analyzed in duplicates of 1 mg and, additionally, 2 μg in quadruplicate. A standard curve was generated by plotting the log of the known copy number of target DNA in standards versus the $C_T$. The amplification plot of each specimen from normal donors or from patients with lymphoma was visually inspected to determine which specimens were positive. A sample was considered to be true positive when both mbr bcl-2/IgH and β-actin amplifications were observed *(see* Fig. 4a,b). In contrast, it was considered negative only if β-actin was amplified without amplification of mbr bcl-2/JH in the same reaction tube *(see* Fig. 4c,d).

Using linear regression between $C_T$ and the amount of target DNA in the standard samples, an equation was derived for each experiment, which was used to quantitate the number of cells in positive samples. Results are expressed as numbers of mbr bcl-2/IgH cells per 2 μg total DNA analyzed, which is equivalent to 240,000 cells. Samples that were determined to be negative on the basis of visual inspection of the amplification plot were considered to have zero number of IgH/bcl-2 targets.

We quantitated the absolute cell number of cells with t(14;18) in 392 DNA samples. As shown in Table 3, when 1 μg of genomic DNA was tested in duplicate, 22% of normal blood donors had detectable t(14;18) in their peripheral blood. When 10 μg of genomic DNA was tested, this number was increased to 40%. In contrast, 44% of specimens derived from untreated or treated patients with follicular lymphomas and 50% of those derived from other lymphomas had detectable IgH/bcl-2 amplicons. To rule out contamination, the products of real-time PCR from normal donors and follicular lymphoma patients carrying the JH/bcl-2 MBR rearrangement were also analyzed using Southern analysis. The expected 100- to 300-bp amplicons were obtained when resolved on 1.5% agarose gels. Hybridization of amplicons with an internal bcl-2 oligonucleotide probe also verified product specificity. The size of the amplicons varied from normal donor to normal donor and from patient to patient (data not shown), but these amplicons were of identical size for all positive reactions for a given positive subject. Quantitation of cells with IgH/bcl-2 revealed that patients with follicular lymphoma had 100- to 200-fold more cells compared with normal blood donors and patients with other lymphomas. However, patients with nonfollicular NHL had significantly higher numbers of circulating t(14;18) cells than normal blood donors ($p = 0.0003$ with Kruskal–Wallis test). From the

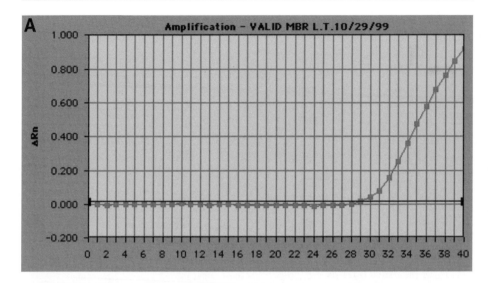

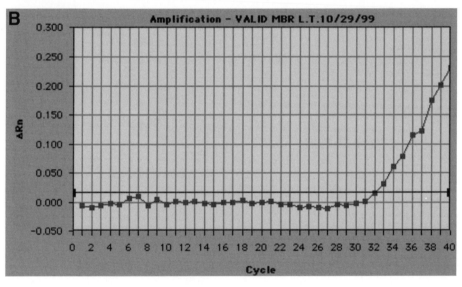

**Fig. 4.** Analysis of DNA from patients with follicular lymphoma: **(a)** IgH bcl-2 at MBR; **(b)** β-actin amplification of specimen a.

133 specimens from patients with lymphoma who had detectable IgH/bcl-2 amplicons, only 52 specimens (39%) had cell numbers higher than the statistical upper limit seen in normal blood donors, defined as the mean plus two standard deviations.

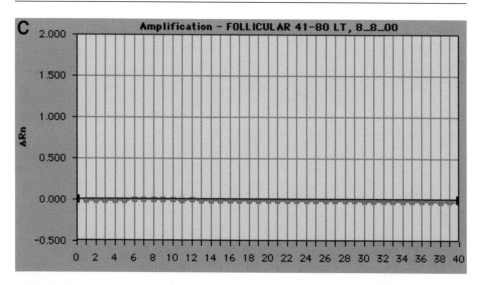

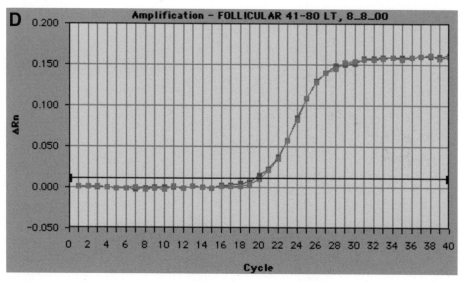

**Fig. 4.** *(continued)* **(c)** germ-line IgH-bcl-2 at MBR; **(d)** β-actin amplification of specimen c.

## CONCLUSIONS

Real-time PCR is emerging as a convenient, accurate, and sensitive method for the detection of t(14;18) in blood or marrow of patients with follicular lymphoma. Many variations of the technique have been reported. Our technique

## Table 3
## Quantitation of t(14;18) in Normal Blood Donors and Patients with Lymphoma

| Individuals tested | DNA tested | Subjects tested | Positive subjects | % Positive | Cells/μg DNA Mean ± SD | Range | Subjects with more cells than upper normal limit[a] |
|---|---|---|---|---|---|---|---|
| Normal donors | 2 μg[b] | 102 | 22 | 22 | 0.6 ± 2.7 | 0–17 | 3 |
| Normal donors | 10 μg | 102 | 41 | 40 | 0.8 ± 2.3 | 0–17 | 2 |
| Follicular lymphoma pts. | 2 μg | 203 | 89 | 44 | 107.3 ± 588.2 | 0–6769 | 40 |
| Nonfollicular lymphoma pts. | 2 μg | 87 | 44 | 50 | 9.7 ± 64.5 | 0–598 | 9 |

[a]The upper normal limit is defined as the mean plus 2 standard deviations and is 6 cells for 2 μg of tested DNA and 5.4 cells for 10 μg of tested DNA.
[b]This consists of two duplicate reactions of 1 μg and four reactions of 2 μg each for a total of 10 μg.

allows the amplification of an internal β-actin sequence, which confirms both the presence of amplifiable DNA and the proper performance of the amplification reaction in a particular tube. We have confirmed the presence of t(14;18) in blood of normal blood donors and in blood and marrow of patients with follicular and other lymphomas. The levels were much higher in follicular lymphoma patients than in other lymphomas, and those were, in turn, much higher than levels observed in volunteer blood donors. This technique is currently used to determine the clinical significance of circulating tumor burden at presentation and during therapy of patients with follicular center cell lymphomas.

## REFERENCES

1. Bieche I, Olivi M, Champeme MH, Vidaud D, Lidereau R, and Vidaud M. Novel approach to quantitative polymerase chain reaction using real-time detection: application to the detection of gene amplification in breast cancer, *Int. J. Cancer*, **78** (1998) 661–666.
2. Dölken L, Schuler F, and Dolken G. Quantitative detection of t(14;18)-positive cells by real-time quantitative PCR using fluorogenic probes, *Biotechniques*, **25** (1998) 1058–1064.
3. Raeymaekers L. Quantitative PCR, in *Clinical Applications of PCR*. Dennis YM (ed). Totowa, NJ, Humana, 1998, pp. 27–38.
4. Lie YS and Petropoulos CJ. Advances in quantitative PCR technology: 5' nuclease assays, *Curr. Opin. Biotechnol.*, **9** (1998) 43–48.
5. Gibson UE, Heid CA, and Williams PM. A novel method for real time quantitative RT-PCR, *Genome Res.*, **6** (1996) 995–1001.
6. Heid CA, Stevens J, Livak KJ, and Williams PM. Real time quantitative PCR, *Genome Res.*, **6** (1996) 986–994.
7. Oka S, Urayama K, Hirabayashi Y, Ohnishi K, Goto H, Mitamura K, et al. Quantitative analysis of human immunodeficiency virus type-1 in asymptomatic carriers using the polymerase chain reaction, *Biochem. Biophys. Res.*, **167** (1990) 1–8.
8. Billadeau D, Quam L, Thomas W, Kay N, Greipp P, Kyle R, et al. Detection and quantitation of malignant cells in the peripheral blood of multiple myeloma patients, *Blood*, **80** (1992) 1818–1824.
9. Orlando C, Pinzani P, and Pazzagli M. Developments in quantitative PCR, *Clin. Chem. Lab. Med.*, **36** (1998) 255–269.
10. Yunis JJ, Oken MM, Kaplan ME, Ensrud KM, Howe RR, and Theologides A. Distinctive chromosomal abnormalities in histologic subtypes of Non-Hodgkin's lymphoma, *N. Engl. J. Med.*, **307** (1982) 1231–1236.
11. Bakhshi A, Jensen JP, Goldman P, Wright JJ, McBride W, Epstein AL, et al. Cloning the chromosomal breakpoint of t(14;18) human lymphomas: clustering around JH on chromosome 14 and near a transcriptional unit on 18, *Cell*, **41** (1985) 899–906.
12. Tsujimoto Y, Cossman J, Jaffe E, and Croce CM. Involvement of the bcl-2 gene in human follicular lymphoma, *Science*, **228** (1985) 1440–1443.
13. Tsujimoto Y and Croce CM. Analysis of the structure, transcripts, and protein products of bcl-2, the gene involved in human follicular lymphoma, *Proc. Natl. Acad. Sci. USA*, **83** (1986) 5214–5218.
14. Cleary ML, Smith SD, and Sklar J. Cloning and structural analysis of cDNAs for bcl-2 and a hybrid bcl-2/immunoglobulin transcript resulting from the t(14;18) translocation, *Cell*, **47** (1986) 19–28.
15. Cleary ML, Galili N, and Sclar J. Detection of a second t(14;18) breakpoint cluster region in human follicular lymphomas, *J. Exp. Med.*, **164** (1986) 315.

16. Tsujimoto Y, Finger LR, Yunis J, Nowell PC, and Croce CM. Cloning of the chromosome breakpoint of neoplastic B cells with the t(14;18) chromosome translocation, *Science*, **226** (1984) 1097–1099.

17. Ngan BY, Nourse J, and Cleary ML. Detection of chromosomal translocation t(14;18) within the minor cluster region of bcl-2 by polymerase chain reaction and direct genomic sequencing of the enzymatically amplified DNA in follicular lymphomas, *Blood*, **73** (1989) 1759–1762.

18. Cotter F, Price C, Zucca E, and Young BD. Direct sequence analysis of the 14q+ and 18q– chromosome junctions in follicular lymphoma, *Blood*, **7** (1990) 131–135.

19. Kneba N, Eick S, Willigeroth S, Bolz I, Herbst H, Pott C, et al. Polymerase chain reaction analysis of t(14;18) junctional regions in B-cell lymphomas, *Leuk. Lymphoma*, **3** (1990) 109–117.

20. Cleary ML, Galili N, and Sklar J. Detection of a second t(14;18) breakpoint cluster region in human follicular lymphomas, *J. Exp. Med.*, **164** (1986) 315–320.

21. Klein G. Comparative action of myc and bcl-2 in B-cell malignancy, *Cancer Cells*, **3** (1991) 141–143.

22. Luthra R, McBride JA, Cabanillas F, and Sarris A. Novel 5' exonuclease-based real-time PCR assay for the detection of t(14;18)(q32;q21) in patients with follicular lymphoma, *Am. J. Pathol.*, **153** (1998) 63–68.

23. Olsson K, Gerard CJ, Zehnder J, Jones C, Ramanathan R, Reading C, et al. Real-time t(11;14) and t(14;18) PCR assays provide sensitive and quantitative assessments of minimal residual disease (MRD), *Leukemia*, **13** (1999) 1833–1842.

24. Voso MT, Pantel G, Weis M, Schmidt P, Martin S, Moos M, et al. In vivo depletion of B-cells using a combination of high-dose cytosine arabinoside/mitoxantrone and rituximab for autografting in patients with non-Hodgkin's lymphoma, *Br. J. Haematol.*, **109** (2000) 729–735.

25. Estalilla OC, Medeiros LJ, Manning JT, and Luthra R. 5' to 3' exonuclease-based real-time PCR assays for detecting the t(14;18)(q32;21): a survey of 162 malignant lymphomas and reactive specimens, *Mod. Pathol.*, **13** (2000) 661–666.

26. Donovan JW, Ladetto M, Zou G, Neuberg D, Poor C, Bowers D, et al. Immunoglobulin heavy-chain consensus probes for real-time PCR quantification of residual disease in acute lympho-blastic leukemia, *Blood*, **95** (2000) 2651–2658.

27. Ferre F. Quantitative PCR, in *The Polymerase Chain Reaction*. Mullis KB and Gibbs R (eds). Boston: Birkhäuser, 1994, pp. 71–88.

# 14 Monitoring Follicular Lymphoma by Polymerase Chain Reaction

## Ming-Sheng Lee and Fernando Cabanillas

During the last three decades, evidence firmly establishing the close association of nonrandom karyotypic abnormalities with particular types of human cancers has been increasing. The importance of these observations is underscored by the revelation that several oncogenes are mapped to the regions known to be involved in tumor-specific chromosomal aberrations. For lymphoid malignancies in particular, the first consistent karyotypic abnormality was observed in Burkitt's lymphoma (1). Approximately 75% of Burkitt's lymphomas display the characteristic t(8;14) translocation and the remaining 25% show either the t(2;8) and the t(8;22). The common feature of these translocations is the involvement of chromosome region 8q24, where the c-myc oncogene resides. Breakpoints on the counterpart chromosomes occur within either the immunoglobulin heavy-chain (IgH) gene locus at 14q32 or one of the immunoglobulin light-chain gene loci at 2p11 or 22q11. Many other cytogenetic aberrations in lymphoid neoplasia appear to follow a similar rule, such as the t(11;14)(q13;q32) in mantle cell lymphoma and the t(14;18)(q32;q21) in follicular lymphoma.

The chromosomal translocation t(14;18)(q32;q21) is one of the most common karyotypic abnormalities in non-Hodgkin's lymphomas. It occurs in approx 85% of follicular lymphomas (FL) and 20% of diffuse large B-cell lymphomas (1). This translocation results in the fusion of the bcl-2 gene residing at chromosome 18q21 and the immunoglobulin heavy-chain gene (IgH) residing at chromosome 14q32 (2–4). By means of Southern blot analysis, it has been shown that the breakpoints on chromosome 18q21 in about 70% of FL fall within a 2.8-kb EcoRI–HindIII restriction fragment named the major translocation cluster region (MBR) (5–7). DNA sequencing of several representative cases reveals that the breakpoints actually are tightly clustered within 150 bp of each other. The breakpoints on chromosome 14q32 are also very consistent, always occurring at the 5' end of one of the J segments of the IgH gene (8,9).

From: *Leukemia and Lymphoma: Detection of Minimal Residual Disease*
Edited by: T. F. Zipf and D. A. Johnston © Humana Press Inc., Totowa, NJ

Tight clustering of the breakpoints at both genes enables the use of two universal primers for amplification of the hybrid bcl-2/IgH DNA sequences by polymerase chain reaction (PCR) in different patients. Because it amplifies only the hybrid DNA of the translocation, PCR permits the detection of one abnormal cell among several hundred thousand normal cells *(10–12)*. Owing to its high sensitivity and specificity, PCR is a powerful tool for detecting minimal residual disease (MRD).

The clinical value of the PCR assay in the detection of small numbers of occult t(14;18)-carrying cells in FL has been extensively examined by many different investigators. Although they appear normal by standard morphological examination and Southern blot analysis, many blood or bone marrow samples obtained from patients in the early stages of disease or in clinical remission have been clearly identified by PCR as positive for the t(14;18)-carrying cells *(13–15)*. Persistent PCR positivity in patients in remission helps explain the continuous late recurrence typical of FL. To determine if t(14;18)-bearing cells persist in patients with follicular lymphoma in long-term complete remission, Price et al. examined patients who had been in remission for more than 10 yr *(15)*. PCR positivity was observed in six of eight patients who initially presented with stage III or stage IV disease. However, it is not known whether these patients who were PCR positive and in long-term complete remission had previously achieved a molecular response and, later, relapsed molecularly. This could explain the long remission in spite of their positive PCR. In contrast, none of seven patients with stage I or II disease had t(14;18)-carrying cells detectable by PCR. PCR negativity in this subgroup of patients is consistent with the low risk of relapse, even though we do not know whether this PCR negativity is the result of the number of t(14;18)-bearing cells falling below the detection sensitivity or to true complete freedom from residual disease.

Utilizing PCR to monitor residual disease in FL in an earlier study, Cabanillas et al. compared the effectiveness of tumor eradication by a new intensive therapeutic regimen named alternating triple therapy (ATT) (adriamycin/cytoxan, ara-C/platinum, and mitoxantrone/procarbazine-based combinations given sequentially in alternating fashion for 12 cycles) to either standard CHOP (cytoxan, adriamycin, vincristine, and prednisone) or CVP (cytoxan, vincristine, and prednisone) *(16)*. A total of 272 blood samples obtained at different times of treatment were analyzed: 111 on ATT and 161 on CHOP or CVP. The results were correlated with the type of treatment regimen and the time when samples were obtained. A high percentage of PCR negativity indicative of absent or extremely low residual tumor burden was achieved by the new intensive chemotherapy. In contrast, most patients treated with CHOP or CVP therapy showed persistent PCR positivity. Sequential follow-up studies were available in 37 patients with median follow-up of 34 mo: 21 received ATT and 16 received CHOP or CVP. Molecular complete response (CR) (as defined by achieving PCR negativity at any time) was attained in 17 of 21 (81%) patients on ATT versus 5 of 16 (31%) patients on CHOP or CVP ($p < 0.01$). None of the 22 patients achieving molecular CR relapsed. In contrast, of the 15 patients who failed to achieve molecular CR, 6 relapsed. These findings suggest that PCR negativity is indicative of very low residual tumor burden and, thus, of a low probability of imminent disease recurrence.

To further investigate the prognostic value of assessing molecular response in indolent follicular lymphoma, investigators at M.D. Anderson Cancer Center conducted a study of 194 patients who had assessable t(14;18)-carrying cells (17,18). The median follow-up was 29 mo (range: 6 to 91 mo). The molecular response rate was noted to progressively increase from 37% at 3–5 mo of therapy to 66% at 15–19 mo of therapy. Failure-free survival (FFS) rates correlated with molecular response rate at each of the first three PCR determinations (at 3–5 mo, 6–8 mo, and 9–14 mo). Patients who were PCR negative tended to have longer FFS than nonresponders. The differences in FFS were more pronounced at the later time-points, suggesting that determination of molecular response may be more clinically meaningful after the first 9 mo of therapy. More specifically, there was a substantial failure-free advantage for patients with evidence of molecular response within the first year of therapy (4 yr FFS: 76% vs 38%; $p < 0.001$). Late failure also occurred more frequently in the molecular non-responders. Furthermore, by multivariate analysis, β2-microglobulin ($p < 0.01$) and molecular response ($p < 0.001$) were the most important variables associated with outcome. When these two determinants were combined, three prognostic groups emerged: (1) low β2-microglobulin and molecular responders, (2) low β2-microglobulin and molecular nonresponders, and (3) high β2-microglobulin and molecular nonresponders. There were no high β2-microglobulin and molecular responders. The 4-yr FFS of these three groups were 86%, 65%, and 23%, respectively ($p < 0.0001$).

The significance of molecular response to central lymphatic irradiation in FL patients with stage I–III disease has also been investigated (19,20). A striking and intriguing finding is the high CR rate for patients who were PCR negative. A total of 33 patients (4 stage IA, 8 stage IIA, 19 stage IIIA, and 2 stage IIIB) were studied. Twenty-one patients had assessable t(14;18)-carrying cells for longitudinal follow-up. A total of 287 PCR results were available: 64 from bone marrow and 223 from peripheral blood. Median follow-up was 44 mo (range: 12–67 mo). There was a clear and steady trend toward conversion to PCR negativity (51% for bone marrow and 68% for peripheral blood at 3 yr), whereas the actuarial proportion of patients free from relapse at 3 yr was 87%. Persistent PCR-positive samples at 3 yr appeared to occur more frequently in patients with initial adverse International Prognostic Index (IPI): 10% for IPI = 0, 31% for IPI = 1, and 63% for IPI = 2. Moreover, IPI was the only statistically significant predictor for relapse: FFS of 91% at 3 yr for IPI < 2 and 75% for IPI = 2 ($p = 0.024$, log-rank test).

Application of the PCR assay in the bone marrow transplant setting was initially reported by Gribben et al., who assessed the immunological purging of marrow by PCR in patients with relapsed FL after an ablative regimen of cyclophosphamide and total-body irradiation *(21)*. A total of 114 patients were studied. In 57 patients, no lymphoma cells could be detected by PCR. The remaining 57 patients had PCR-positive marrows after purging. Correlating the PCR results with FFS, Gribben et al. observed that the FFS was significantly increased in those patients transplanted with PCR-negative marrow ($p < 0.00001$). The observation had been expanded recently to 153 patients with longer clinical follow-up *(22)*. At marrow harvest, only 30% of patients were in CR and overt bone marrow (BM) infiltrate was present in 47%. The FFS and overall survival were estimated to be 42% and 66% at 8 yr, respectively. Patients whose marrow was negative by PCR after purging experienced longer freedom from recurrence than those whose marrow remained PCR positive ($p < 0.0001$). Continued PCR negativity in follow-up marrow samples was also strongly predictive of continued remission. The 12-yr survival from diagnosis for these 153 patients was 69%. Inasmuch as the median survivals from diagnosis from first recurrence in patients with advanced FL were 8 and 5 yr, respectively, myeloablative therapy followed by autologous marrow transplant may prolong overall survival.

However, a somewhat contradictory observation regarding autologous bone marrow transplantation has been reported from St. Bartholomew's Hospital *(23)*. Ninety-nine patients with FL received ablative high-dose therapy as consolidation of second or subsequent remission. Bone marrow was treated in vitro with anti-B-cell antibodies and complement. Sixty-five patients remained alive with a median follow-up of 5.5 yr. Four early deaths and 10 late deaths occurred, and 12 developed either secondary myelodysplastic syndrome (s-MDS) or acute myeloblastic leukemia. FFS and overall survival rates at 5 yr were 63% and 69%, respectively. PCR negativity during follow-up was associated with a significantly lower risk of recurrence ($p < 0.001$) and death ($p < 0.02$), whereas the PCR status of the reinfused bone marrow did not correlate with outcome. Retrospectively, although prolonged FFS can be achieved with autologous bone marrow transplantation, there is, as yet, no survival advantage compared with conventional treatment. The incidence of s-MDS is of increasing concern in this setting.

The use of combined high-dose chemotherapy and allogeneic stem cell transplantation is associated with a high risk of treatment-related mortality and morbidity. Investigators have begun to employ nonablative conditioning regimens to decrease toxicity while achieving engraftment of an allogeneic blood stem cell transplant and allowing a graft-versus-malignancy effect to occur. Khouri et al. reported a pilot study of 10 FL patients in whom nonablative doses of fludarabine, cyclophosphamide, and rituximab were given prior to allogeneic peripheral blood stem cell transplantation *(24)*. All patients achieved engraftment of donor cells with minimal toxicity. The medium number of days with severe neutropenia was six. Only two patients required platelet transfusions and no manifestations of nonhematologic toxicity exceeded grade 2. Of the eight patients with assessable t(14;18)-carrying cells before transplant, seven achieved molecular remission in 3 mo, and in the remaining one, the marrow converted to PCR negativity at 7 mo. Strikingly, all patients were alive, and none had disease recurrence with a median follow-up of 16 mo.

Although eventual translation into improved overall survival remains to be seen, the association of a molecular response with prolonged FFS appears to be a uniform finding in many different studies and in many different treatment settings. Therefore, as a therapeutic guideline, elimination of cells bearing the t(14;18) is highly desirable and should be attempted. However, the fate of patients with PCR-positive marrow after therapy appears to vary: some relapse and others remain in remission for a prolonged period. Perhaps combining a biologic assay with PCR might help assess the proliferative activity of the residual t(14;18)-carrying cells and thereby help predict imminent relapse more accurately. It also raises an interesting question as to whether quantitative monitoring of the residual lymphoma cells would improve predictive capability of the eventual clinical outcome. PCR technology now permits real-time quantification, so the goal is technologically feasible.

## ACKNOWLEDGMENT

This work is in part supported by the Leukemia and Lymphoma Society of America.

## REFERENCES

1. Yunis JJ, Oken MM, Kaplan MI, et al. Distinctive chromosomal abnormalities in histologic subtypes of non-Hodgkin's lymphomas, *N. Engl. J. Med.*, **307** (1982) 1231–1236.
2. Tsujimoto Y, Finger LR, Yunis JJ, and Croce CM. Cloning of the chromosomal breakpoint of neoplastic B-cells with the t(14;18) chromosomal translocation, *Science*, **226** (1984) 1098–1099.
3. Bakhshi A, Jensen JP, Goldman, et al. Cloning the chromosomal breakpoint in follicular lymphoma and demonstration of a breakpoint clustering region near a transcriptional unit on 18, *Cell*, **41** (1985) 899–906.
4. Cleary ML, Smith SD, and Sklar J. Cloning and structural analysis of cDNA for bcl-2 and a hybrid bcl-2/immunoglobulin transcript resulting from the t(14;18) translocation, *Cell*, **47** (1986) 19–28.
5. Tsujimoto Y, Cossman J, Jaffe E, and Croce M. Involvement of the bcl-2 gene in human follicular lymphoma, *Science*, **228** (1985) 1440–1443.
6. Weiss LM, Warnke RA, Sklar J, and Cleary ML. Molecular analysis of the t(14;18) chromosome translocation in malignant lymphoma, *N. Engl. J. Med.*, **317** (1987) 1185–1189.
7. Lee M-S, Blick M, Pathek S, et al. The gene located on chromosome 18 band q21 is rearranged in uncultured diffuse lymphomas as well as follicular lymphomas, *Blood*, **70** (1987) 90–95.
8. Tsujimoto Y, Gorham J, Cossman J, et al. The t(14;18) chromosome translocations involved in B-cell neoplasms result from mistakes in VDJ joining, *Science*, **229** (1985) 1390–1393.

9. Bakhshi A, Wright JJ, Graninger W, et al. Mechanism of the t(14;18) chromosomal translocation: structural analysis of both derivative 14 and 18 reciprocal partners, *Proc. Natl. Acad. Sci. USA*, **84** (1987) 2396–2340.
10. Lee M-S, Chang K-S, and Cabanillas F. Detection of minimal residual cells carrying the t(14;18) by DNA sequence amplification, *Science*, **237** (1987) 175–178.
11. Crescenzi M, Seto M, Herzige BP, et al. Thermostable DNA polymerase chain amplification of t(14;18) chromosomal breakpoints and detection of minimal residual disease, *Proc. Natl. Acad. Sci. USA*, **63** (1988) 4869–4873.
12. Ngan B-Y, Nourse J, and Cleary ML. Detection of chromosomal translocation t(14;18) within the minor clustering region of bcl-2 by polymerase chain reaction and direct genomic sequencing of the enzymatically amplified DNA in follicular lymphomas, *Blood*, **73** (1989) 1759–1762.
13. Berinstein NL, Reis MD, Ngan B-Y, et al. Detection of occult lymphoma in the peripheral blood and bone marrow of patients with untreated early-stage and advanced-stage follicular lymphoma, *J. Clin. Oncol.*, **11** (1993) 1344–1352.
14. Lee M-S, Chang K-S, Cabanillas F, et al. Minimal residual circulating cells carrying the t(14;18) are present in patients with follicular lymphoma and diffuse large cell lymphoma in long term remission, *Blood*, **72(Suppl. 1)** (1988) 247.
15. Price CGA, Meerabux J, Murtagh S, et al. The significance of circulating cells carrying the t(14;18) in long term remission from follicular lymphoma, *J. Clin. Oncol.*, **9** (1991) 1527–1532.
16. Cabanillas F, Lee M-S, MaLaughlin P, et al. Polymerase chain reaction (PCR): an effective way of monitoring response in follicular lymphoma, *Proc. Am. Soc. Clin. Oncol.*, **12** (1993) 365.
17. Lopez-Guillermo A, Cabanillas F, McLaughlin P, et al. The clinical significance of molecular response in indolent follicular lymphomas, *Blood*, **91** (1988) 2955–2960.
18. Lopez-Guillermo A, Cabanillas F, McLaughlin P, et al. Molecular response assessed by PCR is the most important factor predicting failure-free survival in indolent follicular lymphoma: update of the MDACC series, *Ann. Oncol.*, **11(Suppl. 1)** (2000) 137–140.
19. Ha C, Cabanillas F, Lee M-S, et al. Serial determination of the bcl-2 gene in the bone marrow and peripheral blood after central lymphatic irradiation for stages I–III follicular lymphoma: a preliminary report, *Clin. Cancer Res.*, **3** (1997) 215–219.
20. Ha C, Cabanillas F, Lee M-S, et al. The significance of molecular response of follicular lymphoma to central lymphatic irradiation as measured by polymerase chain reaction for t(14;18)(q32;q21), *Int. J. Radiat. Oncol., Biol. Phys.*, **49** (2001) 727–732.
21. Gribben JG, Freeman AS, Neuberg D, et al. Immunologic purging of marrow assessed by PCR before autologous bone marrow transplantation for B-cell lymphoma, *N. Engl. J. Med.*, **325** (1991) 1525–1533.
22. Freeman AS, Neuberg D, Mauch P, et al. Long-term follow up of autologous bone marrow transplantation in patients with relapsed follicular lymphoma, *Blood*, **94** (1999) 3325–3333.
23. Apostolidis J, Gupta RK, Grenzelias D, et al. High dose therapy with autologous bone marrow support as consolidation of remission in follicular lymphoma: long-term clinical and molecular follow-up, *J. Clin. Oncol.*, **18** (2000) 527–536.
24. Khouri IF, Saliba, Giralt SA, et al. Nonablative allogeneic hematopoietic transplantation as adoptive immunotherapy for indolent lymphoma; low incidence of toxicity, acute graft-versus-host disease, and treatment-related mortality, *Blood*, **98** (2001) 3595–3599.

# 15 Editors' Notes

## FLOW CYTOMETRY (CHAPTERS 1, 2, 8)

By the end of the 1990s, the number of fluorescent markers that were available to detect cellular proteins had grown to, at least, 11, This increase was the result of developments in laser technology, fluorochrome chemistry, optical hardware, and data analysis software. These advances, accompanied by technical advice, are presented in the excellent review article of Baumgarth and Roederer *(1)*.

We present a brief overview of the fluorochromes: their excitation and emission properties and the types of lasers used for their excitation. To this end, a brief introduction to the nomenclature for the various fluorochromes is given for those unfamiliar with the field. These fluorochromes are summarized in Table 1. The first group of fluorescent dyes are the *small organic molecules* that are easily conjugated to antibodies. These include fluorescein isothiocyanate (FITC), Texas Red (TR), Alexa 595 (A595), Cascade Blue (CasB), and Cascade Yellow. Next are the *single-protein molecules* requiring more complicated conjugation procedures: phycoerythrin (PE), allophycocyanin (APC), and peridin chlorophyll protein (PerCP). Finally, the *tandem dyes* are covalently linked combinations of donor and acceptor molecules that can then be conjugated to antibodies. Thus, Cy5PE, Cy5.5PE, and Cy7PE are the result of a combination where PE is the donor and either Cy5, Cy5.5, or Cy7 is the acceptor dye.

## LIMITED DILUTION CALIBRATION (CHAPTERS 3 AND 4)

Although the comment that when the starting number of cells positive for minimal residual disease (MRD) is very low or very high gives rise to potential errors in estimation of the number of target cells, this effect is minimized by using a nonlinear calibration model instead of the simpler, better known linear calibration model using limited dilution *(2)*. The statistics of the problem are binomial in that the problem is to estimate the proportion of cells (e.g., $1:10^4$ cells) in the sample that have the particular rearrangement of interest. The limiting dilution assay is constructed by taking a known concentration of cells reactive to the MRD technique (e.g., $10^7$ cancer cells or the equivalent amount of DNA), separating into 10 equal aliquots of, say, $10^6$ cells. One aliquot of the 10 is set aside to be further diluted. Each full-strength aliquot is tested using the MRD reaction.

From: *Leukemia and Lymphoma: Detection of Minimal Residual Disease*
Edited by: T. F. Zipf and D. A. Johnston © Humana Press Inc., Totowa, NJ

Table 1
Fluorochrome Dye Characteristics

| Dye | Excitation wavelength (nm) | Emission wavelength (nm) | Laser commonly used for excitation |
|---|---|---|---|
| CasB | 407 | 440 | Krypton @ 407 |
| Cas Y | 407 | 545 | Krypton @ 407 |
| FITC | 488 | 525 | Argon @ 488 |
| PE | 488 | 575 | Argon @ 488 |
| Cy5PE | 488 or 532 | 665 | Argon @ 488 or YAG @ 532 |
| Cy5.5PE | 488 or 532 | 720 | Argon @ 488 or YAG @ 532 |
| Cy7PE | 488 or 532 | 785 | Argon @ 488 or YAG @ 532 |
| TR | 595 | 625 | Dye @ 595 |
| APC | 595 | 660 | Dye @ 595 |
| Cy5.5APC | 595 or 632[a] | 705 | Dye @ 595 or HeNe @ 632 |
| Cy7APC | 595 or 632[a] | 750 | Dye @ 595 or HeNe @ 632 |

[a]Diode laser operating at 632 nm can also be used for excitation.

The 10th aliquot is then divided into 10 aliquots of, say, $10^5$ cells and diluted with nonreactive DNA to make the same amount of DNA as previously tested. One aliquot is set aside for further dilution. The other nine are tested. The procedure can continue until only one reactive cell remains in the aliquot. Typically, the dilution stops when 10 cell equivalents remain, as 1 cell in $10^6$ nonreactive cells will probably not react. At this point, the number of aliquots at each level showing positive reactions are tabulated and correspond to the number of cells in the aliquot. This is tabulated or plotted providing a curve of reaction versus the number of cells in the sample. The correspondence is to a binomial proportion that can also be considered a count. Taswell (2) stated that the proportion is approximated by the Poisson distribution, but the linear prediction model uses standard regression techniques that are correct assuming Gaussian errors. In either case, ultimately, the Gaussian distribution is used to approximate the errors and provide estimates for the slope and intercept, which are inverted using Fieller's theorem (3–7). This method presumes a linear relationship. Because PCR is a geometric process over the amplification time, the observed signal corresponding to the counts is associated with a logarithm (base 10 usually) of the initial number of copies of the rearrangement (positive cells) that are to be amplified by polymerase chain reaction (PCR), say. At low concentration, the nonamplified DNA tends to interfere with the amplifiable DNA causing the signal to "bottom out." There is a real bottom lower than the apparent bottom seen and occurs when no cell out of the total number of cells is positive for the rearrangement. The next possible higher value above 0 is therefore 1 out of the number of cells in the sample. This is typically below the apparent bottom of the calibration since the minimum number of positive cells necessary to provide a nonzero signal is greater than 1, probably more like 25 cells if the total number of cells is $10^6$. On the high end of the curve, where large amounts of amplifiable DNA are present, the curve saturates. These effects produce the characteristic heel and shoulder graph observed and a nonlinear, nonloglinear relationship between the number of positive cells and the output signal.

## MRD-PREDICTING RELAPSE (CHAPTER 6)

This note is in reference to their use of MRD to predict relapse post-BMT (bone marrow transplantation). MRD was calculated at 1, 3, 6, 12, 18, and 24 mo. Of the four patients who relapsed with no MRD detected, one was a sample of poor quality that probably should have been resampled, if possible. Another was a relapse at 19 mo, 5 mo after the previous measurement (approx 14 mo). Another was 65 mo, 41 mo after the previous scheduled measurement (approx 24 mo). The last relapse was a clonal change. The emphasis must be made that if MRD is to be a reliable predictor of relapse, it must be done at regular short intervals (probably < 6 mo), with the minimum interval yet to be determined. The testing must continue for an extended length of time, perhaps 48 mo.

Another concern is that many researchers are using positive/negative status as the criterion for MRD. We and others [e.g., Radich et al. (8)] have seen "positive" MRD patients continue in remission for years. The criterion for relapse should be based on persistent positive rate of change of the disease level over time. The time interval will undoubtedly be short and needs to be determined. Such a procedure is probably required to increase the sensitivity and specificity of the relapse prediction to an acceptable level.

More rapid means of quantitative MRD measurements are now available that should require only a few days for processing. This assumes that the positive clone(s) has been determined before the BMT was performed. The problem of clonal change reported in this chapter is another problem. The need to continue screening for additional abnormal clones is not clear.

Caligiuri suggested that even a continuously positive patient ($>10^{-5}$ on at least bone marrow or blood samples in triplicate) "…may be compatible with long-term remission." This suggests that a semiquantitative analysis with follow-up at regular intervals during remission may be able to discriminate between continuously positive patients remaining in remission (complete clinical remission [CCR]) and those that relapse. Caligieri also stated that MRD after BMT may or may not relate to disease-free survival (DFS), overall survival (OS), or just relapse. A positive MRD might indicate a noncancerous clone. Thus, a positive or negative status may not be sufficient to determine relapse but require an increase in observed levels. In several studies in this book, the use of BMT did not yield a negative MRD. This should be of some concern to clinicians. MRD might be used as a measure of the completeness of the BMT, if the MRD is negative in the donor. However, a positive MRD may be merely an indication of residual marrow stem cells after BMT and not necessarily a concern for treatment if the graft versus tumor effect is sufficient to maintain control over the residual disease. Indeed, the residual disease seen by the more sensitive MRD techniques may reflect residual disease under control of the immune system or reflect a quiescent clone or stage of the disease.

This may also indicate a strategy (1) for those who "convert" from positive to negative, the interval between successive MRD follow-up may be lengthened, (2) for those who continue positive, a closer follow-up than (strategy 1) should be followed to detect the increase that may precede a clinical relapse, and (3) for those who have increasing MRD, a salvage, or successive therapy might be initiated early (prior to clinical relapse) with potential positive benefits.

## NOTES ON THE SENSITIVITY REQUIRED FOR DISEASE MONITORING

From the preceding section, we see that the more sensitive MRD techniques may be reaching the sensitivity level where they are measuring as positive disease that either will not relapse as a result of immune system control or changes in the disease will relapse very slowly, reflects a nonmalignant subclone, or, possibly, is the result of nonspecific reactivity to the MRD procedure. This effect needs to be studied more thoroughly. It appears that perhaps a level of sensitivity around 1 cell in $10^6$ may be sufficient to reach this level. When in doubt that the level has been reached, a semiquantitative method should be used rather than positive or negative readings.

## STATISTICAL METHODS USED IN THIS BOOK (CHAPTER 2)

Statistical methods used include several standard statistical methods. For proportions such a the proportion of MRD positive or the proportion relapsed in a particular group, chi-square test of association or Fisher exact probability statistics are generally used where proportions are compared. Campana also uses the proportion ± the standard error (SE). This can be confusing. If we are looking at a binomial probability such as a proportion, say $p$, based on, say, $n$ observations (positive/negative, relapse/nonrelapse), the SE is exactly $[p(1-p)/n]^{1/2}$. If we are talking about a set of proportions and the mean of the set, then the SE is the SE calculated from the sample variance and is based on the number of proportions compared. If other factors are to be compared to the proportions (e.g., age, presence of a particular marker, etc.), logistic regression is generally used (9).

If time to a recognizable event (e.g., length of remission from remission induction or the end of treatment to relapse) is to be compared between two or more groups, Kaplan–Meier survival curves are usually calculated and compared using the log-rank or generalized Wilcoxon test. If other factors are to be compared to the time to event (e.g., age, presence of a particular marker, etc.), proportional hazards (Cox model) regression is generally used *(10)*.

## NOTE ON BATCHES OF REAGENTS (CHAPTER 1)

Variations in fluorochrome dyes and other reagents used in these involved assays vary from manufacturer to manufacturer and lot to lot within a manufacturer. Changeover from batch to batch requires recalibration using standards and aliquots of samples run at the time of changeover with both the old batch and the new batch. This should be done along with periodic control runs during a batch.

## NOTES ON SAMPLE SIZE CONSIDERATIONS

The chapters in this book are necessarily methodological in tone and present data to support and illustrate the methods proposed. As such, the power of the individual studies may not be sufficient to properly test for prediction of relapse, DFS, or OS. The field of MRD research is ready for more substantial trials of the methods suggested in this book following a general outline of testing to see if (1) MRD predicts relapse in several diagnostic groups and (2) MRD can be used to determine those patients who can benefit in early salvage or successive treatment before the relapse becomes clinical. Such sample size determinations need to be made within the context of a proper, well-designed clinical trial using standard power calculation software (e.g., DSTPLAN at www.odin.mdacc.tmc.edu).

## GENERAL NOTE ON NEGATIVE VERSUS POSITIVE AS A CRITERION OF RELAPSE

In several chapters in this book, the issue of how to determine a positive relapse has been presented. Lo Coco describes this as the sensitivity of the assay and asks if the level is in the range $10^{-3}$–$10^{-4}$ or $10^{-5}$–$10^{-6}$. Cross presents a "cumbersome" method of defining relapse and questions whether a threshold above which relapse is certain could not be defined. Lee and Cabanillas are concerned with the variable results achieved in the literature using positive and negative. Gribben questions whether molecular CR should be the goal. He used both peripheral blood and bone marrow and found different thresholds. Multiple positive events have been tried and referred to as successful (see Cross).

## REFERENCES

1. Baumgarth N and Roederer MA. A practical approach to multicolor flow cytometry for immunophenotyping, *J. Immunol. Methods.*, **243** (2000) 77–97.
2. Taswell C. Limiting dilution assays for the determination of immunocompetent frequencies, *J. Immunol.*, **126** (1981) 1614–1619.
3. Creasy MA. Limits for the ratio of two means, *J. Roy. Statist. Soc. B*, **16** (1954) 186–194.

4. Fieller EC. Some problems in interval estimation, *J. Roy. Statist. Soc. B*, **16** (1954) 175–185.
5. Finney DJ. *Statistical Methods in Biological Assay*. London: Griffin, 1971, pp. 27–35.
6. Wallace D. The Behrens–Fisher and Fieller–Creasy problems, in *R.A. Fisher: An Appreciation*. Fienberg SE and Hinkley DV (eds). New York: Springer-Verlag, 1991, pp. 119–147.
7. Zar JH. *Biostatistical Analysis*, 4th ed. Upper Saddle River, NJ: Prentice-Hall, 1999.
8. Radich JP, Gooley T, Bryant E, Chauncey T, Clift R, Beppu L, et al. The significance of *bcr-abl* molecular detection in chronic myeloid leukemia patients "late," 18 months or more after transplantation, *Blood*, **98** (2001) 1701–1707.
9. Hosmer DW Jr and Lemeshow S. *Applied Logistic Regression*. New York: Wiley, 1989.
10. Collett D. *Modelling Survival Data in Medical Research*. Boca Raton, FL: Chapman & Hall/ CRC, 1999.

# INDEX

## A

Acute lymphoblastic leukemia (ALL),
adult minimal residual disease,
    assays, 100–102
    childhood testing comparison
        with adults for predictive
        value, 110–113
    clonality assessment, 103, 104
    cure rate, 97
    markers,
        molecular markers, 98
        patient-specific markers, 98,
            100
    oligoclonality, 104
    outcomes from monitoring,
        allogeneic stem cell trans-
            plantation patients, 107,
            108
        high-risk group, 105, 106
        independent predictor of
            outcome, 110
        low-risk group, 106, 107
        study design, 104, 105
    rationale for monitoring, 102,
        103
    real-time quantitative polymerase
        chain reaction, 102
    relapse prediction, 108–110
    testing factors,
        bone marrow testing for
            extramedullary relapse,
            112
        harvested bone marrow
            specimens, 112
        peripheral blood versus bone
            marrow samples, 111

timing of testing, 111, 112
    VH gene usage, 104
bone marrow transplantation, *see*
    Allogeneic stem cell
    transplantation
bone marrow versus peripheral
    blood for residual disease
    detection, 30
flow cytometry,
    antibody panels, 25–27
    data collection, 24, 25
    error sources, 27, 28
    marker selection, 25
    multicolor analysis, 23
    polymerase chain reaction
        comparison, 27, 31, 32
    precision, 24
    sensitivity, 24
immunophenotypic classification
    of cells, 22, 23
minimal residual disease,
    assay criteria, 21, 22
    definition, 98
    prognostic value, 37, 38
polymerase chain reaction of
    clonal markers,
    antigen receptor gene rearrange-
        ments, 38–41, 100
    comparative hybridization, 41, 42
    competitive polymerase chain
        reaction, 42, 43
    fusion gene limitations, 38
    limiting dilution assay, 43
    real-time quantitative polymerase
        chain reaction,
        advantages, 47